Under the Medical Gaze

UNDER THE MEDICAL GAZE
Facts and Fictions of Chronic Pain

Susan Greenhalgh

University of California Press

Berkeley   Los Angeles   London

University of California Press
Berkeley and Los Angeles, California

University of California Press, Ltd.
London, England

© 2001 by the Regents of the University
of California

Library of Congress Cataloging-in-Publication Data

Greenhalgh, Susan, 1949—.
    Under the medical gaze : facts and fictions
of chronic pain / Susan Greenhalgh.
        p .   cm.
    Includes bibliographical references and index.
    ISBN 0-520-22397-7 (cloth.: alk. paper)
ISBN 0-520-22398-5 (pbk.: alk. paper)
    1. Greenhalgh, Susan, 1949—Health.
2. Chronic pain—Patients—United States—
Biography.   3. Arthritis—Patients—United
States—Biography.   4. Fibromyalgia—
Patients——United States—Biography.
5. Physician and patient.   6. Diagnostic
errors.   I. Title .

RB127.G745   2001
616'.0472'092—dc21
[B]   00-048890

Manufactured in the United States of America

9 8 7 6 5 4 3 2 1 0

10 9 8 7 6 5 4 3 2 1

The paper used in this publication meets the
minimum requirements of ANSI / NISO Z39.48-
1992(R 1997) *(Permanence of Paper).*♾

For Marge and Cy

Contents

List of Tables and Figures / ix
Acknowledgments / xi

Part One: Understanding Chronic Pain
Preface / 3
Problematique / 18
Prologue: Finding Dr. Right / 57

Part Two: Doing Biomedicine
1   The Initial Consultation: The Making of a "Fibromyalgic" / 67
2   Medicating the "Fibromyalgic"–Arthritic Body / 87
3   Producing the Good Patient / 113

Part Three: Doing Gender
4   A Most Pleasant Patient / 141
5   Silent Rebellion and Rage / 163
6   A Depression Worse than the Disease / 176

Part Four: A Losing Battle to Get Better
7   Struggling to Make the Treatment Work / 193
8   "Accept It!" Alternative Medicines Offer Medicine
      for the Mind / 212
9   A Life Shrunk, a Mind Gone Nearly Mad / 226

Part Five: Rebellion and Self-Renewal
10   A Second Opinion: The Unmaking of a "Fibromyalgic" / 245
11   The Final Meeting: A Tale of Decline and a Denial / 257
12   Out from under the Medical Gaze / 275

Part Six: Narrating Illness, Politicizing Pain

Conclusion: Re-viewing the Medicine of Chronic Pain / 291
Epilogue: Speaking of Pain—On Stories,
    Cultural Recuperations, and Political Interventions / 323

Notes / 325
References / 345
Index / 365

Tables and Figures

Tables

1 Diseases Diagnosed / 72
2 Medications and Their Uses and Side Effects / 96
3 The American College of Rheumatology 1990 Criteria for the
   Classification of Fibromyalgia / 277

Figures

1 S. G. Well-Being Chart / 167
2 Patient Success in Controlling the
   Symptoms of "Fibromyalgia" / 208
3 An Emotional Free Fall / 239
4 Smythe Patient Handout / 283

Acknowledgments

Writing this book has involved intellectual and personal odysseys that were as exciting as they were unexpected. Thinking through the workings and effects of biomedicine provided an opportunity to extend to the individual body ideas about the operation of professional discourses and systems of control and about the gendered nature of power that I have applied elsewhere to the social body, or population, as a whole. This project has also been therapeutic in the broadest sense. The assistance and support that so many people rendered along the way helped not only to fashion a book but also to recreate a body and a self. Few words can convey the depth of gratitude I feel toward the colleagues, friends, family members, and physicians who have been involved in this project.

A number of colleagues in anthropology, sociology, and medicine read virtually the whole manuscript for me. Adele Clarke, Kay White Drew, Val Jenness, Arthur Kleinman, Karen Leonard, Bill Maurer, Art Rubel, and Ed Winckler provided detailed editorial and interpretive comments that helped me to sharpen the writing and to clarify the arguments. Susan DiGiacomo, Sharon Kaufman, and Ginny Olesen, who reviewed the book for the Press, provided new references and posed provocative questions. Sandra Harding and Sara Kramer read parts of the manuscript and offered piquant critiques that forced me to see problems I had not wished to see.

Through their bodily ministrations and associated conversations, rheumatologist Sara Kramer, neurologist Denise Barbut, and opthamologist Edward Wong offered models of physician empathy and partnership relations with patients that can hardly be surpassed. They represent biomedicine at its best. Adel Fam, Hugh Smythe, and Frederick Wolfe, all specialists in fibromyalgia, provided generous help in sorting out the facts from the fictions surrounding that condition.

I owe a deep debt of gratitude to my family, especially to my mother, whose loving cards and caring conversations sustained me in a difficult time; to my sisters, Cindy and Jo, whose countless phone calls and unconditional support mattered more than they can know; and to my father, whose concern and comments helped to strengthen my self and my writing. I am indebted also to Debbie Barrett, Nancy Naples, Kathy Radke, and Nancy Riley for giving so unfailingly to a friend in need.

Special appreciation goes to Karen Bohan, whose understanding of the human condition and powers of empathy helped bring me back to the world of the living; to Adele Clarke, whose honest reactions to an early draft greatly strengthened the manuscript; to Frances Benson, who took time from her editorial work at Cornell University Press to encourage a writer she had never met; and to Jen Heung, whose subtitle now graces the book's cover.

Discussions with Mike Burton, Liisa Malkki, and many others who have shared with me their personal experiences of illness and health care helped me to see how pervasive the problems documented in this book are. A seminar at the MacArthur Foundation gave me a welcome chance to share this work at an early stage. Emily Martin and Rayna Rapp provided precious words of encouragement along the way.

Finally, at the publication stage, Ethel Churchill offered valuable suggestions on how to proceed. Rob Borofsky helped get the book published. Mimi Kusch was the ideal copyeditor. And Naomi Schneider, my editor at the Press, helped in countless ways to bring this project to fruition.

Part One | Understanding Chronic Pain

Preface

An epidemic of chronic pain stalks America today. Nearly half of all Americans suffer from one or more chronic conditions, including illnesses and impairments, and the number is growing.[1] Even as tens of millions struggle with such established chronic diseases as arthritis, diabetes, hypertension, and heart disease, millions more are afflicted with the new chronic conditions of late-twentieth-century civilization.[2] The past two decades have brought a dizzying number of such ailments: chronic fatigue syndrome, repetitive strain disorder, Gulf War syndrome, environmental hypersensitivity, and, among the newest entrants, fibromyalgia. Although the symptom mixes vary, these disorders share many features. All lack a known organic basis and are difficult to diagnose. All lack a recognized cause but are worsened by stress. All are syndromes of related symptoms rather than true diseases. All are chronic and treatable to a certain extent, but incurable. Most target women in larger numbers than men.

In a culture that worships science, it is to scientific (or conventional) medicine that we first turn for help. Women desperate for someone to acknowledge and alleviate their suffering go to their doctors to name and ease their new pains. Professionally obligated to heal and motivated by humanitarian impulses, our doctors try to live up to our expectations. Although the treatment of chronic pain is one of scientific medicine's most visible failures, in a time of shrinking resources, medical specialists are only too happy to have a new domain in which to apply their skills. Research scientists develop diagnostic criteria for a new syndrome, clinical scientists work out treatment protocols, and a new group of specialists emerges with a guaranteed stable of patients for life. Before long, a bona fide new disease has entered the medical and cultural mainstream. In this way, distress is transformed into disease, and the "diseasing" of social life moves ineluctably forward.

Most of us think that medicine can reveal the truth of our bodies because medicine is a science that claims to have direct, privileged access

3

to the truths of nature. But does scientific medicine convey The Truth or only *a* truth of our bodies? In recent years growing numbers of scholars in the humanities and social sciences have maintained that medicine's truth is only one truth. Moreover, they contend, it is a partial, interested, and value-laden truth that conceals these weaknesses in the discourses of scientific objectivity and in the rhetorics of physician heroism.

These limitations of the scientific approach to healing matter, because scientific medicine wields prodigious power over our lives. This power is produced by the workings of the "medical gaze," a term coined by the French philosopher Michel Foucault.[3] Through the knowing gaze of the physician, medicine claims to "see" diseases that lie deep within the body, bringing them into being as objects of consciousness and intervention. This distinctive way of seeing permits the doctor to know and label our diseases and, on those grounds, to orchestrate interventions in our bodies, with effects that spill over into our lives. How medicine works—what it can and cannot do—affects every one of us, and some of us deeply.

In the medical profession today, there are encouraging signs of greater openness to criticism and growing willingness to address the shortcomings of the scientific, or "biomedical," approach to illness. There is more talk than ever of holistic approaches to healing, partnership relations with patients, and open disclosure of medical mistakes. Yet change has been late and limited. Today medicine at large remains aloof from the more radical critiques of the humanists and social scientists. For good institutional, economic, and legal reasons, most physicians remain inside the discourses of scientific medicine, unable or unwilling to see that their scientific worldview is but one among others. The public actively participates in the mythmaking. We marvel at medicine's high-tech "breakthroughs," while readily forgetting its low-tech mistakes—the wrong leg amputated, the wrong part of the brain excised, and so on. We are awestruck by its promises to overcome human biology and reengineer our genes, neglecting the social, economic, and cultural costs involved. We know the larger system is troubled, but we trust our individual doctors because they have taken the Hippocratic oath—above all, do your patient no harm. And we trust because we have little choice in any case. Many forces have begun to chip away at the power and authority of biomedicine, but its mystique retains a powerful hold on the public and the profession alike. The need for critique remains great.

This book deepens the critique of the humanists and social scientists by moving into the inner sanctum of scientific medicine, the examining room, to discern how medicine does its work in a real-life clinical encounter between physician and patient. My vehicle is the auto-ethnography. The working tool of anthropologists, *ethnography* interweaves fine-grained description with close analysis to create a compelling portrait of a small but closely observed slice of social life. In *auto*-ethnography, the writer is also a participant in the domain of life observed. (I say more about this genre in the next chapter.) The ethnographic core of this book is a case study of one intense doctor-patient encounter that lasted for more than eight months in 1996. This medical encounter carries special interest, because it had all the ingredients of a medical success story— an able doctor, an eager patient, goodwill on both sides—but instead turned into a medical nightmare. In a nutshell, it is a story of a passionate specialist who, through creative interpretation of the diagnostic criteria for a newly emerging chronic disease, convinced both himself and his patient that she had a painful, essentially untreatable lifelong muscle condition called fibromyalgia. Events later proved that she did not. The story traces the effects of this simple idea—that the patient "had fibromyalgia"—on the patient's inner world, bodily health, and overall well-being. To give away the end of the story at the beginning, the effects were nearly ruinous: the patient began to think of herself as a seriously sick person, she grew morbidly depressed, her physical condition worsened, and she started to slip into a mental fog until, nearing the edge of the abyss, she consulted another physician who discovered the mistake and urged that she take steps to undo the damage. When faced with these facts, the diagnosing doctor would acknowledge neither that his patient's life had come undone nor that he had contributed to her deteriorating state.

One might be tempted to tell this story as a medical morality tale of a bad male doctor doing evil to a good female patient. (Indeed, a female doctor even comes to the rescue.) This book strenuously resists this temptation. Whose behavior deserves praise and whose condemnation is far from clear. Not only did the doctor do some good, but the patient actively (if unwittingly) participated in the near destruction of her life. In the end there are no heroes or villains in this story. Quite the contrary, everyone in it was trapped in the same larger systems of power, which for a very long time no one could see and no one could undo.

In this book I try to unravel the tangled threads that led such a promising medical relationship to produce such catastrophic effects. Part of my task is to write a medical whodunit—to sift through the technical details of multiple disease entities, a multifaceted treatment plan, and a panoply of prescription drugs, all with complicated side effects and interactions, to figure out how things got so far off track. In particular, I need to solve the mystery of how the patient could manifest so many symptoms of a disease she didn't even have. (Clue: she had another disease. Second clue: the treatments for one disease had mysterious effects on the other.) As an avid reader of Patricia Cornwell, Amanda Cross, Sue Grafton, and other women mystery writers, I take up this task with relish, albeit with less writerly skill than these popular authors.

As a student of culture and politics, however, my major concern is to show what this case reveals about the workings of power and culture in the biomedical domain. Although I do not claim that one episode can reveal the workings of a whole culture, I do maintain that some of the most subtle seductions and dangers of our hypermedicalized culture can be grasped only through meticulous attention to the minutiae of specific doctor-patient relationships such as the one described in this book. In trying to understand how things could go so awry, I looked closely at three dimensions of contemporary medicine that are highlighted by the critiques of the humanists and social scientists: the workings of science, gender, and popular cultures of illness. I posed three sets of questions of the case material. First, what is the work of scientific medicine, how does it do this work, and what are the effects for the patient who is the object of medical attention? Second, how does gender affect the power dynamics and outcomes of the biomedical encounter? What exactly goes on in the examining room when the physician is male and the patient female? And third, what alternative discourses on the suffering body and its healing are available in the cultural repertoire? Do the alternative and New Age medical discourses that saturate our culture today help the person in pain or do they only worsen the suffering? Or is the answer perhaps some of both?

In taking up the task of political and cultural analysis I build on the work of many others. Growing scholarly literatures—in gender studies, medical anthropology and sociology, and cultural studies of science and technology—have revealed the complex workings of the discourses and practices of biomedicine and their specific effects on women's lives. But there is still a great deal we do not know. This case takes us into new territories that remain sketchily mapped at best. These include the realm of rheumatological medicine, which treats primarily women but remains unexplored by feminist scholars; the psychological dynamics of patienthood; the intimacies of the doctor-patient relationship; and gendered forms of patient resistance to physician power. We also probe newly emerging "postbiomedical" discourses on the social sources of chronic pain and psychosocial routes to healing it. I hope this book will have something new to contribute to those bodies of work from which I learned so much.

In writing this book I have a rather large agenda of empirical, theoretical, and political goals. Descriptively, I want to shed light on a darker side of medicine that tends to get lost in the shadows of triumphal narratives of doctors performing medical miracles and of patients achieving personal victories in the face of serious illness. While such stories are inspiring, we need to pay more attention to medicine's failings. When doctors unwittingly produce bad outcomes and see them as good, we have a rare opportunity to see the inherent weaknesses of the larger system of which these doctors are a part.

My second goal is to improve our understanding of the workings and effects of biomedical power. Because I was the patient whose life came unraveled, I came to know in a very immediate way the shortcomings of existing cultural, literary, and feminist critiques of science and medicine. At the time of the medical encounter I was well versed in the critique of science, yet that critique did not protect me when I most needed its help. (Feminist theory did, however, provide crucial tools for resistance.) My experience as a long-term patient amply supports the weight now given to discourse in the cultural critique of biomedicine. At the same time, it suggests that students of the biomedical encounter would gain deeper insight by probing even more fully than they have into the rhetorics of medicine, the inner world of identity or selfhood, and the deep, psychologically rooted limits on women's resistance in face-to-face encounters with male physicians. Without ignoring discourse, this book gives these latter elements increased prominence, in a way that I hope will enrich our understanding of medicine and improve the fit between sociomedical theory and reality. This book also goes beyond the critique of biomedicine to probe the social roots of chronic pain and therapeutic alternatives that rely on neither the body-cure of conventional medicine nor the mind-cure of some alternative medicines but rather on a broader set of strategies that address the sociopolitical sources of the pain.

My aims are also expressly political. Throughout the centuries women in sexist societies have expressed the pain in their lives in the form of bodily ills. From witches to hysterics to fibromyalgics, women have been harmed or incited to harm themselves for deviating from expected gender norms. For this destructive pattern to be undone, women's pain must be politicized. I intend this book as a political intervention on three levels: the plight of the individual patient, the discourse about one particular chronic pain condition, and the culture of medicine at large. One of my political goals is to alert patients who are unfamiliar with social studies of biomedicine to the power dynamics in their medical encounters. Another is to draw attention to an emerging new domain of power, the "disease of fibromyalgia," which is now seen by patients and physicians alike as a liberating force for women in pain. A third is to provide elements of a critique of the biomedicine of chronic pain that I hope others will build upon and put to work in the service of creating better and more just forms of medical practice.

I wrote this book for students of medicine, gender, and power in contemporary American life. I also wrote it for physicians and patients. Of all these groups, I most hope to reach the biomedical community. Unfortunately, many physicians are like the doctor described in these pages: they tend to protect themselves from hard truths, to refuse to hear that they might have caused harm while they were trying only to do good. My hope is that other doctors, perhaps some less bewitched by the charms of science, might read this book and find in it a cautionary tale of how powerful is the word of the physician and how biomedicine can go very wrong, *especially* when it is confident that it is unequivocally right.

In the remainder of this preface, I provide some background material to the story that follows. I begin by sketching in key features of the disease that will be featured in these pages, fibromyalgia. (Although technically fibromyalgia is a syndrome, for ease of communication I follow common parlance and refer to it loosely as a "disease.") Next I introduce the materials that I used in writing the book. Finally, I outline the chapters that will follow and caution against some readings of the story that I hope to discourage.

The Biomedicine of Fibromyalgia

The last two decades have brought growing interest in fibromyalgia, the name given to a painful disorder of the musculoskeletal system. Arthritis affects the joints of the human skeleton. Fibromyalgia, by contrast, affects the muscles and other fibrous tissues, creating sensations that range from nagging to burning to agonizing pain throughout the body.[4] "My body is screaming!" is how some patients describe the feeling. A syndrome of related symptoms, fibromyalgia, known also as fibromyalgia syndrome (FMS), is often accompanied by severe fatigue, disturbed sleep, morning stiffness, headaches, irritable bowel syndrome, and other debilitating symptoms.[5] Fibromyalgia is similar in many respects to chronic fatigue syndrome; indeed, it has been called the CFS of the 1990s. The two conditions differ in one major regard, however: in sufferers of chronic fatigue syndrome lassitude is the dominant symptom, whereas in sufferers of fibromyalgia pain predominates. In some patients fibromyalgia is only mildly disruptive, but in others it is incapacitating, forcing them to scale back their lives and abandon careers to take care of their bodies. For these people the illness experience can be one of "absolute devastation."[6] Although fibromyalgia is not progressive, with no cure in sight it is considered a chronic condition likely to last a lifetime.[7]

Fibromyalgia is a puzzling disorder whose cause remains unknown. Researchers are continuing their search for an organic basis for the symptoms, but so far efforts to discover a distinctive physiological or psychological pathology have brought little success. Currently, research covers a wide spectrum of possible factors, from metabolic dysfunction, viral infection, immune system dysfunction, and genetic disorder to injury, trauma, victimization, and prolonged stress.[8] With so little known about causation, effective treatment for the condition has remained elusive. Although there is no consensus on the optimal "management" of fibromyalgia, current thinking stresses the use of medications for sleep and pain, combined with exercise and behavioral therapies such as restriction of activities that exacerbate the pain.[9]

Specialists in the condition estimate that a significant minority of American adults—2.4 percent of the general adult population and 10 to 20 percent of rheumatological patients—suffers from fibromyalgia.[10] People of Caucasian descent are more likely than others to be diagnosed with the condition. The disease is seven times more common in women than in men: overall, 3.4 percent of women but only 0.5 percent of men are diagnosed with fibromyalgia. While women of all ages suffer from the symptoms of the disorder, fibromyalgia tends to strike middle-aged and older women the most. The highest rates are found among women who are fifty or older; in this group between 5.6 and 7.4 percent of women are diagnosed as fibromyalgic.[11]

Fibromyalgia in its current configuration is a young disease. Although the condition was named as early as 1927 (*fibro* for fibrous tissue, *my* for muscle, and *algia* for the condition of pain), for most of the twentieth century fibromyalgia scarcely existed as a clinical or research entity. In 1977 two Canadian researchers published a seminal article proposing diagnostic criteria.[12] This article revived interest in a condition, fibrositis, that had been known for centuries but had languished in biomedical obscurity. The term *fibromyalgia* is now preferred to *fibrositis*, since inflammation (*itis*) is generally not present. For proponents of the syndrome, a key step in the growing recognition of the disease occurred in 1987, when the *Journal of the American Medical Association* published an editorial describing fibromyalgia as a common cause of pain that is marked by a constellation of characteristic symptoms.[13] A committee was then formed to define it. Gaining the endorsement of the American College of Rheumatology, the committee published its working definition of the syndrome in 1990.[14] Since then, clinicians and researchers have shown growing interest in the condition. Yet some remain skeptical about whether it really is a new disease—or even a disease at all.[15]

Growing attention to the disease in the medical community has sparked popular interest in fibromyalgia. As word has spread, many women (and some men) are seeing it as the source of their pain. After years of being told they were hypochondriacs or chronic complainers, growing numbers of people are demanding the diagnosis, relieved at last to have a medical name, with its presumption of biological defect, for their suffering.[16] Responding to this demand, a new group of specialists has emerged to treat these patients. The doctor we will meet below— whom I call "Dr. D."—was one of those eager to serve as an expert in this new disorder. Trained by a prominent specialist in fibromyalgia, this doctor harbored no doubt that fibromyalgia was a biologically based disorder that afflicts countless numbers of women, all of whom would benefit from receiving the diagnosis ("knowing the truth") and coming under the care of a specialist such as himself. Awed by her doctor's apparent scientific prowess, the patient we study followed him in believing that fibromyalgia is a true illness and that she "had" it. It was only after the long encounter with the physician was over and she began to read the biomedical literature on her erstwhile disease that she realized that fibromyalgia was a poorly understood, highly controversial, syndrome that lacked even a definitive diagnostic test. "Fibromyalgia" was merely a convenient label for a collection of diffuse symptoms that, had history been different, could have been given a different label or no label at all.

Lest I be misunderstood, I am not suggesting that fibromyalgia is not a real and painful condition. Readers who have, or suspect they have, fibromyalgia know only too well how palpable and debilitating the symptoms of that syndrome can be. As if the physical pain were not bad enough, many if not most have also suffered the psychological anguish of having their complaints dismissed and being told they were simply malingering. The last thing I want to do is to worsen anyone's distress by conveying the impression that the pain of fibromyalgia is not real. To the contrary, in writing a book dealing with fibromyalgia, my intentions are not only to underscore the corporeal reality of that syndrome but also to publicize the daily heroism of those who, through no fault of their own, find themselves having to create meaningful lives within physical limits that would strain the endurance of the strongest among us. Although my relation to fibromyalgia is unusual—after all, I was misdiagnosed—I hope that my disturbing experience, once properly dissected, may help those for whom the diagnosis is appropriate to become more savvy and more wary about the process of becoming a "fibromyalgic."

The historical and clinical features of fibromyalgia noted above make it a fascinating domain in which to study how scientific medicine does its work. The newness of the disease, the still-being-worked-out character of the diagnostic procedures, the lack of effective treatment—these and other aspects of the disease demand resourcefulness on the part of the physician facing a patient who exhibits fibromyalgia-like symptoms. How does he turn the person who finds her way to his doorstep into a patient, someone who has the kinds of problems he is set up to treat? How does he create the scientific facts of the case—diagnosis, prognosis, treatment plan—and knit them into a clinical tale of the nature of the problem and its optimal solution? How does he persuade the patient that his account of her fibromyalgia is true and objective and in her best interest? Finally, how does he get his treatment plan to work? In looking for answers to these questions we will learn much about how scientific medicine works. We are fortunate to have Dr. D. as our clinician. He not only rose to the challenge, he had everything down to a fine art.

A Word on Materials

This book draws on a rich body of primary materials that document the course of the doctor-patient interaction and its daily effects on the patient during the eight months that "S." was a patient of "Dr. D." The most important of these materials are a medical diary and a medical chart, both created and maintained by the patient. Although these materials have now become the empirical basis for a critique of biomedicine, the reader must realize that, at the time, the patient's sole motive in keeping these records was to improve her health. She wanted desperately to get better and spent countless hours every week using her chart and diary in an attempt to reason out how things could be getting worse despite massive efforts to make them better. Writing about the experience and exposing these shameful parts of her life for all to see was the furthest thing from her mind. The notion of writing a book occurred to her after the long ordeal had come to a close with no sense of closure. It lacked closure because her doctor refused to credit her account of how her life had come undone as a result of his interventions. The desire to speak her own voice and be heard, coupled with the worry that other patients might be suffering as she had, led her to make her story public in a book that I hope will bring wider scholarly and public attention to the problems of doctor-induced illness and medical devastation of the patient's inner world.

The medical diary is a computerized account of every doctor's appointment and all but one telephone conversation that took place during the eight months of treatment. This was an unusually high-contact medical relationship, involving six office visits ranging from two to five hours in length and twenty-two phone conversations running perhaps from fifteen to forty-five minutes. Doctor and patient spoke by phone two times a week during the first two months and once or twice a month thereafter. In most cases the patient took paper-and-pencil notes during the appointments and conversations, then entered them, along with other observations, into her computer file later in the day. The second major source of information is a ten-item chart in which the patient recorded daily changes in her medical regime and physical and emotional well-being. (This chart is described in detail in chapter 5.) These two sources of information give us a rare opportunity to trace the ethnographic links among physician interpretations and orders, doctor-patient interactions, and patient reactions daily for eight months. In her effort to make sense of her suffering, the patient also created a miscellany of computer files, notebooks, and handwritten notes. Though seemingly trivial, these pencil scribblings and electronic jottings will provide us with crucial evidence of the patient's deteriorating mental state and of what happened to turn things around.

These materials differ from the ethnographic field notes that usually form the basis of anthropological studies. Because in this case the recorder of the field notes was one of the individuals in the ethnographic encounter, the notes and other materials she produced were also active agents in the interaction itself. Like commodities, which, anthropologists have shown, have social lives, these writings were effectively characters in the medical drama, with social lives and social effects all their own.[17] The chart, for example, was not simply a passive record of "physician inputs" and "patient outcomes." Quite the contrary, it took on a life of its own, entering into the doctor-patient relationship in unexpectedly lively and contestatory ways. In the patient's hands the chart served as a technology of knowledge creation and as a weapon in the political battles with her doctor over who could represent her body and what counted as medically relevant knowledge. In the end the chart literally saved her life, and both sets of materials gave her the means with which to write this analysis of what happened.

For Dr. D.'s reading of S.'s case and his medical philosophy more generally, I have relied primarily on S.'s notes on their conversations, but supplemented them with two other documents in which Dr. D. speaks for himself.[18] One is a typed report he placed in S.'s patient file after the initial consultation. The second is a tape recording of a public lecture on fibromyalgia that the doctor gave in May 1996. The views that D. presented in these sources are virtually identical to those that S. ascribed to him in her diary, suggesting the credibility of the diary as a source of information on the doctor's medical opinions. While I have faithfully recorded everything that transpired in the doctor-patient relationship, to protect Dr. D.'s privacy I have altered certain features of his identity. These changes are relatively superficial ones that have no effect on the medical issues addressed in the book.

In addition to these primary ethnographic materials, I have used three other sets of written materials to illuminate the social, cultural, and biological contexts of the medical encounter. Letters, e-mails, and other communications with family and friends help to reveal the social context of illness. The written items also include a sampling of the rapidly growing number of books written for the layperson in the area of alternative medicine. These include works on stress reduction, meditation, "spontaneous healing," and sundry other topics. Such books, which can be found in the health, psychology, and self-help sections of bookstores across the country, provide fascinating insight into cultural constructions of health and illness in America today. Finally, I have drawn on technical studies of fibromyalgia to reveal biomedical understandings of the disease and its optimal treatment. I have also mined technical writings for evidence of the social construction and contested nature of the disease within the medical profession. My coverage of the biomedical literature is selective, dealing with aspects of the disease of particular relevance to this project. Encounters with the biomedical community also included correspondence with leading specialists on fibromyalgia; these letters too have become documents for ethnographic use. Like the chart, these social, cultural, and technical materials were far from inert. Throughout the eight-month episode they actively shaped the patient's understanding of her situation and, in turn, conditioned the way in which the medical encounter unfolded.

A Look Ahead and a Caution

The book contains twelve ethnographic chapters. These are framed by a problematique, a prologue, a conclusion, and an epilogue. The problematique, which follows this preface, lays out the book's central questions and the analytic approaches taken to answering them. A central task of the problematique is to locate my ideas within the existing scholarly literatures on social and scientific aspects of medicine, women's psychology and gender identity, and the cultures of alternative medicine. Readers who want a better understanding of their own experiences as patients or physicians should find much of interest in these discussions. To make them accessible to a wide range of readers, both scholarly and general, I have tried to avoid specialist jargon and to place all references to the scholarly literature and discussion of strictly academic matters in the endnotes. Nevertheless, some readers may find that there is more than they want to know here about the workings of science, gender, and illness cultures. I invite these readers to bypass the problematique, turning directly to the story of the ill-fated medical encounter that begins in the prologue, "Finding Dr. Right." This prologue provides a brief history of the patient's ills before she became a "fibromyalgic" and the social context in which these ailments emerged. This context helps to explain why the patient became so enamored of Dr. D.

The twelve chapters in Parts II–V that form the heart of the book relate the patient's eight-month experience as a "fibromyalgic" and her six-month struggle to recover from it. These chapters move chronologically. They begin in March 1996, when the patient fell under the "gaze" of biomedicine and end in May 1997, when she finally wiggled out from under that gaze and, as her defiant slogan puts it, "quit the body job." The chapters are divided into four parts, each examining a major analytic dimension of the medical encounter.

Part II explores the workings of biomedicine during the initial months of the medical encounter. What happened during those early spring months set the stage for everything that was to transpire during the following summer and fall. Chapter 1 tells the story of the initial consultation. It shows how, in five short hours, a skilled practitioner deployed the discourses and rhetorics of medical science in a way that transformed the patient's bodily identity from "a person with arthritis" to "a fibromyalgic-arthritic patient." Chapter 2 takes the reader into the realm of rheumatological drugs, detailing the doctor's pharmacological discourse—or drug talk—and its effects on patient and doctor alike. The effects on the patient included not only relief from her initial symptoms but also the emergence of a complex of new symptoms that her doctor ascribed to her "fibromyalgia." Chapter 3 traces the rhetorical production of patient compliance, revealing how the patient was both sweetly seduced and blatantly bullied into acquiescing to the medicalization of her body.

Part III probes the workings of gender in the medical encounter. Chapter 4 depicts the patient's relationship-first approach to getting good care and how it led her to create a compliantly pleasant outer self while silencing an inner self that was full of doubt and anger. Chapter 5 documents the silent rages the patient felt and the secret rebellions she mounted in a desperate yet fruitless attempt to resist her doctor's intrusions into her life. Chapter 6 lays out the painful psychological consequence of "fighting like a girl": a deep, enervating depression that became far worse than the bodily disease.

Part IV narrates the consequences of the interlacing of science and gender that unfolded during the summer and fall, with a brief detour into an encounter with alternative medicine. What they add up to is a losing battle to get better. Chapter 7 discloses how, following her doctor's orders, the patient turned her life into an object of medical scrutiny, surveilling herself closely and cutting out all activities that seemed to make the "fibromyalgic" pain worse. During the summer she also dipped into the literature on alternative and New Age medicine in the hope of finding a way to ease the new symptoms. Chapter 8 delves into some of the books she read and some of the mind-cures she tried before realizing that they were making things worse, not better. Chapter 9 describes a life shriveled and shrunk as the patient eliminated all sources of pleasure from her life in a desperate attempt to rid herself of the "fibromyalgia." This chapter also recounts the hair-raising developments of mid-fall, when the patient's mind began to fog up and malfunction, bringing her close to the edge of a psychological abyss.

Part V tracks the patient's long-forestalled rebellion against her doctor and the project of reconstructing the self she launched to heal the wounds that medicine had inadvertently inflicted. Chapter 10 tells the story of the patient's late-fall visit to her previous rheumatologist in which she discovered that her transformation into a "fibromyalgic" was a huge mistake. Chapter 11 narrates how the patient found her voice again and staged a final, high-drama meeting with her doctor in which she mustered the courage to tell him what had happened, only to hear him deny her pain and disclaim responsibility for everything that had gone wrong. Chapter 12 documents the patient's six-month journey to bodily recovery and the useful if sobering lessons she learned along the way. The book's conclusion addresses each group of imagined readers separately to tell them—that is, you—what I hope you will take away from the book. An epilogue suggests that storytelling by the ill is one of the most promising paths to changing the culture and politics of chronic pain.

The reader should be forewarned that, because S. was in the process of relocating from the East Coast to the West Coast when the story takes place, the action unfolds in no fewer than four states: New York (where S. originally lived and worked), California (where she found a new job and home), Washington (where D. practiced medicine), and Maine (where S. spent a summer). S.'s numerous moves and complicated communications will be sorted out as the story progresses.

There are two types of readings of this story that I hope to discourage. Some readers who identify primarily with the doctor will see S.'s anger at Dr. D. as excessive, sufficient cause to dismiss this book as "doctor bashing." *Please do not do this.* The anger displayed in this book is the patient's anger, which she recorded in her diary at the time of the medical encounter. It is not the author's anger. My task as author is to make that anger comprehensible. As author, I have taken great pains to distance myself—whom I refer to as "I"—from the patient, known here as "S.," to portray Dr. D. in the most favorable light possible. My aim here is not to criticize the doctor but to understand why the sort of medicine he practices too often falls short of its goals. This book challenges physician readers to see beyond the training that taught them to discount patients' ideas and feelings to a recognition that patients possess valid knowledge and legitimate emotions that might prove useful to them in their efforts to create more humane and effective forms of medical practice. Moreover, unlike most patient accounts of medical errors, which blame the doctor and exculpate the patient, in this book the former patient takes full responsibility for her part in the undoing of her health. Physician readers should welcome this more balanced approach to understanding medical mistakes.

Other readers who identify primarily with the patient may be frustrated and angry at S. for her persistent passivity in the face of threat and her staying sweetness in the face of abuse. These readers will be tempted to dismiss her as having too many faults to speak for the plight of the ill. *Please do not do this.* Of course S. had faults; everyone has faults. I, the author, am also angry at S., my former self, for "allowing" her life to come undone. I actively dislike—and hope I have now jettisoned—those aspects of her personality that caused her to write patient "love letters" to the doctor who was unknowingly devastating her health. My task as author is to step outside this patient's personality to show that its passivity and pleasantness were not so much individual flaws as products of the conditions of gender and chronic illness in American culture. It may be painful to acknowledge this, but in our culture women are too often confined within psychological prisons that make them greet their abusers with smiles. What is unusual about S. is not that she was pleasant, but that she escaped from the prison of pleasantness to recount how it felt to be locked up. And she escaped because that passivity and pleasantness were mostly on the surface; when we peer inside we will see that S.'s inner world was home to a titanic struggle for agency and voice. Indeed, there were two S.'s; fortunately, the more politically aware and assertive one won the struggle.

S.'s be-nice-and-obliging approach to her doctor was equally a product of the conditions of chronic illness. Unfortunately, it is hard to convey a sense of those conditions to people who have not endured this kind of debilitating pain. Words simply cannot describe the brutal realities of unending pain and fatigue. Such pain forces the mind to attend to the body, robbing people of their faculties for rational judgment and blinding them to the structural sources of their distress. Nor are there words to explain how the never-ending problems of chronic illness frustrate family and friends, leaving the chronically ill person isolated from her social network and pathologically dependent on the doctor, who alone in the world holds the hope that things can be made right. In this situation, creating a good relationship with that doctor becomes a life-and-death matter, a desperate attempt to prevent the only lifeline back to the world of the living from snapping in two. This book challenges readers who are sometimes-patients to move beyond their personal experience of illness as something that can be cured to understand how it feels to be sick with an illness that will never go away.

Problematique

It was a slight slip, really—a misdiagnosis of an emergent chronic-pain syndrome. But when the misdiagnosis was followed by a raft of new symptoms, what started out as a little mistake grew bigger. The new symptoms were misinterpreted as part of the disease and then mistreated with a therapeutic plan that did not fit the problem. When the mistreatment failed to work and the debilitating new symptoms grew worse, threatening the patient's mind, dreams, and life, she went nearly mad. By the end of the eight-month ordeal, a small mistake by a doctor had undone the patient's life.

What went wrong? How could medicine, which is supposed to eliminate pain, end up creating it instead? Since the time of Descartes, the work of scientific medicine has been depicted by a metaphor of repair: the body is a machine, the physician a mechanic who fixes its broken parts.[1] Contemporary wags have likened the doctor's work to that of the automobile mechanic who fixes the carburetor and gets the vehicle back on the road. But this humble metaphor does not capture what transpires when the physician undertakes to treat a patient. The physician's work is not merely restorative, but also productive: he creates fears and hopes, images and identities, perhaps even side effects and symptoms that did not exist before. The repair analogy is also too optimistic, for although the doctor is supposed to fix body parts, he may inadvertently break them instead. The pill, given for the headache, produces stomach pain as well; the biopsy needle, aimed at the liver, punctures the bowel instead. Finally, the artisanal image is anachronistic, for the critical tools of the physician are no longer the physical implements of the mechanic; rather, they are the cognitive and linguistic tools of the scientific-professional expert. Today it is not the stethoscope or scalpel that does the fundamental work of medicine; it is the ideas, conveyed in words, that persuade us that what is done is right and good. Our repair metaphor is not just wrong; it is also dangerous because it is part of a powerful mythology that clouds our perception. It keeps us from seeing the real work of medicine and its interventions in our identities, our emotions, and our lives. Metaphors matter more than we think.

Michel Foucault, the French philosopher and social critic, grasped these points well. In his 1963 study, *The Birth of the Clinic,* he described the penetrating "gaze" of scientific medicine and how it gradually gained sovereignty over the care of the ill.[2] Following new codes of scientific medicine in which the disease, not the patient, was the object of knowledge, the gaze of the physician gave him the power to know and name the patient's disease and, on that basis, to organize massive interventions in his life.[3] "The eye that knows and decides, [is] the eye that governs."[4] The patient comes to the doctor for help, but finds himself first transformed into an object of science and then reduced to a disease, an "endlessly reproducing pathological fact."[5] The process is jarring and violent, all the more so because the medical gaze denies its violence, claiming beneficence instead: "[T]o look in order to know . . . is not this a tacit form of violence, all the more abusive for its silence, upon a sick body that demands to be comforted, not displayed?"[6] Although the patient remains a silent cipher in the *Clinic,* Foucault's historical study remains one of the most incisive accounts of the conceptual nature of medicine's power and the disruptive effects of scientific medicine on the patient's inner world.

With the rise of social studies of medicine, much has been written about the disjunction between the physician's narrow view of his task as finding and fixing disease, and the patient's larger view of her illness as part of a life that needs to be put in order.[7] But less has been written about what happens to the patient, not only physically, but also philosophically and psychologically, when her worldview is disturbed, her body and life rearranged according to the rules of an esoteric system she neither understands nor influences.[8] The effects of this system on the inner world of the patient is a central focus of this book. To understand how a discipline of the body can deeply intervene in the mind and emotions, it is necessary to re-view the work of scientific medicine. Metaphors like that of the humble auto mechanic train us to *not see* the kinds of conceptual and linguistic tools that the physician uses all the time and the extrabodily effects of these tools on the object of his attentions. A major task of this book will be to look beyond these commonsense metaphors to see how the creation of metaphors and stories is part of the work medicine does. The book's central analytic task is to dismantle the pervasive myths surrounding medicine to discover how medicine works and with what effects on its objects. I maintain that the key to the workings of medicine is its "scienceness," its character as the clinical branch of science focused on the human body. Drawing on critical studies of science and medicine, I argue that scientific medicine is a powerful cognitive, linguistic, and material apparatus of social control whose power over us lies ultimately in a set of discourses, or understandings, about the suffering body and its healing. It is these discourses, which are enacted and concealed through rhetoric, that explain both the bodily effects, intended and unintended, and the "spillover effects" into the rest of our lives.

One of the ways scientific medicine keeps its myths mythic is by doing its daily work in private, behind the closed door of the examining room. It is in the private space of the doctor-patient relationship, out of earshot of professional peers and regulatory agencies, that the patient is turned into an object of medical scrutiny, his problems medicalized for his doctor to fix. This book provides an unusual opportunity to peer into an examining room and eavesdrop on what transpired during one long and lively doctor-patient interaction. Our access to this space is granted by the author, who was the patient in the medical encounter. Because she kept copious records of the experience, we have detailed information on much of what was said and done and with what consequences for the patient's body, mind, and emotions over the full eight months of the interaction.

What gives this single case broader interest is that the illnesses in question were chronic. Medicine has made brilliant advances in the diagnosis and cure of acute illness. In the identification and treatment of chronic illness, however, it has made at most modest gains.[9] Yet chronic illness is pervasive, diminishing the daily lives of huge numbers of Americans.[10] In *The Illness Narratives,* a knowing book about chronic illness, the anthropologist and psychiatrist Arthur Kleinman warned sharply that: "[T]he medical profession is dangerous for such patients."[11] I will have more to say about these dangers shortly. For now it is simply important to note that, in examining chronic illness, we will see medicine operating in the face of one of its greatest challenges. The study of chronic illness exposes both the weaknesses of scientific medicine and the dangers that medicine poses for patients.

Scientific medicine does not do its work in a social and cultural vacuum. Although science often claims to be uncontaminated by such forces, an impressive body of sociological and anthropological research has shown that every medical encounter is shaped by the social location and cultural beliefs of the particular patient and doctor involved. This case gives us an opportunity to investigate the shaping roles of two features of the social and cultural landscape that are generally salient in the medical encounter: gender relations and the cultures of illness. Gender dynamics influence who has voice and power in the medical encounter. From novels to personal narratives to social surveys, many sources suggest that when the doctor is male and the patient female, the patient experience can be trying. At its worst it can be hellish. This case will add layers of new meaning to the concept of a patient hell. Both cultural beliefs about illness and popular cultural alternatives to scientific medicine color the patient's views of the causes of illness and the therapeutic alternatives to conventional treatments. The case explored here will reveal how New Age and other alternative medicines that promise the sick person help and empowerment can end up hurting and disempowering her instead.

The particulars of this case make it especially suitable for studying the interrelations of science, gender, and popular cultures of illness. The doctor involved was ultrascientific, followed most of the rules of scientific medicine to the letter, and played his role as scientist of the body with utmost seriousness and sincerity. New models of physician empathy and egalitarian doctor-patient partnerships had not found their way into his practice. For her part, the patient was both an avid believer in scientific medicine and an eager consumer of the cultures of alternative medicine. Her gender identity was complex and contradictory, embodying the norms both of feminism and of white middle-class femininity (these latter, unconsciously). Although the consequences of the biomedical intervention were extraordinary, what took place during the eight-month encounter was but the ordinary workings of science, gender, and illness cultures. In this problematique I explain what I mean by the normal workings of medical science, gender relations, and illness cultures and introduce the constructs I use in the analysis that follows. In the final section I describe the book's genre, auto-ethnography, and its intellectual and political significance.

Science as Storytelling, Clinical Medicine as Science

Most of us, laypeople and scientists alike, think of science as representational—that is, as something that tells us the real truth about the natural world, without artfulness or expressivity. We also think of the truths of science as objective, disinterested, and value free. We think, that is, that the methods of science insulate it against the intrusion of the scientist's interests and values. It is on these bases that we have granted science its extraordinary cultural authority and social power over our lives.

The Stories That Science Tells

In his provocative study, *Science as Writing,* physicist-turned-literary-critic David Locke upends our comfortable assumptions.[12] He presents a compelling case that science is not representational, but expressive—artful, affective, and artificial. Our image of science as a conveyer of disinterested, value-free truths, he contends, is a product of an official rhetoric that draws attention away from the interests and values that inform the making of science and from the gaps and weaknesses that inhere in the methods by which scientific truths are obtained. Our supposedly artless science, he wants us to believe, is artfully constructed.

Why should science need to indulge in artifice? Because the natural world that scientists study is bafflingly complex and chaotic. Any number of interpretations might be right, depending on what part of the whole the scientist looks at, from what perspective, and for what purpose. Moreover, the methods of science, sophisticated though they are, have not been made error free. These methods are more like sieves, full of tiny holes through which human error can leak to infect the creation of scientific facts. "[I]n truth," Locke writes, "about much of what they do, scientists are uncertain . . . Things *seem* to happen . . . but they cannot always be sure. Or they are sure, but mistaken."[13] Not only error but also the values and interests of the scientist can seep through the sieve's holes to affect the making of scientific truth. But if we knew that science was error prone, it would not be Scientific Truth but merely scientific truth, one possible truth among others. If we knew that science was tainted by individual interests or values, it would no longer be a general Science, but merely a particularistic science, say, the science of physicist David Locke working in the Yale University Physics Lab in July 1985. If Science were shown to be only a collection of particular sciences, then the edifice of its power and authority would come tumbling down, the esteemed scientist reduced to the humble producer of partial and particularistic truths. For science to do its work, these aspects of the scientific project must be hidden—not only from the layperson but also, and more important, from the scientist himself.

Given the impossibility of eliminating human influence and technical error, Locke continues, the actual work of science is not so much to tell The Truth but to tell a truth and then to dress it up as The Truth. More specifically, the work of the scientist is to create a set of scientific facts and to compose these facts into a story about the natural world. The scientist must then persuade us, the public, that the story is good and true and untarnished by his values and interests. Once we are persuaded that his story is correct, he or someone else (the engineer, the industrial scientist) can then apply his ideas to the world to achieve the ultimate end of science: to improve the working of nature itself.

The Science That Clinical Medicine Enacts

In this book I argue that this storytelling approach to science, which has been applied to a number of *research* sciences, can also illuminate the work of the *clinical* science of medicine.[14] Calling the doctor's account of the patient's ills a story draws attention to the fuzziness of the boundaries between fact and fiction. Like fiction, medical facts are not discovered but humanly constructed. Stories are also compelling in ways that decontextualized facts are not. It is by weaving his handcrafted facts into a meaningful story that the physician tries to get the patient to accept those facts as true. In recent years some humanistic and social scientific students of medicine have begun to portray medical work as the telling of stories, or "clinical tales," in the felicitous phrase of Oliver Sacks.[15] But the rhetorical aspect of narrativizing to which Locke calls attention— in the crass language of our consumerist culture, the selling of the stories—has received less notice in studies of medical storytelling.[16] Moreover, existing work on medical narratives, which is scattered across a variety of disciplines, tends to portray storytelling as *the core task* of doctoring. This weight placed on narrative no doubt reflects the interest of the medical humanities and social sciences in language and communication. But there is much that goes on in clinical medicine that remains unspoken. If we view clinical medicine as a science, it becomes apparent that storytelling is only one of a larger set of scientific practices that the physician-scientist undertakes in his work on the patient-object.[17] I argue that we need this larger view of medicine as science if we are to see the full impact of a medical encounter on the patient. We also need this enlarged view if we are to understand how medicine can inadvertently make mistakes and injure patients and then somehow make both the mistake and the injury disappear from view.

For insight into how clinical medicine operates as a science, I draw on two literatures that have developed in the borderlands between sociology and anthropology: constructivist perspectives on medicine and practice approaches to science. These two literatures are now coming together and revealing that the power of scientific medicine to alter our bodies, identities, and lives exists on a scale previously unimagined.[18] Our commonsense notion of illness is that it is a real, biological entity that medical science discovers, names, and treats. In the last two decades constructivist perspectives on illness have undermined these everyday beliefs by showing that illness is not so much a real phenomenon—although it has biological bases and produces genuine discomfort—as it is a phenomenon that is *made real* by the operations of medical science. It is "socially constructed," or brought into being, by the specific practices, technologies, and styles of reasoning by which it is studied and represented by researchers and diagnosed and treated by clinicians.[19] Although all diseases are socially constructed in this sense, the constructedness of illness is easiest to see in psychosomatic disease. One of the most arresting illustrations of this process is anthropologist Allan Young's study of "post-traumatic stress disorder," in which memories of trauma produce psychiatric symptoms.[20] Young's historical study shows how PTSD was newly invented, slowly endowed with facticity, and eventually accepted as real not only by researchers and clinicians but also by patients and the public as well. Although I do not trace the process here, over the last two decades fibromyalgia was brought into being and "made real" in the same sorts of ways. (The preface highlighted some key dates and developments in the social construction of fibromyalgia.)

In this book I will show how a similar process of social invention of disease occurs in the microsetting of the doctor-patient encounter.[21] In the typical case, a patient visits a doctor with a fairly clear-cut complaint, the doctor follows standard procedures to attach a disease label to it, they treat it according to established practice, and the symptom goes away. Here is medicine at its best. The case examined in this book is not typical, though such cases may be more numerous than is commonly thought. In this case, a patient came to her doctor with a clutch of enigmatic complaints, the doctor used scientifically prescribed techniques to affix a diagnosis to it, they treated the diagnosed condition according to standard protocol, and a bevy of new symptoms associated with that disease materialized in the patient's body. In both cases, disease can be said to be socially or clinically constructed, that is, made an object of observation and intervention by the discourses, technologies, and practices of biomedicine. Yet in one case the symptoms disappear, in the other they appear de novo. In the latter case, in which the symptoms somehow emerge out of the clinical encounter, perverting the goals of medicine, we can say that the disease is clinically manufactured. Why did one doctor cure the disease while the other created it? The answer lies in the adequacy of the social construction, or the goodness of the clinical tale.[22]

And the reasons one story was exemplary and the other deficient lie in differences in the tidiness of the patient body and differences in the susceptibility of the scientific procedures and thought processes to human error, interests, and values. I return to these points below.

To see how illness can be clinically manufactured, I view clinical work as a kind of laboratory science in which the physician-scientist uses the conceptual, linguistic, and material tools available in his examining room "laboratory" to do the basic-science work of deciphering which disease(s) the patient has and the applied-science work of treating them. In taking this approach I am following the lead of sociological and anthropological students of science, such as Bruno Latour, Karin D. Knorr-Cetina, Sharon Traweek, and Nelly Oudshoorn, who have viewed science as a practice and scientists as practical reasoners who create the facts in a highly prestructured setting.[23] The well-established discourses, rhetorics, and procedures of science shape and narrow the range of facts that can be created, and then shape and narrow the way the facts are represented to other scientists and the public at large. The doctor-as-lab-scientist approach dovetails with the "dense pragmatic perspective" of sociologists such as Isabelle Baszanger, who focus on the everyday routines by which clinicians operationalize theoretical knowledge and mobilize technical resources in organizing clinical courses of action.[24]

Although Foucault's influence on my thinking may not be perceptible to some readers, his penetrating vision of the nexus of language, knowledge, and power in modern life is deeply embedded in the intellectual infrastructure of this book. Key Foucauldian themes I advance include the discursive and productive nature of modern power, the centrality of scientific discourses and practices in constituting modern subjectivities, the social and historical constructedness of the body and illness, and the ubiquity of resistance to power.[25]

How Biomedicine Works

I now step back from the literature to show how I weave together Locke's ideas on stories, errors, and error-camouflaging rhetorics, medical constructivist notions of illness as a social construction, and science-as-practice images of the doctor as working scientist. The result is a wide-angled view of clinical medicine that takes us behind the myths to see how medicine routinely makes mistakes that have serious consequences for patients and then just as routinely makes us think that it has not.

Medical Myths and Medical Tasks

Medicine is a special branch of science because its objects are not lizards or quarks but human beings—you and me. When *we* are the objects of scientific scrutiny, which story science tells matters more to us, since the story can result in personal pain or pleasure. In addition to the mystiques of truth and objectivity that it shares with science generally, clinical medicine is haloed by another mystique: that it can do no harm, only good. This happy idea is reflected in the Hippocratic oath, which all physicians take and all patients know, if not by name, then at least in substance: Above all, do no harm. Based on these beliefs—truth, objectivity, and good—we as a society have given scientific medicine the exclusive legal right to name and treat illness.[26] On the basis of these beliefs, we as individuals allow doctors to define our problems and to alter our bodies with chemical and surgical interventions.

Does scientific medicine deserve the power and authority it now possesses? That is a big question that we cannot answer right away. Let us start with a smaller question: How does clinical medicine actually work? Most of us go to the doctor expecting him to help us fix our problems. But if we follow the logic outlined above, our doctor's project is more complicated than that. Thinking of medicine as a science and of science as storytelling, we might say that the project of clinical scientific medicine involves four tasks.

The clinician's first task is to turn the person who comes into his office into an object of medical scrutiny: a patient. This involves medicalizing her problems—defining them as bodily pathologies—because this is the type of problem the doctor is set up to treat. Of course, people who consult a medical specialist already see themselves as prospective patients whose problems are medical. Yet medicalization is not complete until the doctor turns the anticipatory patient into the type of patient he is prepared to treat. In turning the patient's problems into diseases, especially of the sort he is trained to manage, the doctor is simply constructing for himself a "do-able" problem, a task all scientists face in their work.[27]

Second, the clinician must translate the disorganized details of the patient's suffering body into the "scientific facts" of the case—the diagnosis, prognosis, and treatment plan—and weave them together into a compelling story about what is wrong and what must be done to right it. Theoretically, the clinical story should also include the cause of the diagnosed disease.[28] Yet in chronic illness, our focus here, the cause is often obscure, leading physicians to soft-pedal or even skirt the issue in their clinical tales.

Third, the doctor must convince the patient that the story is true, objective, and efficacious. That is, he must persuade the patient that the story is complete and error free, unaffected by his values and interests, and will work to ease her pain. Fourth and finally, he must put the prescribed treatment into effect to improve on the suffering body by alleviating the symptoms of the illness he has diagnosed (which may or may not be what ails the patient). These four phases might be called those of patient construction, storytelling, persuasion, and treatment.

Discourses and Practices

The tools the clinician brings to this four-part task are the discourses, practices, and rhetorics of biomedicine. Together they make up a powerful conceptual, linguistic, and material apparatus that shapes the story that is told, the treatment that is used, and, in turn, the bodily outcome of the medical encounter. The most straightforward of these tools are the material practices of biomedicine. These include clinical practices (the physical exam, diagnostic testing, and so forth), treatment practices (the administration of drugs, procedures such as injection and surgery), and many more. These bodily practices are most prominent in the patient construction and treatment phases.

These material practices are the most familiar of the clinician's techniques; they are what we normally think of when we think about how the physician does his work. But they are not the most important implements in the physician's tool kit. The most consequential tools are conceptual and linguistic. These are the instruments with which he creates his story and persuades the patient that it is true and good and viable. The most crucial of these tools are the discourses and rhetorics of biomedicine. Let us begin with the discourses.

The major item in the biomedical tool kit is a powerful set of discourses that together form the worldview of the biomedical practitioner. This worldview is sometimes referred to as "the biomedical model."[29] In the medical social sciences the term *discourse* is employed in two ways. Some scholars use it to mean serious talk between doctor and patient about illness and the body.[30] Others imbue it with a more Foucauldian meaning.[31] In this book I use *discourse* in the Foucauldian sense to mean an historically specific body of knowledge (*the* discourse of biomedicine) that is made up of groups of statements (specific medical discourses) that limit what can be said, written, and thought about illness and its treatment at a particular time. Although these statements are part of physician (and patient) talk in this ethnography, what makes them discourses is not their spoken character, but their role as key components of the larger body of biomedical knowledge.[32] Each of these specific discourses embeds one or more underlying assumptions about how biomedicine works. These assumptions almost always go unstated, with the result that practitioners see their worldview not as one perspective among many but as the sole truth about the suffering body and its healing. In Foucauldian terms, for physicians the truth is a function of what can be said, what is discursively possible.

While each branch of medicine has its specialized discourses, all practitioners of scientific medicine share a general biomedical discourse. Common use of this discourse ensures that physicians work in a roughly similar fashion regardless of their specialty.[33] Over the last decade social scientific and humanistic students of biomedicine have carefully dissected the biomedical model and laid bare its fundamental tenets. As a result, we now have a clear picture of the mind-set of most working physicians.[34] For present purposes we can describe the specific discourses that physicians routinely use in terms of four sets of ideas, each of which performs a different conceptual function in the larger body of biomedical knowledge:

1. The discourse of *objectification* splits the patient into two parts, the "objective" body and the "subjective" mind and emotions, declaring the body the sole object of interest and the physician the expert on that body.

2. The discourse of *quantification* turns the patient's bodily signs and symptoms into a set of numbers so that the only information that counts is that which can be quantified.[35]

3. The discourse of *pathologization* makes disease, not health, the object of attention and affixes a set of disease labels to the patient's ills.

4. The discourse of *amelioration* downplays the issue of cause, focusing instead on the urgency of treating the disease, thereby improving on nature itself.

These discourses inform all four phases of the biomedical endeavor, but they are particularly important in the patient construction and storytelling phases. For example, in turning the sick person who sits before him into a patient he can treat, the physician confines his attention to the body (objectification), turns the symptoms and signs he notes into numerical measures (quantification), and attaches disease names to the ills he discovers (pathologization). In creating the facts of the case and assembling them into a larger story, he uses the numbers he has gathered to fashion a diagnosis and prognosis (quantification) and then outlines the treatment program that must be undertaken if the patient is to get better (amelioration).

Clearly, the discourse has a marked effect on the story that is told. A patient presenting a certain set of symptoms would have quite a different story told about her if she were consulting a practitioner of, say, Chinese or Ayurvedic medicine or any variety of more homegrown alternative medicines. It makes little sense, then, to talk about right and wrong stories, since a story that is wrong from the perspective of one discourse might be right from the vantage point of another. One can, however, talk about good and bad stories. Good stories are ones that fit the case: They describe the patient's signs and symptoms and specify a treatment that works. Bad stories are ones that do neither.

When a biomedical practitioner tells a good story, the strengths of conventional medicine's radically materialistic approach to illness become manifestly clear. By limiting their attention to the physical body and approaching its dysfunctions through systematic and scientific investigation, physicians can often isolate the physical causes of a bodily complaint and ease the symptoms through bodily intervention. Medicine at its best is a marvelously effective discipline.[36] But when the clinician tells a bad story, the limits of biomedicine's discourses stand out with equal clarity. Unfortunately, it is the bad stories and the limits of medicine that must preoccupy us here.

Prone to Error

The physician must convince the patient that his story is true and objective, but a second look at these discourses belies the idea that a biomedical story can be completely either. Perhaps most obviously, a biomedical story must be partial rather than complete, since the discourses of medicine by definition exclude affective and mental components of illness and signs or symptoms that cannot be quantified. A story created from these assumptions may be not only partial, but even poor. The story might be weak because the discourse of objectification makes the doctor the expert on the patient. Although the patient's knowledge might contain crucial clues to what is wrong, the discourse has made that knowledge at best ancillary, at worst extraneous to the process of fact creation. Errors can also creep into the specification of the treatment, for the discourse of amelioration sidesteps the question of cause. When the cause is not identified, the treatment might address the wrong problem and fail to heal the patient's ills. This line of argument might strike the reader as silly or far-fetched, but I will show that these sorts of slips are part and parcel of normal medical practice.

The probability that a practitioner of biomedicine will tell a bad story is significantly heightened when the patient has a chronic illness. In chronic illness many of the symptoms are vague and nonspecific (aches and pains, fatigue and sleeplessness), increasing the likelihood of misdiagnosis.[37] Because the symptoms of chronic illness respond to stress and other social forces that wax and wane, the past pattern of disease may not foretell the future, raising the risk of a flawed prognosis.[38] In chronic illness the problems that exacerbate symptoms lie partly if not largely outside the body, in what students of social medicine call the patient's "lifeworld." When these causes are not addressed or are misunderstood, the likelihood that the treatment will be misguided and ineffective is enhanced. Although he did not use this language, the creation of bad stories is part of what Kleinman meant when he said that biomedicine is dangerous for the chronically ill.[39] What makes it hard to recognize this danger is that the physician has done his best to tell a good story according to the rules of biomedicine. The problem is not an incompetent or malevolent doctor, but a narrow and reductionist set of rules. Biomedical stories are very often bad stories for chronic patients.

It is not only the discourses of biomedicine that can result in ill-fitting stories. A large literature on medical mistakes shows how the messiness of the patient body and the still imperfect methods of scientific medicine can also weaken the stories medicine tells, especially about chronic illness.[40] This emphasis on mistakes may sound overly critical to the lay reader, but that is because the public has been kept uninformed about the true extent of error in medical work. Although few records of medical mistakes are kept, and those that are maintained focus on "serious harm," experts have long believed that iatrogenic, or doctor-induced, injury constitutes a "problem of enormous proportion."[41] A late-1999 National Academy of Sciences report documenting the deaths of 44,000 to 98,000 people a year from mistakes made in hospitals alone both confirmed the experts' suspicions and suggested that such numbers, frightful though they are, represent only the tip of the iceberg.[42]

In the cases of mistakes linked to bodily and methodological problems, it is less the truth than the objectivity of the story that is compromised. Let us consider the two types of problems separately. First, the
patient body is inherently disorderly and chaotic. It comes to the clinician not as a neat collection of diseases, but as a tangle of aches and pains,
complaints and cries, in which past and present are jumbled up together.
When a number of different stories might fit the situation, the interests
and values of the clinician can creep in to color his judgments about the
best diagnosis and prognosis for the case.[43] These influences sneak in subtly, unconsciously. Consciously, the clinician's aim is only to do his level
best to identify and treat the patient's diseases.

Objectivity is also compromised by the regrettable fact that the methods available to diagnose disease, forecast its future, and alleviate its symptoms remain inexact. In taking the patient's history, for example, the clinician might neglect to ask about something that would be crucial in
detecting the patient's disease. In the physical examination of the patient's
body, a slight slip of the fingers to the right or left of the diseased organ
might result in an overlooked tumor. Similarly, minute changes in the degree of pressure exerted might affect which anomalies of the body are
brought to light. Though useful protocols have been worked out, pok-
ing and prodding remains an art as much as a science. This treatment of
methodological problems has been illustrative only. Yet this tiny handful
of examples hints at the sorts of weaknesses in the science of clinical medicine that make the task of the physician difficult. Methodological gaps,
combined with the messiness of the human body, act to compromise truth
and objectivity, leaving room for human error or individual interests to
creep in to shape the story that is told. When error and interest enter in,
the result can be weak, even bad, stories that do not fit the case.

The Work of Rhetoric

I have argued that, given this room for slippage, making mistakes is as
much a part of medicine as getting it right. Sociologist Marianne A. Paget
puts it pointedly when she writes that medicine is an "error-ridden activity."[44] To do his job effectively, however, the physician must believe
he has gotten it right, or at least as right as is humanly possible. Psychologically, it is difficult to admit error; it is harder still to see that one's
stories have been subtly colored by one's values and interests.[45] In *The
Healer's Art,* Eric J. Cassell, a physician himself, argues that the physician hides his doubts and fears behind a shield of invincibility and then

forgets that it is only a shield.[46] As important as convincing himself, the physician must convince his patient that his story about his body is right. He must persuade his patient that errors have not been made, that the clinical tale is true and objective, and that the treatment plan it includes will work to alleviate the patient's pain.

This work of persuasion is accomplished with the tools of rhetoric. The rhetorics of biomedicine perform heroic tasks, but they are the unsung heroes of medicine. Because the physician must believe in what he has done, he must use these slight turns of phrase, these subtle modulations of the truth, blindly, unconsciously, without seeing what they do. As a result, the everyday rhetorics of medicine tend to go unrecognized as professional tools.

Social scientists and humanists have shown that physician talk is full of colorful rhetoric, especially of a metaphorical sort.[47] Our interest here lies in how these linguistic devices work: how they fit into the physician's larger science project and with what effect on the object of scientific inquiry and intervention. It may well be that the more new, disputable, and/or error-prone the field of medical activity is, the more imperative is the use of a rhetoric of science to establish the field's credibility and legitimacy. If that is the case, we would expect the biomedicine of fibromyalgia to be especially replete with science rhetoric. Work on rhetoric in science at large suggests how this persuasional talk might be constructed. Evelyn Fox Keller, the biophysicist-turned-science-critic, has described the "rhetorics of domination, mastery, coercion" over nature that lie at the heart of the scientific project.[48] David Locke has teased out the rhetorics of reification by which scientists make things that are only probably true seem definitely true.[49] Both these linguistic devices were deployed by the scientist-physician examined in this book. Yet this was just the beginning. Because he was a skilled rhetorician, we can draw on his persuasive vocabulary to create a longer list of rhetorical devices that, following Locke, we can call the doctor's "personal rhetorics."[50] Some if not all of these devices also function as "official rhetorics" of biomedicine as a whole. Here, however, I am concerned with their use as the personal rhetorics of an individual physician. The list I have drawn up includes six persuasional devices frequently employed by the physician featured in this book. Some of these usages are common and probably form part of the personal rhetorical tool kits of the majority of clinicians. A few (especially numbers four and five) may strike readers as odd or extreme. Use of these verbal tactics is probably quite rare.

These six linguistic techniques can be divided into three classes according to the primary uses to which they are put. (Most have more than one use; the discussion below focuses on the main one.) The first two rhetorical devices emphasize the objectivity of the clinical work, drawing attention away from any partialities, ambiguities, or holes in the procedures through which the interests or values of the clinician might enter:

1. *Scientism:* Everything that is said and done is rational, objective, logical—in a word, scientific.
2. *Reification:* Things that may seem uncertain or unknowable are real, knowable, and known.

The next two devices stress the truth value of the story and the efficacy and infallibility of the medical project. They divert attention away from the possibility that the disease might be unconquerable or that the doctor might make a mistake:

3. *Domination:* Medicine gains mastery over nature by discovering its secrets, determining its limitations, and intervening to fix them.
4. *Biomedical infallibility:* Medicine and its practitioners virtually never make mistakes; any problems that arise are the result of a bad body or bad attitude on the part of the patient.

The last two usages stress the beneficial nature of the treatment for the patient. These rhetorics deflect attention away from the possibility that the doctor might inadvertently do harm:

5. *Physician heroism:* The doctor is a medical miracle maker who conquers illness and improves on nature itself.
6. *Patient benefit:* Everything that is done is for the benefit of the patient; the physician derives no benefit other than personal satisfaction from anything he does.

Such rhetorics are usually harmless. Indeed, from the doctor's point of view, such exaggerated claims can prove helpful, even necessary, in getting a reluctant patient to comply with unpleasant treatments that the doctor knows—or thinks—will work. But use of this kind of rhetoric poses dangers for the chronic patient. Because of a history of ills that are never healed, many chronically ill people go through life with a deep yearning to find a doctor who can fix what is wrong. This longing for help, along with the sadness and inner turmoil that are always part of chronic illness, leave the chronic patient emotionally vulnerable to the rhetorical appeals of a doctor who claims to be more scientific, more heroic, more infallible than his peers.[51] The social isolation of the chronic patient, a result of needing more support than most friends and family members can bear to give, increases the susceptibility to the judgments of the doctor, who may be the only person in the patient's social world who can always be counted on to care about her problems.[52] When the rhetoric turns out to be just that, and the ills remain unhealed, the patient ends up in deeper psychic pain and social isolation than ever.

Medicine often gets it right and heals the patient. When the illness is acute, this is probably the norm. However, when the illness is chronic, biomedicine often if not usually gets it wrong, and the patient does not get substantially better. To understand these cases, we need to grasp how the making and concealing of mistakes, small and large, is built into the workings of biomedicine. This little subplot within the larger drama of medicine is hard to see because the clinician himself does not see it. What I have depicted as rhetorics many physicians see as gospel truth: their work is scientific, they rearrange nature to the good, they make few mistakes, they are godlike healers, everything they do is in their patients' best interest. It is not surprising that they think these things, since these are the very attitudes that were inculcated in them in medical school.[53] But as observers rather than practitioners of medicine, we can and must step outside the biomedical discourse. We must get behind the rhetorics of physician infallibility and patient benefit, because unquestioned clinician belief in them is dangerous. Blind faith in these rhetorical exaggerations is perilous, because it can justify abuse and coercion in the name of patient benefit.[54] In addition, it fosters an unhealthy dose of hubris that makes it difficult for practitioners to acknowledge that they can make mistakes, let alone to take responsibility for their actions when things go wrong.[55] Although these problems can arise in any medical situation, they may be more probable, or at least more protracted, with chronic illness, which by definition is more stubborn and resistant to physician interventions. Finally, these rhetorics are harmful because they prevent us from seeing what actually happens to the chronic patient, especially inwardly, when she enters a long-term biomedical relationship.

Inner Disruptions

One of the most powerful myths of medicine is contained in the Hippocratic oath. Its no-harm ethic only makes sense if we accept the discourse of objectification by which medicine treats the body alone. Once we step outside that discourse, we are forced to acknowledge that the body is ineluctably connected to the mind, the emotions, and the larger life of the person. Personal experience tells us that any intervention in the body inevitably affects these other domains of existence. Despite the seriousness of these consequences for the patient, few have ruminated on this set of problems. One who has is the physician Eric J. Cassell. In a penetrating essay on suffering, Cassell has described how medical care can actually *cause* suffering by treating only the body while ignoring that care's often destructive interventions in the patient's personhood, or sense of self.[56] Any aspect of the person—from social roles to relationships, emotions, and so on—can be disrupted by illness and by health care, leading to a kind of existential suffering that is different from, and more devastating than, bodily pain. This kind of damage is likely to be especially great in chronic patients, whose sense of self is fragile and constantly under assault from symptoms that come with no warning, disrupting life plans and creating pervasive uncertainty about the future.[57]

For this sense of self that is vulnerable to biomedical disruption, we can coin the term *bodily identity* to distinguish it from the gender identity that will be discussed below. Because identities are multiple, these and still other identities coexist in the same person. At the most general level, bodily identities fall into two classes: "normal" and "stigmatized," or "ill." Erving Goffman's work on stigma suggests that most people probably struggle to retain a "normal" bodily identity.[58] A sense that one's body falls within the range of what is "normal" is worth fighting for, for once that identity is "spoiled" by a biomedical label, one is subject to all the problems of the stigmatized—from discrediting and discrimination by others to feelings of shame and inferiority that come from within.

From a broader perspective outside the worldview of biomedicine, what becomes clear is that the potential for disruption to the patient's inner world is built into the biomedical project. A closer look shows that it inheres in every phase of that project. Let me explain by example. In the patient-construction phase of the medical endeavor, the patient's mind and emotions are severed from the body, that body reduced to a disease that the physician alone can fathom. The physician claims to intervene only in the body, but in conceptually sawing off the body from the rest of the person and ripping the right to know that body out of the hands of the person inhabiting it, he intervenes in the mind and emotions just as surely as if he were an executioner of the self. This is strong language, to be sure, but it is warranted if the speaker is a patient. The transformation from a person into a patient leaves the patient traumatized, yet with no guidance on how to recover. That trauma is philosophical, emotional, and even political—for ultimately this is about power.[59] The trauma deepens as the encounter proceeds. The diagnosis and prognosis conveyed in the storytelling phase are not mere labels for a disease and its future course; because they are weighted with personal and cultural meanings, they are interventions in the patient's self. As Kleinman has put it, "[M]eaning arrives with a vengeance together with the diagnosis . . . once applied to a person, [it] spoils radically that individual's identity and is not easily removed."[60] Depending on how dismal the diagnosis and prognosis are, they may be highly disruptive, forcing massive changes in the patient's sense of her self and her future. The persuasion and treatment phases have similarly disturbing effects that I invite readers to imagine for themselves.

When the story the doctor tells is a good story and the treatment works to alleviate the pain, these inner disruptions are temporary and readily forgotten in the joy of improved health. When medicine works this way, the patient's attention can stay focused on the benefits of medicine's reductionistic approach to disease. But when the story is bad and the symptoms persist or even worsen, the philosophical and emotional traumas become protracted, eating away at the patient's inner self. Unless the patient finds a way to cope with them—say, by giving up hope of getting better or by transcending them spiritually—over time these inner injuries can become as debilitating as the bodily injury caused by the disease. This, I believe, is the plight that many chronic patients find themselves in when they go to the doctor for help but get little. They suffer a double dose of pain, the first physical, the second psychic. This is precisely what happened in the case that we explore in depth below. Out of the discourses of biomedicine, the doctor fabricated a bad narrative that served his professional interests—although he remained unconscious of these interests to the end—but did not fit the patient's case. With the rhetorics of biomedicine, he persuaded the patient that the diagnosis was correct. From the material practices of biomedicine, he fashioned a treatment program that produced the symptoms to go with the diagnosis. The medical manufacture of illness not only worsened the patient's bodily conditions; it also undermined her bodily identity, her emotional equilibrium, and her life projects. Yet when she discovered the damage, there was no one to help her undo it. Biomedicine had washed its hands of responsibility for its mistakes, leaving it to the patient and to other social institutions to fix what had been broken. I return to these issues of medical error, responsibility, and reform in the conclusion.

A Word on Managed Care

Although my central concern in this book is the scienceness of medicine, I cannot leave this discussion of established medicine without mentioning one aspect of the larger institutional context that profoundly affects the way in which it treats chronic illness (and, indeed, all illness): the recent spread of managed health care. Potentially risky for any patient, managed care poses particular dangers for the chronically ill, whose extensive needs simply cannot be met by an organization driven by an ethos of economy and efficiency. Although I will not analyze its role, managed care was a critical if silent actor in the drama that unfolds below, affecting doctor and patient alike. I return to the significance of managed health care in the conclusion.

Gender Troubles in the Doctor-Patient Relationship

Few of us think of ourselves as having "relationships" with our doctors. Yet we do, and they are complex, power-laden ones. When the doctor is male and the patient female, this is especially the case. In the medical setting gender often works to amplify the voice and power of the physician. The patient is doubly silenced and subordinated, first in the hierarchy of science and then again in the hierarchy of gender. Her life and happiness depend urgently on a successful treatment of her ills, but it is her doctor, not she, who controls the means to ensure one.

We owe our awareness of these gender troubles in the doctor's office to the women's health movement. In the late 1960s and early 1970s, groups of women across the country began to gather to compare notes about their experiences of medicine and many other matters. They discovered, in the words of the best-known group, a shared "frustration and anger toward specific doctors and the medical maze in general."[61] These sorts of frustrations gave birth to the women's health movement which, in the ensuing decades, has been instrumental in raising women's consciousness about the "condescending, paternalistic, judgmental and non-informative" manner in which doctors, in particular obstetrician-gynecologists, treat women patients and the consequent dangers attending women's health.[62] Among its accomplishments, the movement has stim-

ulated scholarly research on the political dynamics and bodily consequences of the interactions between male doctors and female patients.
Despite the growing numbers of women in medicine, male physician and
female patient remains the modal medical relationship.

Power and Sexism in the Examining Room

Medical sociology reveals how the hierarchies of science and gender overlap in the examining room, leaving women patients in positions of little
power. This sociological work is important, because it is based on relatively large samples, giving us the big picture of what transpires in the
modal medical relationship. This research suggests that male doctors tend
to treat women differently and in a more dehumanizing fashion than they
treat men.[63] While there are certainly many male physicians who treat
female patients with respect, the sociological record suggests that women
experience a remarkable degree of verbal abuse and personal degrada-
tion at the hands of male clinicians.[64] Yet for a number of complex reasons, women rarely talk back to their doctors. The studies of doctor-
patient conversations conducted by Sue Fisher and Alexandra Dundas
Todd, among the largest to date, contain virtually no cases of women
openly challenging their doctors.[65] Today, as the larger social climate becomes more critical of institutionalized medicine, and medical information spreads on the Internet, more and more patients seem to be willing
to confront their doctors. Yet the balance of power in the doctor-patient
relationship remains highly asymmetrical.

This is not to suggest that women are simply passive victims of biomedical power. (It goes without saying that male doctors are not all active agents of biomedical domination either.) Women have their own
needs and interests, which they actively promote in their medical encounters. Because these concerns and requirements vary with factors such
as age, class, ethnicity, and illness, women's political responses to their
physicians vary widely.[66] Some women feel comfortable and comforted
allowing a male authority figure to take care of them. These accommo-
dating patients do not regard their doctor's "Now, dear . . . " comments
as demeaning and in general are happy to comply with doctor's orders.
Others hear the same words as sexist or condescending and resist male
medical authority in whatever ways they can. Perhaps the majority of
these rebellious patients remain silent and compliant in the examining
room, exercising their power at home by refusing to follow the doctor's
directions or simply by not going back.[67] A small and probably growing

minority has the courage to challenge the doctor in the medical inter-view itself, but they rarely succeed in changing his mind. In one study, argumentative patients only ended up feeling powerless, producing long silences in the consultation that were "too often punctuated with barely restrained sobs."[68] Unfortunately, when communication is so one-sided, the medical outcome often suffers.[69]

The sociological research documents the power and sexism that per-vade the medical encounter and the varied ways in which women pa-tients respond. Although we know *how* women react in medical settings, we know less about *why* they usually comply with but sometimes resist biomedical power. To understand the dynamics of compliance and re-sistance, we need a more in-depth understanding of how the encounter with masculinist medicine looks from the perspective of the patient. Here the work of ethnography is helpful.

Medical anthropologists such as Emily Martin and Rayna Rapp have ethnographically opened up the world of the woman patient, docu-menting complex patterns of acceptance and, more rarely, rejection of the demeaning metaphors and seductive but disruptive technologies of biomedicine.[70] Anthropological work on women's reactions to the med-icalization of their problems more generally reveals mixed and unstable responses, ranging from selective compliance to selective resistance, with the dominant mode of response a kind of pragmatic ambivalence.[71] Few anthropologists, however, have studied the workings of power in the doc-tor-patient relationship, an arena in which the power of biomedicine can be found in one of its most concentrated forms. To understand the gen-dered dynamics of compliance and resistance in this pairing of "intimate adversaries," in Todd's fitting phrase (just how fitting, we shall see shortly), we need to extend to this new domain the kinds of questions anthropologists have asked in other settings: How do women patients approach the problem of getting good medical care? Beyond passively resisting, what positive strategies do they adopt to get the help they need and to oppose unwanted intrusions into their lives?

The work of Martin, Rapp, and many others has underscored the im-portance of difference, in the sense of the *social difference* of race and class, in women's proclivity to accept or reject medicine's offerings. While emphasizing the instability and flux of patient politics, this body of re-search has shown that, in general, white middle-class women are rela-tively accepting of biomedicine, while women of color and less economic privilege adopt more oppositional stances.[72] Social difference is indeed important, but there is another difference that may be equally significant.

This is the *inner difference* and inner instability that may lead a single patient to collude with biomedical power at one time and to challenge it at another. To understand this inner difference of multiple selves, we need to ask new questions about the patient's interior life. What is the psychological reasoning behind women's tactics of collusion and contention? What emotions impel their use? For answers to questions like these, we need to find a way into the innermost world of the patient. Yet what goes on in this domain is so private and so personal that it may be simply inaccessible to conventional anthropological and sociological research, reachable only through autobiographies or auto-ethnographies such as this one.

A Reflexive Look into the Patient's Inner World

Because so little is known about these inner landscapes of compliance and resistance, I began this part of my inquiry with some introspection. How, I asked myself, did an extended biomedical encounter look through the eyes of the patient? What was she trying to achieve in the interaction? How did she go about pursuing her ends? What was the emotional economy of the interaction with the doctor? Appropriate to a subject about which little is known, the exploration was unapologetically inductive. In looking reflexively at S.'s approach to the long adventure with Dr. D., I found, to my personal chagrin, that, to the patient, the doctor-patient relationship was first and foremost a *heterosexual relationship* in which the suffering body became a good excuse to see the doctor. This view of the doctor-patient interaction as a sociosexual relationship differs radically from the conventional biomedical picture of the doctor-patient relation as a technical, technology-mediated quest to repair a broken body.[73] It also departs from dominant sociological portraits of the encounter as a power struggle between competing interests (in the political economic view) or as a collusive negotiation of the disciplinary power of medicine (in the Foucauldian view).[74] But the differences do not end there. As a male-female relationship, in which the gender identities of the parties loomed large, the doctor-patient interaction studied here contained elements not only of the sexual politics brought out so well by the sociological research but also of veiled sexual desire. Far from being a peculiarity of this patient or this doctor, the element of desire, or personal feelings, is probably often present in cross-sex (or, for lesbians and gays, same-sex) medical encounters, especially long-term interactions in which chronic patients tend to be involved.[75] In this case, the longing for a good relationship entwined itself with the longing for a well body, producing a degree of emotional investment in the relationship that was far greater than one would expect from existing work on the medical encounter.[76] And when things began to go wrong, the emotional aftershocks—from depression to betrayal to anger—were as intense as the longing and hope that had preceded them. These emotional oscillations were as much a defining feature of the medical encounter to the patient as were the vagaries of the body. To capture these dimensions of the medical experience, which were central to the production of rebellion, we need to enlarge our array of concepts to include self, relationship, and emotion. And to develop these constructs, we need to broaden our conceptual terrain to embrace the fields of women's psychology and feminist theory.

The centrality of identity, feelings, and connection to the patient's experience of the medical encounter led me back to the field of women's psychology, the long-abandoned focus of my study and research as an undergraduate. In their work on women's morality, socialization, and depression, described in detail below, Carol Gilligan and her colleagues Lyn Mikel Brown and Dana Jack have collectively sketched out important elements of the psychodynamics of women's self in relationships with others. Their picture of these dynamics provides a veritable road map to the psychosocial odyssey on which the patient studied here embarked and to the emotional peaks and valleys she traversed along the way. Although this body of work has been subject to extensive critique in the women's studies literature, it contains important insights and implications that have been overlooked by earlier readings of it as theoretically outdated and politically problematic.[77] New readings of the Gilliganian corpus, on which I draw below, stress its radical implications for theories of identity and morality.[78] In this book I highlight those insights that illuminate issues of gender identity. Gender identity is the core construct around which issues of emotion, relationship, and politics all cluster. Although Gilligan's principal concern was women's morality, not identity, here I appropriate her and her colleagues' work for my own purposes, placing it within a theoretical literature that provides ways to avoid the intellectual problems that their critics have worried about.

Gender Identities: The "Discursive Self" and Its Resistant Potential

Questions of identity, self, and subjectivity—all of which refer to our understanding of who we are and how we live our lives—have been central concerns of feminist theory for the last two decades. Probably the dominant view today, and the one most useful for our purposes, follows Foucault and other poststructuralist thinkers in holding that there is no authentic, core, or essential self.[79] Rather, the self is a "discursive construction" that is actively constituted by individuals out of the discourses, or scripts, available in their environment. For this self, which she brings to theoretical life in her book *Moral Voices, Moral Selves,* feminist theorist Susan J. Hekman has coined the term *the discursive self.*[80] At any given time, Hekman explains, we are confronted with an array of discourses of selfhood, scripts we are expected to follow. We can either adopt the subjectivity that is offered to us or assemble a different identity from other discourses that are rooted in alternative social institutions and practices.[81]

For women living in a patriarchal world, the dominant discourses on subjectivity are those of femininity. These scripts on femininity are numerous and vary with social situations. Conveyed in the schools, the media, and many other social institutions and practices, the dominant discourses on femininity urge us to be motherly, wifely, and caring at home, professional but not bossy at work, and sexy but not aggressive in romantic encounters. The dominant script on the feminine self-in-relationship is the pleasant, compliant self that is elaborated in the work of Gilligan and her colleagues. The predominance of this script in our culture undoubtedly explains why so many of Gilligan's critics note that, despite their intellectual reservations, they find her model intuitively appealing because it "feels" right.[82] In this book I want to honor that intuition and to suggest that the felt appeal of the model stems from its invisible presence in many domains of social life—including the medical encounter. Indeed, I will argue that this model of feminine identity delineates the self that many women patients unconsciously embrace in their relationships with their male physicians. What Gilligan and her colleagues tend to overlook, however, at least in their early, best-known work, is that scripts on femininity are written not for women as a generic category, but for women of particular races, classes, sexualities, and so forth. Thus, as the critics have noted, the "feminine" self in the world of Gilligan, Brown, and Jack is best described as the self of "mainstream" white, middle-class, heterosexual women.[83] Women of other races, classes, and sexualities are offered other scripts on femininity to follow. Later work by Brown, Gilligan, and their colleagues recognizes and explores these differences.[84]

Although one identity tends to predominate at a given time, our gender identities are not unitary, coherent, or fixed, as the earlier psychological work seems to imply.[85] To the contrary, they are usually multiple, often contradictory, and always in process, being constructed and reconstructed in ongoing power-laden social interactions in which the subjectivities of the parties are constantly open to contestation. Gender is not only something one *is*, then, but also something one *does* in interaction with others. It is, in the words of sociologists Sarah Fenstermaker, Candace West, and Don H. Zimmerman, a "situated accomplishment" produced in everyday interactions.[86] The central question here is which gender identity or identities emerge from the negotiated power dynamics of the medical encounter. We return to this issue shortly.

For both Foucault and feminist theorists of the self, identity is intimately tied to power. On the one hand, since our identities are fashioned out of extant discourses, in the mere act of creating our identities we subject ourselves to the power of those discourses. Thus, for example, when we unconsciously follow the good-girl routines set out for us in the dominant discourses on femininity, we become subject to the power of feminine ideals—which are rooted in the dominant institutions and practices of our society—to constitute our subjectivities and, in that way, define our lives. On the other hand, as Foucault famously wrote, power also produces resistance to domination. We are capable of resisting power because we are self-creating subjects who piece together elements of identity out of the discursive tools available. "The resistant subject," Hekman explains, "is one that refuses to be scripted by the dominant discourse and turns instead to subjugated knowledges . . . [or marginalized subjectivities] . . . to fashion alternative discourses of subjectivity."[87] Indeed, Hekman continues, the history of the women's movement is precisely the history of women refusing to be scripted feminine and "claim[ing] the right to adopt subjectivities . . . that grant them equality, rights, and justice before the law."[88] The discourses of feminism also provide individuals with discursive tools that enable them not only to claim new identities but also to critique the existing power structures and to take political action to change them. Simply by rejecting one identity and claiming another, women can resist domination. Such "discursive resistance" is real resistance, but when it is accompanied by political acts, it can also stimulate larger political change.

In their work on women's self-in-relationship, Gilligan and her colleagues have provided an elaborate psychological map of a dominant script on femininity written for mainstream women. In the following section I lay out the main elements of the dynamic and show how they powerfully illuminate the psychodynamics of the "feminine" self that the patient studied here put forward in her relationship with her doctor. This work supports and deepens the sociological notion of limited resistance by showing how women collaborate in and contribute to their own oppression in the biomedical encounter. But there was another, "feminist," self in this doctor-patient relationship whose psychodynamics are not captured in the work of the psychologists. It was this self, fabricated from the discourses of feminism, that broke through to anger and open revolt against biomedical power. A later section describes this more resistant "feminist" self and how it gave birth to political action.

The "Feminine" Relational Self
and the Psychodynamics of Patient Compliance

Research on women's psychology has revealed the deep costs imposed on women's inner selves by the still-sexist society in which they must live. Gilligan's landmark study, *In a Different Voice,* began with the well-established notion that, in a society in which achievement in the public domain has historically been a male prerogative, women's fundamental self is relational. That is, it is based on intimate relations with others, especially men.[89] Because that sense of self is threatened by separation and aggression, women try to avoid isolation and to prevent aggression through activities of care that make the social world safe. Out of this psychology of relationship is born an "ethic of care" in which the good or moral woman is one who cares for others, ensuring that no one is hurt. For this gift of care, she expects to be loved and cared for in return.

The developmental roots of this ethic are explored in Brown and Gilligan's study of adolescent development, *Meeting at the Crossroads: Women's Psychology and Girls' Development.*[90] For girls, they show, early adolescence is a time of crisis. In a world that devalues them, girls learn to silence themselves. Rather than risk conflict that might sunder their relationships, leaving them alone and powerless, they split their selves into an "authentic" inner self that no longer speaks and a pleasing but "false" outer self that reflects what others want them to be: "good girls" on their way to becoming "perfect women." In accordance with poststructuralist notions of identity, many readers have challenged the authors' claim that girls have authentic and inauthentic selves.[91] I understand Brown and Gilligan to mean true and false in an *experiential* rather than in an *essential* sense. To the girls they worked with, the voices that were silenced *felt* genuine, because they articulated the girls' innermost sentiments. To say that a given self *feels* authentic is not the same thing as claiming that a given identity *is* authentic.[92] Because it implies the existence of essentially true and false selves, however, in the ethnography below I avoid the terms *authentic* and *inauthentic*. I retain the phrases "silencing the angry self" and "creating a falsely pleasant outer self," however, because they capture crucially important psychological dynamics.

The psychological costs of adopting that pleasant outer "feminine" self are steep indeed. In her study of women and depression, *Silencing the Self*, Dana Jack has shown how the ethic of care can hurt women by making them vulnerable to depression.[93] In muting their own needs and attending to others', women become deeply confused about where their own self leaves off and the selves of others begin. The blurring of boundaries between self and other reduces their ability to recognize abuse and leaves them at risk of depression when they discover that they have lost their most fundamental possession: their sense of self.

In this book, I contend that many women (at least mainstream white, middle-class, heterosexual women) take this feminine identity and its relational reasoning into the biomedical encounter, where they put it to work in their quest to get the best medical care they can out of a system in which they are doubly silenced and disempowered. The strategies they use in their relationships with doctors are remarkably similar to those described by Gilligan, Brown, and Jack. Because the stakes are both emotional and physical, however, the consequences of caring too much are more devastating in the medical setting. This "psychomedical perspective" is useful because it provides a framework that makes psychological sense out of many of the findings of the medical sociologists. It is important because it suggests a new and disturbing set of consequences that flow from the potent mix of medicine and gender.

In generalized form, the psychomedical dynamic I postulate is as follows. When the medical stakes are high (as, for example, when the illness is serious or longstanding), many women can be expected to take a relationship-first approach to their health care. (Men may emphasize relationships with their doctors, too, but the psychodynamics of the process and the nature of the relationships they construct are likely to be different. This is a fascinating subject which, unfortunately, I cannot pursue here.[94]) It is important to remember that this relationship-first approach is not followed by every woman patient in every doctor's visit. When the health problem is relatively minor or temporary, the patient's attention is likely to remain focused on fixing the problem, not on creating a relationship. But when the illness is serious or of long duration and/or involves major psychological problems, a different set of emotional—and thus also relational—dynamics comes into play.[95] It is in these circumstances that women "do gender" by enacting a feminine identity of the sort described above. Emotionally vulnerable and dependent, the seriously ill patient has little choice but to place her trust in her doctor. And, indeed, many very ill patients (and some not-so-ill ones as well) derive comfort and reassurance from allowing themselves to become completely trustful of and dependent on their physicians.[96] But how do they ensure that the doctor will not betray that trust? They do so, I contend, by investing heavily in the relationship with him. While women undoubtedly create special relationships with both male and female physicians, my concern here is with the connections they form with male health care providers. In these connections, the fundamental assumption is that if they form a warm, trusting relationship with their doctor, he will take care of their bodily needs. According to this relational logic, safety and health lie in a good relationship. Accordingly, women set about creating that good relationship, modeling it on the class of "intimate relations with men." In this model, the woman must create an outside or public self that is compliant and pleasing to the doctor. This self is guided by an ethic of care in which making the doctor happy may become as important as, if not more important than, taking care of the self. Making him happy may mean silencing their critical concerns, suppressing their anger, and preserving the hierarchy of power in which the doctor makes all the decisions about their care. Though this strategy makes psychological sense given the social cards women have been dealt, it is patently risky. When carried to an extreme, it leaves women unable to communicate their worries, unprotected against their doctor's mistakes, and at risk of a depression that can become more debilitating than the disease.

The "Feminist" Self and the Politics of Patient Resistance

The patient whose psychological makeup we will dissect below provides a textbook case of the compliant "feminine" self, its relational reasoning, and the heavy costs that reasoning imposes. But this case also contains elements of a different, contradictory gender identity—a different way of "doing gender"—that provided the emotional and intellectual wherewithal to talk back to and even openly to rebel against medical authority. This identity, which the patient saw as "feminist," was scripted out of notions of equality and justice and critiques of patriarchy advanced by feminist scholars and activists over the last three decades. Such understandings also served as political tools that in the end enabled the patient to challenge and dethrone her doctor. At any given time one gender identity tended to predominate and to shape the emotional, relational, and political dimensions of the self the patient presented to the doctor. While one identity dominated at a particular time, elements of both subjectivities were always present. Even when the "feminine" self held sway, the warring "feminist" self was actively struggling to gain expression.

By recognizing the existence of this other, partly submerged identity, we are able to see antagonistic emotions and forms of resistance to biomedical power that remain invisible in work on women's subjugation in the medical encounter. In the case examined here, these political resources include a muted anger that the patient rehearsed in her mind but could not yet openly express and tactics of subversion that remained invisible to the doctor but over time empowered the patient.[97] What tied these tactics of resistance together was their silent character, their deployment in private writings and conversations that the doctor could not see or hear. Although the work of Gilligan and her colleagues tends to equate silence with powerlessness and psychological pathology, more recent thinking in feminist psychology recognizes that silence contains multiple meanings, which are anchored in different subject positions. Maureen A. Mahoney argues that silence can be a "psychological space of resistance and negotiation" in which "the capacity to speak out with confidence and authority" is nurtured.[98] Although these episodes of nonspeaking are experienced as times of shame, confusion, and anxiety, Mahoney contends, far from being pathological, refusals to speak publicly can be healthy responses to being controlled as well as rich states of developmental growth.[99] In this ethnography, silent forms of resistance, rooted in the patient's "feminist" identity, provided crucial emotional and intellectual resources that enabled her openly to challenge the doctor when the time was ripe. Although suffered in confusion and distress, the patient's secret resistances became crucial pathways to public protest and personal power.

Recognizing the multiple, contradictory, and processual character of patients' gender identities, and the relational, emotional, and political entailments these gender identities involve, suggests new ways of understanding power and resistance in the biomedical encounter. The focus on gender identity extends our grasp of power's workings by showing that the politics of both compliance and resistance is rooted in an inner terrain—that of selfhood—that students of biomedical power have scarcely begun to explore. These larger implications of the analysis of patient identity and politics are explored in the book's conclusion.

Cultures of Illness, Cultures of Blame

Biomedicine operates within a larger culture that today is obsessed with illness and the body. Spread by the media, books, and everyday conversations, popular beliefs about bodily suffering powerfully shape the sick person's understandings of why he is ill and what he should do to get better. The effects of these ideas are often more powerful than biomedicine recognizes and more insidious than alternative medicine, a major purveyor of these notions, intends.

In her influential essay, *Illness as Metaphor*, philosopher Susan Sontag drew attention to our culture's long-standing tendency to metaphorize illness.[100] Through metaphor, the culture has turned a bodily disorder into a moral matter in which outward signs of disease are seen as evidence of inner flaws. Psychological theories of illness, she argued, are punitive, for they blame the patient for being ill—"she deserves it," "she's one of life's losers"—and make her responsible for getting better. In the past few decades, not only illness but also health has become a moral matter. Whether promoting exercise, health foods, or other "wellness behaviors," health crusaders portray the pursuit of a healthy lifestyle as a moral duty, the achievement of good health an "affirmation of a life lived virtuously."[101] Written twenty years ago, Sontag's critique of our moralization of illness has even more bite today, when the metaphorizing she described has become a veritable industry: Alternative Medicine, Inc.

In recent years the public has grown deeply dissatisfied with mainstream approaches to chronic illness. But it has not given up hope for a cure to chronic pain. Building on this wellspring of public interest, alternative approaches to healing have flourished, becoming some of the major articulators of our cultural discourses on illness. Although many widely divergent alternative approaches exist, the ones that have gotten the most attention are not the well-established therapies such as Chinese and Ayurvedic medicine but the less proven self-help and New Age approaches whose manifestos crowd the shelves of bookstores around the country. These approaches are the focus of attention in this book.

Virtually all holistic approaches hold that the mind and body are deeply interconnected and that our thoughts and emotions powerfully affect our physical selves. Although framed as a critique of, and alternative to, mainstream medicine, holistic medicines are oddly similar to conventional medicine in important ways. Both neglect structural sources of pain—whether political, economic, environmental, or social—treating illness as an individual problem whose roots lie close at hand. Both overstate the extent of individual control, neglecting the powerful cultural and psychological forces that shape individual behavior and that place much of what we do beyond our immediate control. Both are therapeutic discourses that focus on treatment while slighting the question of cause. The self-help and New Age approaches share these features of alternative medicines generally, but they push the philosophy more toward the mind than the body in the mind-body duality. If scientific medicine promotes the body-cure, many of the self-help and New Age medicines advance the mind-cure, which holds that by changing our thoughts and attitudes we can change the state of our bodies. Like scientific medicine, these medicines are reductionistic, tracing illness to body *or* mind but neglecting the ways in which body and mind work together, in interaction with specific social and environmental contexts, to produce disease.

For the chronically ill, these self-help and New Age discourses are highly seductive, for they make sense of senseless pain and promise hope in a situation long bereft of it. But, as Sontag warned, the dangers of being seduced are great, for along with hope and empowerment comes a heavy dose of cultural blame. Today, when alternative therapies are available in every mall in the country, the ill person is blamed not only for getting ill, but if the therapies fail, he is also blamed for not getting better ("he gave up too soon," "he didn't want to get well"). Academic culture critics like Elaine Showalter inadvertently amplify the blame heaped on the sick by the popular discourses. In her much-touted book, *Hysteries: Hysterical Epidemics and Modern Culture,* she attaches terms like *psychogenic* and *psychological plagues* to contemporary epidemics of chronic pain such as chronic fatigue syndrome and Gulf War syndrome.[102] While the psychological dynamics she highlights undoubtedly contribute to these disorders, and the cultural dynamics she exposes turn them into virtual epidemics, Showalter neglects the ways in which biology interacts with psychology to place some bodies at risk, leaving other bodies with the same psychological makeup blissfully pain free.[103] "I don't wish to offend these sufferers," she writes, but then proceeds to do just that by implying that they possess a degree of control over their bodies that no one, sick or well, can achieve.[104] To break the cycle of "hysterical epidemics," she urges, we must "claim . . . our full humanity as free and responsible [human] beings . . . ; we must look into our own psyches . . . for the answers."[105] Showalter's study is part of a new wave of explanatory models of illness that blame the victim for his illness.[106] Many critics, especially in the social sciences, see these new models more as accusation than as explanation.[107] Though making others responsible for their own illnesses helps us deny our own vulnerability to disease and death, it adds to the burdens of the ill. By placing responsibility for illness on the afflicted, the culture compounds the problems of the chronically ill by adding to the misfortune of bodily pain, psychic distress, cultural censure, and social stigma.

The cultural discourses are intended to broaden the discourse on illness, but they may have the paradoxical effect of making the sick, or perhaps only the sickest of the sick, all the more dependent on scientific medicine. Feeling blamed, the ill person can react only with denial of the imputed connection between her mind and her body, her life and her disease. Hence the "longing for organicity," the desperate craving for a biological disease label, that clinicians see in their chronic patients and that cry out from the pages of patient self-help newsletters.[108] These patients—too often labeled "malingerers" and "clinical headaches" by the biomedical community[109]—are the wounded survivors of a culture that blames them for their illness.

Promising help, contemporary cultures of illness place the chronically sick in a trap: they cannot admit that psychosocial factors worsen their illness, because if they do they are blamed for causing their own problems. So they are forced back on biological labels and biomedical practitioners as their only source of solace and relief. By placing personal responsibility on the individual rather than looking at larger structural factors that may lie behind the individual's personality or lifestyle, popular discourses prevent the chronically ill from addressing the problems in their lives that may contribute to their symptoms. The result is a kind of culturally induced paralysis that can discourage the use of helpful alternative therapies and can add psychological distress to the physical pain of being ill.

While much ink has been spilled over these issues by social commentators and medical experts, we know less about how alternative discourses and therapies play out in the lives of real patients. From illness narratives of the chronically ill, we know that struggles with mind-body issues are fundamental parts of the experience of chronic illness in our culture.[110] But even when the use of alternative medicine is a major theme in illness autobiographies, the authors often write as converts to the cause and exude uncritical enthusiasm for the healing powers of mind and emotion.[111] Self-reflective accounts of encounters with alternative medicine are rare. The case reported in this book provides an opportunity to witness critically the effects of some self-help and New Age therapies on the life of a chronic patient who turned to them in desperation when the therapies of biomedicine did not work. It shows how instead of "opening the blocks" to healing, some alternative medicines can block healing instead. But it also shows a way out of the trap, an escape route that avoids both the Scylla of biomedicine and the Charybdis of alternative medicines. The escape route the patient discovered was to locate the problem not in the individual body or personality but in the larger structures of inequality in society, in particular, in the structures of gender inequality. The idea that the production of "fibromyalgia" might be related to struggles over women's place in society has led me, as author, to reflect on and worry about the larger historical implications of the invention of fibromyalgia for women. I share these worries in the book's conclusion.

Auto-Ethnography as Cultural and Political Critique

In presenting my material I have chosen to write an ethnography, the classic genre of anthropology. Today many moving patient testimonials document personal struggles with serious illness.[112] Perhaps because medical anthropology has only recently turned its attention to Western medicine, however, we have few ethnographic accounts of what happens when patient meets doctor.[113] But the ethnographic approach provides unique insights that other approaches—whether survey based, historical, or literary—cannot supply. Through close description and analysis of a small slice of social life, ethnography shows how the culture at large does its work. In this ethnography, I take medicine as a culture and use one intimately observed case to limn the workings of the system as a whole. Here ethnography takes the form of cultural critique.

This book presents not only an ethnography, but an auto-ethnography of a medical encounter.[114] In auto-ethnography observer and observed are one and the same person. Auto-ethnography differs from autobiography in that the focus is not on the writer, but on certain experiences in the writer's life that illuminate important or previously hidden aspects of the larger culture. The emphasis here, for example, is not on the patient herself, but on the patient's protracted encounter with a doctor who fully embodied the scientific approach to medicine.

Avoiding Solipsism

In writing autobiographically one runs the risk of solipsism, or excessive preoccupation with the self. I have sought to avoid this problem through the use of three literary devices. First, as just noted, I have made the empirical focus of the study not the patient, but the doctor-patient relationship and its embeddedness in the larger cultures of medicine and gender. In this way, I have "written culture" while also "writing my (former) self."[115]

Second, I have drawn a clear demarcation between the person observed, whose thoughts, feelings, and experiences are described, and the author-analyst, in whose voice the study is written. To enforce this distinction I have created a literary space between myself as author and S. as patient, using the first-person "I" for the author and the third-person "she" for S. This distance was easy to maintain, since a good part of S.—many of her hopes, dreams, and beliefs—died during the encounter described in this book. In addition to my desire to avoid overly focusing on myself, my creation of two literary figures was motivated by the social facts and some compelling analytic considerations.[116] The social fact is that S. could not have written this book. She was in too much physical and psychic pain even to grasp what was happening to her, let alone to muster the energy necessary to write a book. Only the post-S. I, who was born at the end of the episode, was able to step back and make sense of that encounter and to undertake the long-term project of turning it into a book.

In separating "I" from "S.," I also had two larger analytic objectives. First, a central argument of this book is that S., as a subject with a distinctive sense of her self and its place in the world, was extinguished during the encounter described below. The creation of another self, "I," who succeeded S., underscores the point that biomedicine can profoundly damage, even destroy, the patient's self. Writing about my former self in the third person also enabled me as analyst to adopt a variety of critical attitudes toward S. The ability to mock, scold, grieve for, and sometimes even praise the patient opened up a large volume of analytic space, allowing me to press critical points and to develop theoretical arguments that would have been difficult to advance had I written in the first person. Although these considerations may have led me to exaggerate the difference between the two social beings, the gap is nonetheless real. S. and the I who is writing this book have to some extent different understandings of life, emotional makeups, physical bodies, and even career trajectories. In important ways, S. and I are two different people. Because S. is my former self, and because she lives on in my memory, I am able to use her testimonial as a positioned witness as the basis for this book. As many have suggested, the ability to give testimony to moving or traumatic events is part of what gives auto-ethnographic writing its power.[117] But I as author am able to feature S.'s testimony only because she left diaries and charts documenting her experiences. S. as sentient subject no longer exists.

Third, I have presented the ethnographic materials within a larger structure that is analytical rather than historical or biographical. At the level of the chapter and of the group of chapters, or book part, the central narrative is not the unfolding of a life but the development of an argument.[118] This theoretical framework deflects attention away from the individual life and toward the larger argument being advanced.

In addition to these literary means, I also develop a substantive argument that should help to put any worries about self-centeredness to rest. As elaborated above, I argue that the selves of individuals are not inherent or given, but actively created out of the discourses of the culture. The culture thus defines the possibilities of selfhood that are available to individuals at any given time. If this is so, then when we write about our selves in theoretically sensitive ways, we inevitably write about our culture. The boundary between self and society begins to break down, auto-ethnography blurs into ethnography, and concerns about solipsism should fade away.

Why Auto-Ethnography? Intellectual and Political Significances

Auto-ethnography is an especially productive vehicle for this project. First, because it can offer deep personal insight into the self and soul of the patient, it is uniquely suited to an exploration of the effects of medicine on the inner world of the patient, a central concern throughout this book. Second, because it allows me to use the patient's own contemporaneously penned words to describe her illness experience, the auto-ethnography enables an account of illness and its social origins that remains close to the patient's original experience. Such an account avoids the vexing problems of professional transformation of illness into social science jargon and the consequent dehumanization of suffering and silencing of the afflicted about which medical anthropologists such as Arthur Kleinman, Joan Kleinman, and Susan M. DiGiacomo have expressed concern.[119]

Use of the auto-ethnographic form also carries political significance in the discipline of anthropology of which the reader should be aware. In anthropology, interest in auto-ethnography arose out of a larger disciplinary critique of classic ethnography.[120] Like the science of medicine, the science of classic anthropology posited a distanced observer who, through close observation of a cultural Other, was able to produce the objective Truths of culture. Today many anthropologists see that earlier project as part of the deployment of Western power over other cultures. Moreover, though respecting science, they believe that its truths are always partial and interested, reflecting the social locations and cultural values of its makers. In an effort to reduce power hierarchies and to scale back claims to authoritative knowledge, a new generation of critical anthropologists has turned to alternative forms of ethnography in which to do their work. Although its use remains rare in anthropology at large, and rarer still in medical anthropology, the auto-ethnography is a promising means by which to pursue these political and intellectual ends.[121] The auto-ethnography breaks down the barrier between observer and observed, scientist and object, cultural self and Other, by making them one and the same person (who, however, assumes two different roles). Moreover, the auto-ethnographer does not claim to produce objective truth. With science critics Sandra Harding and Donna Haraway, I fault claims to objectivity by knowledge producers who represent themselves as impersonal, impartial, and impassive—such knowledge makers remain unlocatable and thus not answerable to the consequences of their claims.[122] The alternative to impersonal and irresponsible objectivity is the claim to produce *partial truths* that are rooted in identifiable social locations and that are thus responsible for their assertions. This auto-ethnography claims to tell such a partial truth. It is a "situated" or "positioned" truth reflecting the world as seen by a white, middle-class, forty-something academic woman with a particular history of bodily ills and care. This is very much that patient's story; had the doctor written this book instead, it certainly would have been very different. In using this ethnographic genre, my aim is to furnish a political critique not only of the doctor's brand of medicine but also of science's larger claim to produce objective truth, including claims of this sort by anthropology itself.

Though I have highlighted some of the advantages of the auto-ethnographic genre, there are also drawbacks that need to be noted.[123] My particular positioning with regard to the illness described here has profoundly shaped the interpretations I offer of that experience. Although personal involvement has enabled me to see previously hidden aspects of the illness experience, it may also have restricted my vision in ways I cannot perceive. My intense moral and emotional engagement with the medical encounter featured in these pages may also have tempted me to overgeneralize from my own experience. Although I have tried to minimize these problems by embedding my arguments in the scholarly literatures on chronic illness and biomedicine, such problems are to some extent unavoidable in auto-ethnographic writing.

The Rewards and Risks of Writing about Emotion

Autobiographical writing has also been favored by feminist anthropologists, in part because of its ability to acknowledge and to reveal the role of emotions in the production of anthropological knowledge.[124] In a series of introspective works published over the past decade, Ruth Behar has courageously pioneered this style of "vulnerable writing."[125] In this study I push this process of exteriorizing the interior further by acknowledging the role not only of emotions but also of physical suffering and pain in shaping the creation of anthropological knowledge.

Writing of emotion and pain, however, is risky. In the Western philosophical tradition, emotions are regarded as suspect and their purported opposite, reason, is deemed the sole legitimate faculty with which knowledge may be acquired.[126] Writing emotionally thus leaves one vulnerable to charges of being irrational, particularistic, private, and subjective, rather than reasonable, universal, public, and objective. The risk is especially great for women, since they have long been associated with the emotional, irrational side of these binaries. Writing against the grain, the feminist theorist Alison M. Jaggar argues, persuasively I think, that feminists' concerns about emotionality may be overdrawn. Far from threatening feminist scholarship, she suggests, certain kinds of emotions can play strategic roles in the development of critical social theory.[127] In a thoughtful essay on the role played by emotion in the creation of knowledge, Jaggar argues that the familiar dichotomies set out above are artificial.[128] Although feelings are experienced as private and particularistic, she demonstrates, emotions are actually social constructs taught to new members of society and shared by large categories of people. Moreover, far from being antithetical to knowledge, emotions are necessary features of all knowledge, influencing the values, observations, and thoughts that make up the process of intellectual inquiry. Most scholars, she believes, are unaware of the role of their emotions in their scholarship, because our culture encourages us to control or even suppress our emotions. Jaggar suggests that emotional reactions that fall outside the bounds of convention—what she calls "outlaw emotions"—offer particular promise for feminist theory. Atypical emotional responses, which are usually appropriate to the person's social situation of subordination, can facilitate the building of critical theory by motivating investigations into new issues and by enabling new versions of reality that challenge dominant views.

At the heart of this book lie a handful of emotions that most Americans would probably be happy to dub "outlaw": deep depression about, rather than stoic acceptance of, chronic illness; personal fondness for, rather than cautious reserve toward, a physician; and, later, raging anger at, instead of quiet gratitude toward, the same practitioner. Because of their very unconventionality, these emotional reactions enabled—or rather forced—me to see the political and psychological dynamics of the medical encounter in new, nonconventional ways. These powerful yet perverse emotions not only motivated the writing of this book, they also shaped the theorizing that underlies its arguments. This book suggests that instead of fearing our emotions, we should attend more closely to them, for they have much to teach us about the workings of gender and power in the world in which we live. Having said that, I recognize that reading about these inner landscapes of pain may prove deeply discomfiting to some. This book will challenge readers accustomed to equating scholarship with cool objectivity to recognize that emotions can enrich our scholarly work in unexpected and productive ways.

Finding Dr. Right

By the age of forty S. had a thick medical file. Pieces of her body's history could be found up and down the East Side of Manhattan, from Cornell Medical Center on Seventieth Street to New York University Medical Center forty blocks to the south. Clearly, S. had sought some of the best physicians from the best centers of academic medicine in the city. Her records were also strewn all over the medical landscape, in the offices of neurologists, orthopedists, rheumatologists, physical therapists, and even cosmetic surgeons—so many specialists had she seen looking for help diagnosing and treating the pain in her knees, elbows, neck, and fingers. That the problem was bodily or biological she had no doubt; after all, the swelling and pain were in her joints. The solution, just as obviously, was to find expert medical help: that is what people do when their bodies stop working properly. The decision to medicalize the problem was thus made without even a passing thought.

This prologue recounts some key episodes in S.'s search for the right doctor to treat her ills. The story begins with the quest for a diagnosis and ends with the discovery of a doctor whose promises for treatment sounded too good to be true. It moves from New York City, where S. was employed during her thirties and early forties, to southern California, where she moved in her mid-forties to assume a new position. It is a tale of disillusion, confusion, and desire—disillusionment from encounters with thought-less doctors, confusion over a once-healthy body now out of control, and desire born of worsening health conditions that seemed to spiral ever downward.

East Coast Doctors:
Thoughtless Men and Empathic Women

S. had begun her search for doctor and diagnosis in her mid-thirties, when the joint condition that was later to dominate her life first made itself felt. At the age of thirty-six she had surgery for carpal tunnel syndrome, asking to have both hands operated on at the same time to avoid the necessity of two interruptions to her busy schedule. After that, mysterious symptoms began to appear. A few weeks after the surgery her left knee started to swell, growing so large and painful that she could scarcely walk. S. felt deep in her bones that the two events were connected, that her knee was swelling to protest the surgical assault on her system. Then in her late thirties she injured her neck during a three-day home-painting marathon. The excessive strain on her neck, which had been craned back at a ninety-degree angle while she painted a low ceiling, traumatized her whole upper-back area, causing a searing, spreading pain that immobilized her for months. It was this episode that sent her on a concerted search for medical help.

The process of finding a good doctor had been emotionally traumatizing. Indeed, many of her medical encounters, especially with male physicians, had been degrading and disempowering. A young doctor at N.Y.U. Medical Center had injected her knee with corticosteroids while carrying on an animated telephone conversation with a colleague about another patient. S. felt like a barnyard animal and never went back. A more senior physician, a world-famous neurologist at Cornell Medical Center, had sat her down and said, his voice dripping with scorn, "You are a very pleasant woman," as though pleasantness were a social sin. And that was her diagnosis: even after hearing her account of her neck injury and subsequent pain and conducting a clinical examination, he insisted that there was nothing wrong with her except her personality. S. cried for weeks, unable to understand how being pleasant had caused her body so much pain. And she was still in great pain. Adding financial injury to the emotional assault, he had charged her $500 for the visit.

Feeling wronged, S. wrote a pointed letter to the eminent neurologist. She expressed anger at him for dabbling in psychotherapy when his expertise lay elsewhere and for charging women with somatizing their psychosocial problems while giving men physical explanations for their bodily ills. (She knew three men who had consulted the doctor and received diagnoses of a physical sort.) "In short," she wrote with feeling, "I got much less than my money's worth" (Letter, October 7, 1990).

The noted physician replied by offering to let her consult a colleague in his department, a specialist in the links between neurological and arthritic conditions, at no charge. Because the colleague was a young woman, S. harbored a small shred of hope that the specialist might be more sympathetic and helpful than the male doctors she had seen. After much agonized backing and forthing, S. agreed to see the young neurologist, despite the sickening feeling that overcame her every time she pictured herself returning to the department of neurology at Cornell Medical Center.

The woman doctor was more empathic than S. had imagined possible. She took a brief medical history, conducted a clinical examination, and concluded that S. was probably suffering from psoriatic arthritis, which was now flaring in the neck region because of the recent injury. The diagnosis made eminent sense, since S. had a mild case of psoriasis, the skin condition, and the pattern of joint swelling matched that of the psoriatic form of arthritis rather than the more common rheumatoid arthritis, or osteoarthritis. The young doctor at N.Y.U. had diagnosed psoriatic arthritis several years earlier when she had sought treatment for a swollen knee. Also, in S.'s family there was some history of psoriatic arthritis, which was known to have genetic roots. Since a rheumatologist, not a neurologist, was the proper medical specialist for her condition, S. thanked the doctor for her help, went home, and made an appointment with a woman rheumatologist affiliated with N.Y.U., whose name she had encountered in her medical travels around the city.

Dr. K., a woman about S.'s age, confirmed the diagnosis of psoriatic arthritis and put S. on an antiinflammatory drug to control the joint swelling. (The disease could not be cured, but its symptoms could be controlled.) It was not only the knowledge that she was finally in competent hands that made S. like Dr. K. From the first minutes of the first visit, when the doctor commented on her stylish Joan and David shoes, it was clear that this practitioner would be different. Instead of reducing her to a body and ignoring everything else or, at the other extreme, ignoring the bodily component and blaming everything on her personality, Dr. K. treated her as a whole person, acknowledging that she had a life and a career as well as a disease. Dr. K. believed that the course of the arthritis was largely shaped by biological factors beyond the patient's control, but that stresses in a patient's life could worsen the condition by precipitating flares. Accordingly, Dr. K. often asked about S.'s work and home life, perhaps teasing out stresses that might be exacerbating the symptoms. Instead of hiding her personal life behind her white coat, Dr. K. occasionally shared details of her own life, especially when they related to things that were happening in S.'s world. At those times she broke down the barrier that is usually erected between doctor and patient, knower and known, subject and object of medical science. Although Dr. K. remained distant and professional, and she was always rushed, she created an atmosphere in which S. felt that she could speak the truth of her life and, for the most part, be heard.

During those last few years in New York S. had plenty of stress to talk about. She had grown disillusioned with her once-perfect job in social and policy research. She was having difficulties with her new boss. She had a grueling five-hour-a-day commute. All these factors surely contributed in some indecipherable way to the growing number of flares that materialized in her early forties. The medication Dr. K. prescribed kept things largely under control, but each new flare had to be countered with a new attack of medication. Over the next few years S. found herself taking increased dosages of the antiinflammatory; short-term rounds of Prednisone, a cortisone-based drug; and a powerful new drug, Methotrexate, which is often used in cancer treatment. The potential side effects of all these drugs—on the bones and on vital organs such as the liver and the stomach—were so scary that S. could not bring herself to read the inserts that came with the medicine.

As her forties wore on, the joint swelling was up and down, here one month, gone the next, in this finger one year, in that toe the next. The overall trend, however, seemed forever downward. Things became increasingly serious until S. landed in the hospital for surgery on a thumb joint that had swollen beyond usability. The joint had deteriorated so much that it could no longer be corrected; the operation merely fused the bones to preserve minimal functioning of the thumb. The strong medication, while evidently helpful, was not fully controlling the symptoms. Every half year or so S. had a new swelling, and each new swelling meant an increase in medication and the potential loss, for life, of another joint.

West Coast Doctors: A Dream Too Good to Be True?

When she was forty-five S. moved to southern California to take up a new position as a university professor. Her first rheumatologist was assigned to her by the health-care plan she was required to join because of her preexisting condition. He was a charming man, but an indifferent joint doctor who spent too much time chatting about his cat and other matters of questionable medical significance. When her joints swelled, he put S. on rounds of Prednisone, increasing the risk of bone thinning and eventual osteoporosis.

At forty-six S. was nearing the end of her rope. The stress of coping with a demanding new job in an unfamiliar work environment with little social support was taking its toll. On the scale of life stresses S. was off the scale: she had not just moved three thousand miles to a new part of the country. She had also changed jobs, fields, and types of organizations; disrupted her family life (her husband was still based in New York but had found work in several West Coast cities); and lost the social network that had held her hectic life together in New York. A heavy load of teaching and committee work prevented her from doing her own research and writing, making her feel she had lost her professional and personal identity and thus her very self.

Every stress in her life seemed to write itself out on her body. The connection between life distress and body symptom was now frighteningly close. Two days after a big blowup at the university, her right pinkie ballooned into the classic "sausage digit" of psoriatic arthritis, sending her back to her doctor for yet another round of Prednisone. While the joints of her fingers had been a problem before, now the joints in her feet were swelling as well, making walking difficult. Her ability to sleep was impaired, leaving her physically drained and emotionally weak and, in turn, all the more vulnerable to the stresses of her new life.

Despite S.'s valiant efforts to stay in control, her life was becoming a vicious cycle of overwhelming stress, fatigue, and symptoms. The doctor to whom she had been assigned was not paying attention and seemed insufficiently concerned about the seriousness of her condition. As soon as she was allowed to change health plans, S. switched to a plan that offered freedom in the choice of specialists and immediately began the search for another rheumatologist. This one had to be a woman.

But the search for a woman doctor did not get far. For, quite by chance, around this time S. was put in touch with a fellow sufferer of psoriatic arthritis, and of many other conditions as well. The new friend, Anna, whom we will meet again in later chapters, told her about a doctor (male, unfortunately, and a short flight away in Seattle) with a radically different approach to rheumatological care. Anna had heard about him from her family in Seattle, where she had grown up. According to Anna, who had been seeing him for two years, Dr. D. used aggressive pharmacological intervention—in plain English, strong drugs—to make his patients as close to symptom free as possible. In many of his patients he diagnosed something called fibromyalgia, a condition involving widespread muscle pain and a sleep disorder. He resolved the sleep disorder with medication. This sounded extremely promising to S., for she was having great difficulty sleeping. The thought of getting help with her sleep problem had powerful appeal.

Yet, Anna pointed out, there were also disadvantages to going to Dr. D. These were in addition to the inconvenience and expense of traveling to seem him. First, the doctor insisted on micromanaging his patients' lives, with frequent appointments, endless tests, and other demands that were time consuming and intrusive. Second, he had a "bad bedside manner," a blunt way of putting things that seemed uncaring at best, cruel at worst. In Anna's case, he had put her on a drug that made her gain thirty pounds then endlessly berated her for not being able to lose weight. She felt miserable about this punitive treatment but believed she had no choice but to stay with Dr. D. because, as she put it, he was the only doctor who "would not give up on me." So she stuck it out, despite the abuse.

To S., however, these sounded like small prices to pay for the promise of help with the arthritis and the tantalizing hope of getting some sleep. In her weakened and vulnerable state, with no one to look out for her and nowhere else to turn, S. thought Dr. D. sounded like a dream come true. And it was a dream she could make true. Her new health-care plan covered appointments and lab work with doctors outside the primary service area. And Seattle was one of the cities where her husband had found work. If they coordinated travel schedules, when she visited the doctor she could also spend time with her husband.

Seeking more information, S. called relatives and friends in Seattle, who in turn called people they knew who had serious rheumatological problems. Within a few days S. had learned that Dr. D. had a reputation in Seattle as a committed and thorough specialist. He seemed to provoke strong feelings in people. While a few strongly disliked his style of practice, others adored him, calling him a hero to sufferers of chronic pain. Though he insisted on regular, in-person visits, he was willing to treat patients who lived at a distance, staying in touch with them between appointments by phone. He had contract arrangements with laboratories and radiology centers up and down the West Coast, making it easy for long-distance patients to have their blood work and other tests done near their homes.

This news about Dr. D. was both reassuring and encouraging. Although she was wary of male doctors after so many bad experiences in New York, S. was tempted by the apple of too-good-to-be-true promises. Desperate for relief from her pain and fatigue, hopeful that this new approach might actually help, and believing she had little to lose in any case, S. called Seattle and made an appointment for an initial consultation.

After the consultation S. wrote in her medical diary: "Saw [D.] for first time today. I think my life will never be the same" (Diary, March 8, 1996). That comment was to prove prescient, though in ways she never suspected at the time.

Part Two | Doing Biomedicine

CHAPTER 1 The Initial Consultation

The Making of a "Fibromyalgic"

March 8, 1996, is a day that S. will never forget. To be sure she did not miss her appointment with Dr. D., she flew to Seattle the night before. The appointment was scheduled for 9:00 A.M. S. went into the meeting brimming with anticipation that he would have a new and better treatment for her arthritis. She emerged five hours later in a muddle of shock, fear, and gratitude. She was shocked to discover that she had four more rheumatological conditions, including fibromyalgia, a serious lifetime ailment; fearful about the now terrible state of her health; and grateful for having found a doctor who was willing to help manage her many ills.

What happened during those five hours in the examining room? The new doctor somehow reached into S.'s core being and disrupted her most deep-seated beliefs about her health. He disturbed her understandings of what was wrong with her (diagnosis), how her conditions would develop (prognosis), and what must be done to make them better or, more accurately, keep them from getting worse (treatment plan). In the process of substituting his medical narrative for hers, Dr. D. profoundly altered—indeed, jarringly rearranged—his new patient's bodily identity. Before the appointment S. thought of herself as a person with psoriatic arthritis whose disease was worrying and occasionally debilitating but in the long run no more than an inconvenience in a full and rich life. After the appointment she saw herself as a fibromyalgic-arthritic person whose diseases were serious conditions that would be with her for life and force major cutbacks in her plans for the future. S.'s comfortable sense of her self had been shattered, her plans for her life splintered like so many pieces of broken glass.

How could a single doctor's visit have such a large impact? How could one's sense of self be so radically altered in such a short time? This chapter unravels that mystery. It begins by setting out S.'s raw experience of what transpired, starting with the gathering of her medical history, then moving on to the orchestration of the clinical exam, the announcement of the diagnosis and treatment plan, and finally the disclosure of the fee.

In the second half of the chapter we step back to examine the larger process by which S. was brought under the medical gaze. Dr. D. was a skillful practitioner of the discursive and rhetorical arts. Deploying an impressive array of verbal tactics, he attached a new set of diagnostic labels to S. in a way that made them seem not only plausible but also true and requiring intensive medical treatment of a sort that he was most competent to provide. Implemented through ritualized practices and well-rehearsed rhetorics, the discourses of medicalization—objectification, quantification, pathologization, and amelioration—literally transformed the person who found her way to the doctor's doorstep into "the rheumatological patient." These discourses and the larger story they compose bear close attention, for they hold the clue to everything that later went wrong.

A Life-Altering Event: The Trauma of the Consultation

To S., Dr. D. had the air of an earnest scientist. As he bustled about preparing for his new patient, she studied him carefully for clues about what might be in store for her. The new doctor was heavyset and bespectacled, with long, wavy brown hair that sat untamed on his head. Appropriate to the scientist, he was indifferent to sartorial style, wearing a bland shirt and a dull tie under the white coat of the medical man. Physically, he was unimposing—thick in the waistline, short in height—which may be why S. felt neither threatened nor intimidated by him. And he was quite young—perhaps in his mid-30s—though of course he gave no clues about his age or any other personal matters about which S. was deeply curious. Such a young doctor, she assumed without giving it a thought, would share her liberal, baby-boomer values. These first impressions put S. at ease, giving her hope that Dr. D. would be different from the male doctors she had seen in New York.

The History: An Erasure of the Past

S. had but a moment to register these impressions, for the medical history-taking was soon underway. She had prepared for that. For many years she had been keeping a medical diary, a computerized file in which she recorded all the ups and downs of her bodily conditions and the treatments various doctors had prescribed for them. Before seeing Dr. D. she had spent many hours reviewing her medical records and updating the file. She even printed it out in a handsome font. She took the printed history to the appointment, thinking the new doctor would be keenly interested in her story of her medical past. But he wasn't. The file told the patient's history in the patient's own voice. The doctor wanted to start all over and retrieve the facts in his own format. He handed the printed file back to her, suggesting she might consult it for information (regarding dates, drugs, and so forth) he would ask about. In returning the file to her, he effectively wiped the slate clean, turning S. into a blank slate on which a new story—his own—could be written. Gathering facts for his account, he proceeded to ask his preferred questions, one by one, delving into this episode and that, all in the most minute detail, until everything was covered from the onset of symptoms to the present. In the two hours it took to collect the history, S.'s own version of her bodily past had been erased, his substituted for it. S. was irked by this. But more than miffed she was intrigued and, to tell the truth, amused by some of the questions he was asking. Did she hook her bra in the back or hook it in the front and then turn it around? When she got up at night to go to the bathroom, was it because she had to urinate or because she was awake with nothing else to do? When she took Methotrexate, eight tablets consumed in three doses twelve hours apart, did she take the pills in a sequence of three-two-three or three-three-two?

All this patient attention to detail greatly impressed her. No doctor had ever inquired into so many matters before. A bit of a mad scientist herself—S. loved to keep records of everything—she was happy to find not only a kindred spirit but also a serious and systematic scientist of the body. The doctor's scientific attitude—the sober demeanor, the detailed questions, the careful recording of facts—gave her hope that he might be able to uncover clues about her problems that other doctors had missed. The scientific virtuosity also made her think that the doctor had access to secrets of her body that she herself did not and could not know. Why would he want to know all those particulars unless they would solve the riddles of her bodily ills?

The Clinical Exam: Muscle Pain Where Before There Was None

The doctor's meticulous attention to detail continued into the clinical examination. He studied S.'s skin for evidence of disease process. He checked her grip strength to assess function in her extremities. He brought out a tape measure and measured the length of each leg, looking for discrepancies that might signal skeletal alignment problems. He then turned to her joints, examining them one by one, manually feeling for swelling, bone deformity, and other anomalies. Concentrating on the fingers and toes, he bent this joint and that, up and down, to discover their range of motion and to learn how much pressure applied to which places would cause pain. Every so often the doctor would stop and write down what he had found, using preprinted diagrams of the skeleton to ensure accurate entry of the facts.

S.'s muscles, never before examined by a rheumatologist, now became the object of clinical scrutiny. He pinched her legs and thighs, back and arms, looking for the eighteen "tender points" of fibromyalgia. Much to the doctor's satisfaction, the pinching produced some slight pain, which he duly recorded in his notes. S. was amazed to discover that she had pain in so many places that she had never known about before! Emotionally drained from having had to expose so much of herself to a stranger, S. was relieved when the doctor finished the exam. He picked up her file and left the room, telling her to get dressed.

The Diagnosis: Five Diseases Instead of One

As the minutes ticked by and the doctor did not return, the suspense began to build in S's mind. What had he found? *What did she have?* He had given no hint during the physical exam. S. grew anxious. After a little more time elapsed, Dr. D. came back into the examining room. He sat down, placed S.'s file on the desk in front of him, and looked very solemn. Worried, S. clutched her notepad and pencil and got ready to write down everything he said.

This is what she wrote. It comes from the entry in her medical diary dated March 8. Readers not familiar with these rheumatological conditions can find brief explanations of them in table 1.

Diseases

1. Probably *psoriatic arthritis.* Symptoms are most consistent with this diagnosis. [Doctor] wants to make sure with new blood test.

2. *Degenerative arthritis,* too, that is, secondary osteoarthritis caused by the psoriatic arthritis. [In the] neck especially.

3. *Primary osteoarthritis,* too, especially in knee, thumb cap, . . . feet maybe . . .

4. *Fibromyalgia.* This is the "pain all over" I often feel. Associated with

sleep disturbance: pain produces loss of non-REM [rapid eye movement] sleep, and no deep sleep produces more pain. [The fibromyalgia is a] manifestation of arthritis. Musculoskeletal sites of pain [are] not treated, so [you] get *pain amplification*—diffuse pain . . . Pain pathways are never closed so pain continues to exist, even to spread.[1] Problem exists because primary disease (PA) not treated. Also is *referred pain,* in which pain is referred away from the site of origin . . . [M]essages originating in one joint are sent elsewhere. Everything conspires to increase the pain. PA is the primary trigger. That combined with the osteoarthritis produces fibromyalgia.

5. Also some mild *scoliosis,* or curvature of the spine. Perhaps have always had this. (Diary, March 8, emphases added)

In cool, clinical language, the doctor listed these conditions, one after the other, making no attempt to rank them by importance or to suggest that some were serious while others were not. He spoke as though he were delivering a lecture to a classroom of students, not telling a nightmare story about her life. Nor did the doctor offer any sympathy, any gentle words to reassure her that everything was okay, that despite the number of rheumatological problems he had discovered, her overall condition was not that bad. To the contrary, he seemed to be trying to make it seem as bad as possible. This was troubling. Why had he listed the primary and secondary osteoarthritis as two conditions rather than one? Why had he included scoliosis along with the other diseases when it is merely a skeletal condition that often has no implications for health? He seemed to be trying to find as many physical problems as possible, put labels on them, and then pin these labels onto her.

S. felt terrible. Suddenly she was five times sicker than she had been before. And before she had been already pretty sick. As she struggled to grasp the enormity of the news her mind raced over the diagnoses, trying to understand what each one would mean for her life. The diagnosis of psoriatic arthritis was no surprise; she had known about that condition for years and had found ways to cope with it. The diagnosis of osteoarthritis—primary and secondary, no less—was harder to deal with. While she was aware of the sometime pain in her neck and knees and thumbs, having a technical name for it—osteoarthritis or, much worse, degenerative arthritis—made the problem seem much worse. Now it was no longer just an occasional pain in the neck and knees; now it was a real disease that would require medical attention. Moreover, the term *degenerative arthritis,* which the doctor had introduced

Table 1

Diseases Diagnosed

Disease	Features
Psoriatic Arthritis	A rare form of arthritis found in 5 to 7 percent of people with the skin condition psoriasis and .1 percent of the general population. PA is part synovitis (inflammation of the joint membrane) and part attachment arthritis (inflammation in the joint where the tendon or ligament attaches to the bone). In the majority of cases joint involvement is nonsymmetrical, spotty, and irregular. PA often affects the fingers and produces "sausage digits," fingers or toes swollen uniformly from top to bottom. People with PA usually feel perfectly well; fatigue, morning stiffness, and wasting of bone calcium rarely occur. The prognosis for PA is generally good; only 25 percent of those with asymmetrical PA, the most common kind, develop progressive joint disease.
Osteoarthritis or Degenerative Joint Disease	An exceedingly common kind of arthritis that "almost everybody gets" with age. Among women, 2 percent under age forty-five, 30 percent aged forty-five to sixty-four, and 68 percent over sixty-five have OA. OA involves degeneration of the cartilage that faces the ends of the bones. The joints involved may include finger joints, the neck or lower back parts of the spine, or the weight-bearing joints, especially the knees and hips. Usually only one or a few joints are affected. OA is a mild condition, with the majority of people experiencing no pain, stiffness, or inflammation. In primary OA no predisposing factor is apparent; secondary OA arises from a precipitating condition. OA is often progressive but can also stabilize or even improve.
Fibromyalgia Syndrome	A moderately common condition found in 2.0 percent of the adult population and 3.4 percent of adult women. FM is marked by persistent pain in muscles in all four quadrants of the body. Diagnosis also requires the existence of eleven of eighteen "tender points" detected on palpation by the physician. Symptoms commonly associated with FM include disturbed sleep, fatigue, morning stiffness, paresthesias (abnormal skin sensations), anxiety or other psychological distress, headaches, and irritable bowel syndrome. Although no clear biological abnormality has been found, the pain and fatigue of FM can be very debilitating. FM is not crippling, deforming, or progressive.
Scoliosis	Scoliosis, a lateral curvature of the spine, occurs in roughly 2.0 to 4.0 percent of the child and adolescent population. Of these, roughly 15 to 20 percent require treatment. The most common form, idiopathic scoliosis,

Table 1 (*continued*)

Disease	Features
	is inherited. Mild scoliosis, marked by a curve of ten to twenty-five degrees, produces few if any symptoms. More severe abnormalities, which may produce back-ache and fatigue, are generally corrected in childhood or adolescence with a spinal brace and/or surgery. The prognosis varies with the severity of the deformity and the age at which the abnormality develops. Mild scoliosis is rarely progressive.

SOURCES: Wilson et al. 1991; Fries 1995; Wolfe et al. 1995; Berkow 1997; Taylor 1998

before its synonym, *osteoarthritis,* made it sound like the condition was going to get progressively worse: she would increasingly "degenerate" until all her joints were eroded. This is not what she had come to hear! And the scoliosis—how bad was that? The last thing in the world she needed was back problems!

Of the five labels, the strangest was fibromyalgia. Yes, she certainly had difficulty sleeping, so that part made sense. And the doctor had found all eighteen tender points (on which, more below), so there must be something there. But what was this "pain all over" he was talking about? She had not used those words. Nor did she feel pain all over her body; the pain was localized in a few joints. Why was he putting words into her mouth? But there was no time for questions now. The appointment had already run over its allotted time, and the doctor had not even begun to talk about treatment. That came next.

The Management Plan: A Ten-Part Intervention in the Patient's Life

Dr. D. did not use the word *cure.* Occasionally he referred to the "treatment" of her conditions. But his preferred word was *management,* a not-so-subtle hint that the conditions he had diagnosed would not be going away. The plan he outlined left little room for hope that things would get much better. Quite the contrary, he seemed to be saying that they would get much worse—unless, that is, decisive action was taken immediately and on all fronts. His plan for action called for no fewer than ten interventions in S.'s life. Here they are, as she recorded them in her medical diary on March 8. More information on the drugs, which formed the core of the management program, will be presented in chapter 2. Later chapters will also clarify the meanings of the technical terms. Although

S. was not familiar with these terms at the time, Dr. D., she felt, threw them all out without stopping to explain them.

Management

1. Baseline drug [must be] a good antiinflammatory—Best is endomethicin, i.e., Indocin. This is [the] most effective . . . Problem with Indocin is tolerance. Some people have headaches. Also possible are mental changes—dulling, torpor, not feel like self, irrational decisions. Wants me to try Indocin, try to tolerize to it [for] several days to a week . . . If headache, try Tylenol to relieve it, two Extra-Strength tablets four times a day . . .

2. Methotrexate—good response [so far]. Up to 9 tablets, 3–3–3, or 22.5 mg [a week].

3. Plaquenil—to control swelling . . . [D. says] I actually have serious inflammation that really needs to be controlled. The short-term rounds of cortisone work, but [resort to cortisone] just indicate[s] that the baseline treatment is failing. Plaquenil has the potential to produce serious side effects in the eyes. But these can be avoided with careful monitoring, and if problems arise, if they are caught in time, they can be fixed. Must have opthamologist check each six months. And patient must check each week with Amsler Grid. First need baseline eye assessment . . . Plaquenil takes 6 to 8 to 12 weeks to kick in. Need this to protect against further inflammations . . .

4. [Wear] wrist splint at night—both wrists. Especially right wrist is collapsing both down and in . . . Need to preserve neutral alignment as long as possible.

5. Feet—orthotics. Buy a good walking shoe, . . . [with] lots of room in toes . . . Get one whose insole lifts out; this will be replaced. Buy Spenco insoles at FootLocker. Get Jogger or Cross Trainer, this will be used to replace insole. [Buy] $2 inserts at drugstore. [D. will use these to create metatarsal arch supports.]

6. Must learn to sleep on side or back—Start by getting the right kind of pillow [for which D. provided an order form].

7. Sit-ups— . . . 10 [reps] a day. Leg lifts . . . [also 10 a day]—Necessary to build muscle strength around the knees, which are in really bad shape . . . Gradually will add weights . . .

8. Sleep—[here we need] pharmacological intervention. Elavil . . . for sleep, 10 mg . . . Modifies non-restorative sleep pattern (Stage 3–4 interruption, this is abolished) . . .

9. Menopause [which S. was going through]—[daily calcium] supplementation of about 1000 [mg] is good. Make sure are taking 400 units of

Vitamin D [to facilitate absorption] . . . Need 24-hour urine assessment to make sure calcium is being absorbed properly. Hormone Replacement Therapy—yes, to prevent osteoporosis. Need to worry about [thinning of] bones . . .

10. Carpal Tunnel Syndrome—Okay. No residual problems [from the earlier surgery] . . . Wants to see surgeon's report . . .

Plus: Return in three weeks. [And get all medical records sent or faxed to D. as soon as possible.] (Diary, March 8)

S. was in shock. If her conditions were so serious that all these things needed to be done, clearly she was in terrible shape. Why had none of the other doctors ever told her that her health problems were so grave? Moreover, some of the interventions D. had listed sounded downright dangerous. While she welcomed the suggestions for exercises and mechanical devices that would improve her life, she was worried about the proposed increase in the number and dosage of drugs, many of which posed risk of injurious side effects.

The Bill: A Shock to the Pocketbook

S. had little time to recover from the blow delivered by the doctor's disease-management plan when she was hit by another bomb. Signaling that the appointment was over, the doctor slid a bill across the desk toward her. S. could not believe her eyes: he was charging her $1,000! Perhaps anticipating her reaction, the doctor explained in quiet tones that the charge had to cover all the time he had spent with her. That seemed reasonable enough to S., but the appointments nurse who set up the consultation had told her the visit would cost $350. Trying to hide her dismay, S. casually picked up the bill and attached file, collected all the laboratory slips and X-ray requisition forms the doctor had written out, and calmly walked out of the examination room to the exit counter, where she stood shell-shocked for a few minutes. Then she took out her checkbook and wrote a check to Dr. D. for $1,000.

The Result: An Identity Destroyed and Recreated in Five Hours

S. left the medical center in emotional turmoil. She was shocked at how her view of her life had suddenly become so bleak, fearful about the future of her health, and grateful beyond words for having found a doctor who was not only attentive to every last detail of her bodily state but also willing to help manage her many serious problems. Describing these intensely contradictory feelings in a letter to her parents a few days later, she wrote:

> *19 March 1996*
>
> Dear Mom and Dad,
>
> [T]his guy [D.] is a bit of a nut . . . for thoroughness . . . [H]e diagnosed three new conditions I never knew I had: osteoarthritis, . . . fibromyalgia, . . . and scoliosis . . . Plus, of course, psoriatic arthritis. His hope is to treat all these conditions at the same time, attacking them with serious medicine so that they don't get worse.
>
> The exciting thing is to finally have some doctor take my complaints seriously . . . Of course, there are also down sides to this [new medical situation]. I am thrilled to have someone who will take care of me, or take responsibility for ensuring that I get everything [that modern] medicine can give someone with my conditions. However, to know that I have these conditions is, well, quite depressing. All along I had thought that psoriatic arthritis is something that comes and goes, so that my condition would eventually go away. [Dr. D.] says: not so. Based on the history he has, it seems that my [conditions . . . are] likely to be progressive. This is very dismal news indeed . . .

We see here how readily S. internalized the doctor's narrative about her bodily realities, their likely future course, and necessary treatment. She writes: "someone *with my conditions*," "to know that *I have these conditions*," betraying not a trace of doubt about the correctness of the diagnoses. From a basically healthy person with one rheumatological condition that she expected would come and go and eventually go into long-term remission, she was metamorphosed into an essentially sick person with five chronic conditions that would stay with her for life and probably get worse. The mere *idea* that she was so sick—that her conditions were so numerous and so serious—had invaded her inner world, transforming her view of her self and her future and depressing her spirits.

Creating the Rheumatological Patient: Dr. D. Displays His Skills

What had happened to S.? Quite evidently, she had fallen under the medical gaze. In a series of carefully choreographed rituals of medicalization— the history, the exam, and so on—Dr. D. had turned her into an object of medical scrutiny. He had attached to her new labels—the fibromyalgic, the osteoarthritic, the scoliatic—redefining her as a chronically, seriously, and progressively ill person whose medical management required a comprehensive package of pharmacological and other intrusions into her life that he was best equipped to provide. In creating a patient whose ills "matched" his training and skills, Dr. D. was just doing what scientist-physicians generally do: he was creating a "do-able" problem and, at the same time, gaining patients for his practice (for more, see the Problematique). From these material and discursive elements, he had constructed a new, fully elaborated story about her body—complete with diagnosis, prognosis, and treatment plan—that both required and produced a new identity on her part.

How had the doctor changed her view of her life so quickly, so that after a mere five hours she had begun to view her body and life through his interpretive grid? Dr. D. was not only a good storyteller, he was also an artful practitioner of the science of medicine. In the initial consultation he had skillfully deployed both the discourses and practices of medical science to transform S. not only into a patient but into a willing patient whose emotional state made her *eager* to undergo the agonizing treatment that was to ensue. Dr. D. had turned her into precisely the kind of patient he was set up to treat. That patient was one who believed her body was badly damaged and becoming more so, who depended heavily on the doctor to know and treat her ills, and who trusted his scientific expertise so absolutely that she would never dream he could make a mistake. What other kind of person would put up with what was to follow? It also helped if she had ample time on her hands to make frequent doctor's appointments, each two to three hours in length, and to manage the almost full-time job he had created around caring for her failing body. Remarkably, the doctor could help put time in his patients' hands, too, although that is a story for a later chapter.

Ritualized Practices of Medicalization

The last section hinted at ways in which the ritualized practices of the initial consultation worked to turn doctor and patient into subject and object, knower and known, mind and body of medical science. Here I bring these techniques of medicalization together, emphasizing now the doctor's practices rather than the patient's reactions. I begin with general "patient-construction" practices and then turn to diagnostic practices.

During the medical history taking, S.'s record of her bodily past was erased, with D.'s literally written over it. What counted to her no longer mattered; what counted to him was to count for medical science. In the clinical exam the doctor became the observer, the patient the observed. Lying prone on the clinical table, the patient body became an object of intense scrutiny and detailed inspection. Feeling and measuring, counting and writing, the doctor became the doer of Science and the definer of the truths of her body.

The rituals of the diagnosis—the doctor's departure from the room, file in hand; the long minutes spent in his office; the heroic return and pronouncement of the truths of the body—worked to surround the labeling process with an aura of mystery, of truth being produced in sacred places that only the doctor could enter. Lifted up and away from the messy details of the feminine body-object, the labeling practice was elevated to the level of Science, which only the masculine mind-subject, working in silence and solitude, could perform. As if to say that no truth, no matter how small, could escape the medical gaze, the diagnosis consisted of five items, the management plan twice that. And, if everything else had not yet convinced the patient of the doctor's inestimable authority and expertise, the fee, announced in the closing minutes of the consultation, served as a pointed exclamation mark that the patient could not possibly misread: this doctor's services were worth serious money!

The history taking and physical exam served also as diagnostic practices whose aim was to discover the pathologies of the body, bring to light their manifold signs and symptoms, and attach disease labels to them. But the patient body was inherently chaotic, a disorganized collection of aches and pains, complaints and sorrows. How was the messy stuff of the patient body turned into five neat disease labels? Proceeding like a laboratory scientist, the clinical scientist methodically gathered information from the patient's verbal reports, her body, and her existing medical file. That information was then filtered through the experienced eye and trained mind of the clinician. Weighing it in light of "the literature" and cases of other patients he had clinically observed, he converted the chaos of life into scientific fact.

The diagnosis of psoriatic arthritis was easy to reach, since it had been attached to the patient before. Dr. D. reaffirmed its correctness by observing the characteristic pattern of joint involvement, extracting from the patient the telltale history of joint swelling and surgery, noting the family history of the disease, and examining the X-ray reports of bone deformity in the patient file. With all this evidence, there was a watertight case for this diagnosis.

The diagnosis of fibromyalgia was more difficult, since the patient lacked many of the characteristic symptoms of the disease. She lacked not only the main symptom, widespread pain, but also the headaches, morning stiffness, and paresthesias (numbness, tingling) that afflict the majority of fibromyalgics.[2] Yet there were methods the doctor thought could reveal the existence of the disease in the absence of these symptoms. Most important was the tender-point examination. In this procedure, the doctor was supposed to exert a scientifically specified amount of pressure in palpating eighteen scientifically identified points on the body and then classify the patient's verbal and facial reactions to each pinch as "not painful," "mildly painful," and "more than mildly painful." As Dr. D. saw it, the patient gave "mildly" or "more than mildly painful" responses to all eighteen pinches, clear evidence in his mind of the presence of fibromyalgia. The diagnosis was also based on the patient's oral report of sleep problems and associated fatigue, both common in the fibromyalgic. From her answers to a series of questions—how long had she had these difficulties, what was the characteristic pattern of waking and sleeping, did she feel rested during the day?—he decided that what she called "sleep difficulties" constituted a biologically based "sleep disorder." This disorder, he explained, is characterized by a disturbed brainwave function in which alpha waves interrupt the delta waves of deep sleep, preventing the patient from getting restorative sleep. There were tests that could be done to establish the wave pattern, but he considered them unnecessary; D. believed he knew from experience what the problem was. The results of these two procedures led him to conclude that his new patient had fibromyalgia.

The final three diagnoses—the two forms of osteoarthritis and scoliosis—were derived from visual inspection and manual examination of the patient's skeletal system, which, to Dr. D., showed the characteristic deformities of those afflictions. The deformities were quite mild. Indeed, the radiologist reading the X-rays S. had taken at her primary health care center a week later found her skeletal system to be entirely normal (a fact S. herself did not discover until much later). Of the thoracic spine, where D. had found scoliosis, the radiologist reported: "There is a normal curve without evidence of bone or disc disease or injury. Impression: Normal spine." (Dr. Edward R. Dana Report, March 18, 1996). The radiologist filed precisely the same report on the cervical spine, where Dr. D. had discovered osteoarthritis (Dr. Edward R. Dana Report, March 18, 1996). (With characteristic thoroughness—or hubris—D. would later order copies of the original films, study them closely, and then write his own verdicts on his personal copy of the radiologist's reports.) Although other doctors S. had seen either had not uncovered any spinal problems or had

considered any anomalies they had found clinically irrelevant and unworthy of mention, for reasons he did not share, D. felt it necessary to
report every one of the diseases and conditions he had discovered. In this
way osteoarthritis and scoliosis joined the list, bringing the total to five.

Thus were created the scientific facts of S.'s case. The science of diagnosis was an inexact science that involved a heaping measure of personal judgment. But Dr. D. presented his diagnostic procedures as those
of a precise and revelatory science that disclosed the truths of the patient
body. Here is how he described the results of his handiwork for colleagues
who may later be leafing through S.'s file:

RE: PATIENT: GREENHALGH, SUSAN M.
    I had the pleasure of assessing Ms. Greenhalgh in an extended complex
    high consultation on March 8, 1996 . . .

IMPRESSION:
    Ms. Greenhalgh has skin findings compatible with psoriasis which appears
    relatively mild at this time . . . With regard to her joint symptoms and
    findings, she does have synovitis and dactylitis axial symptoms involving
    the neck and peripheral joint symptoms and findings involving the DIP
    joints, PIP joints, wrists, knees, MTP joints, toe PIP and toe DIP joints. She
    has no clinical history or findings of sacroiliitis. Prior investigation revealed
    on X-ray of the hands and wrists from December 7, 1994, to reveal the
    presence of an erosion at the medial base of the right fifth metacarpal as
    well as in the right ulnar styloid. There is radiographic as well as clinical
    evidence of deformity involving the hands and wrists as well as feet and she
    has had spontaneous effusion of the left second toe PIP joint and surgical
    lesion of the left thumb MCP joint. These findings are compatible with the
    diagnosis of *psoriatic arthritis*. I think it important to rule out other causes
    of inflammatory polyarthritis that may coexist with psoriasis such as
    rheumatoid arthritis. She has no other features to suggest the presence of
    any other connective tissue disease. She indicates that screening for Lyme
    disease previously has been negative. Additionally, she has findings of
    primary and secondary osteoarthritis involving the first CMC joints, DIP
    joints, feet and patello-femoral joints. She has associated *fibromyalgia*
    with accompanying nonrestorative sleep pattern and 18 out of 18 tender
    fibrositic points. She has a *thoracic rotoscoliosis*. (Dr. D. Report, March 8,
    1996, emphases added)

Discourses and Rhetorics of Medicalization

These rituals, while important, were not yet enough to produce the willing patient. The doctor needed to change S.'s understandings of her body,
to convince her that it was in very bad shape and getting worse so that
she would be well disposed, even anxious, to "serve" as his patient and

to accept his plan for medical management as the plan for large portions of her life. This is not to suggest that the doctor was cynically manipulative, deliberately exploiting his patient's physical weakness, emotional vulnerability, and lack of rheumatological expertise to increase his patient load. Not at all. As far as S. could tell, Dr. D. earnestly and completely believed in everything he said. That is why he was so successful in getting his patient to believe it too.

In persuading the patient to accept his view of her life, the discourse of medical science supplied Dr. D. with powerful tools. And the doctor had mastered that discourse well. Let us look again at what he said, thinking of his words and phrases as elements in the larger discourse of biomedicine. In this first consultation the medical discourse Dr. D. deployed did four main things. First, it separated the subjective from the objective, making the doctor the expert on the patient's body, while defining the patient's emotions and ideas as subjective and therefore of no interest to medical science. Second, the discourse quantified the patient's corporeal conditions, turning her bodily sensations, anatomy, and physiology into numbers in the doctor's file. The numbers were useful, but they were incomplete, counting some things but not others. Third, focusing on pathology rather than wellness, it attached new disease labels to the patient, transforming her bodily identity into one of a seriously, multiply, chronically, and progressively ill person. Finally, sidestepping the question of cause, the discourse emphasized treatment and asserted the need for immediate medical attention of the sort this doctor was better equipped than any other to provide. Taken together, these discourses worked to create the rheumatological patient who was fully readied for biomedical intervention. In later conversations Dr. D. would extend the biomedical discourse to embrace the subject of prescription drugs and their use in treating her diseases. Here we concentrate on the "patient construction" and diagnostic discourses that he elaborated during the first five hours of their acquaintance.

Dr. D. was a master not only of the biomedical discourses but also of the *rhetorics* that could make the discourse seem so incontestably right. Dr. D.'s rhetorical flourishes—his word choices, emphases, inflections, and so on—added weight to his words in ways that S. became aware of only as time went by. Given the limits of information (only a few of these stylistic devices had found their way into the early diary entries), this chapter describes just a handful of these devices to give the reader a feel for the doctor's gift for persuasive talk. There will be more on rhetorics in chapter 3.

To repeat, the reader must not think that the doctor was deploying his conversational skills self-consciously. To the contrary, as far as S. could tell her doctor spoke freely, with no awareness of the discursive structure, rhetorical style, or narrative shape of his talk. She came to this conclusion because the doctor often used corny metaphors—a favorite was "you have to prick your finger on a thorn before you can smell the roses"—that were so clichéd she could not help but wince every time he used one. (He stopped using them as time went by.) Presumably, had the doctor been aware of the linguistic features of his speech, he would not have resorted to such trite metaphors.

Objectification. The first and most powerful effect of Dr. D.'s discourse was to separate the objective from the subjective, the body from the emotions and mind, placing feelings and thoughts outside the frame of interest and making the doctor the expert on the body. Throughout the initial consultation the doctor's intense focus on the patient's body provided unmissable clues to the fact that the body would be the central—indeed, virtually the only—object of medical concern. But the doctor did not leave it to his patient's cunning to figure out where he stood on the issue of the "subjective" or emotional component of her health. Although depression is a common affliction of those with chronic rheumatological conditions, Dr. D. declared it off limits in his practice. While acknowledging that many fibromyalgic patients were depressed, he explained, theirs was a secondary depression that emerged because of the primary muscle condition. He would treat the muscle condition, and the depression would go away. (The depression associated with S.'s arthritis was never mentioned because, in D.'s view, fibromyalgia was S.'s main medical problem.)

If the body was to be the exclusive focus of concern, the doctor was to be the unchallenged expert on the body. We have seen how the routines of the medical history and physical exam made Dr. D. the authority on S.'s body. Discursive practices had the same effect of transferring the claim to know the patient body to the physician. In the discovery and designation of the tender points of fibromyalgia, for example, the patient felt no pain on her own, but the doctor was able to produce painful sensations by pinching her in special places. The truth of the designation and the pain was then backed up by offhand references to the authority of the medical literature, which indicated that there were eighteen such tender points, located at this and that place on the body, all of which she "had." The discourse of medicine had attributed muscle pain to a patient who before had none. Similarly, in dispensing the diagnosis of fibromyalgia, the doctor spoke of the "pain all over which [she] feels." Here again, he spoke the discourse of medical science—if she "has fibromyalgia," then she must also "have pain all over"—with little interest in what she actually felt. Here the doctor claimed to represent the patient's bodily condition better than the patient herself could. The doctor, not the patient, became the expert on the patient's pain. This linguistic legerdemain was to prove highly consequential, because the official criteria for the diagnosis of fibromyalgia included not only the doctor's detection of tender points but also the patient's perception of persistent pain in all four quadrants of the body. In making this leap from tender points to diagnosis, the doctor adopted what might be called a creative attitude toward the official criteria. While creativity is often called for in medical practice, this creative move was to have serious consequences. This leap of faith in the presence of his specialty disease—in plain talk, this misdiagnosis—became the pivot of the vicious cycle that will preoccupy us in later chapters. In this cycle S.'s condition spiraled downward, while her doctor continued to insist that she was fine. Again and again he misinterpreted the problems as manifestations of fibromyalgia, when their true cause lay elsewhere.

Quantification. Like all good scientists, Dr. D. loved numbers. He seemed truly to enjoy turning S.'s physical reality into a cluster of numbers, a finite set of "objective" measures that he could use scientifically to assess the state of her health (or, more accurately, her disease). At the first appointment he collected and recorded the baseline numbers: she had twenty-one "active" arthritic joints and all eighteen tender points of fibromyalgia, many of them more than "mildly painful." In Dr. D.'s scheme, the numbers could not lie: S. was in very bad shape. The doctor also collected quantified measures of her grip strength, the length of her legs, and many other things he did not share with his patient. In future appointments he would use these baseline numbers to measure the bodily improvements that had occurred under his regime of medical care.

The clinical results would soon be supplemented by the numbers from the blood and urine work. Dr. D. had a reputation for being "test crazy," according to S.'s Seattle informants, and he lived up to it in treating S. For the initial diagnostic workup the doctor ordered seventeen blood tests and four urine tests. After the first set of tests, regular monthly tests produced thirty-nine numbers or measures. The laboratory reports listed both the normal readings on all these numbers and S.'s readings, with S.'s "abnormals" clearly marked H and L, for high and low. With the collection of these results, S. came to be represented as a set of numbers, of normals and abnormals, in her doctor's file. These numbers would later be used to measure the effectiveness of the drugs. The sedimentation rate, for example, provided an index of inflammation, which some of the drugs were supposed to reduce. The numbers would also be used to check for adverse side effects from the drugs, which often showed up early in biochemical anomalies of the blood. Thus, from the initial consultation onward, the state of S.'s musculoskeletal health was to be represented not so much by how she felt or how she thought she was doing as by how the doctor's numbers were moving.

In general, quantifying signs and symptoms and then collecting numbers on them at regular intervals is a good way of gauging bodily change. But the doctor's numbers counted some things and not others. While including signs of disease that could be assessed in the laboratory or examining room, the doctor's numerical record omitted two classes of symptoms that would be crucial in S.'s case: symptoms the doctor considered important but could not measure (such as the quality and quantity of the patient's sleep) and aspects of S.'s health that only she deemed important enough to merit medical concern (for example, her emotional well-being or her ability to think and write). Over time, these two evaluations of the patient's health—the doctor's numerical record and S.'s lived reality of her body—would produce widely divergent understandings of how treatment was progressing.[3] The two assessments were so different that, to the very end, doctor and patient would never see eye to eye on what happened to S. under D.'s care.

Pathologization. The work of biomedicine is to find things wrong with patients, which practitioners then proceed to make right. Accordingly, medical discourse focuses on disease rather than on health. A core task of biomedicine is to affix disease labels to its objects; the more and the more serious the labels, the greater the scope for medical intervention.

If S.'s experience was any indication, Dr. D. was a masterful labeler of patients. His labeling practices had four attributes. First, his diagnoses were *numerous.* S. had not one illness or even two, but five. We saw above how this number was made to look so large. S.'s sleep problems were relabeled a "sleep disorder," evidence of the presence of "fibromyalgia." Osteoarthritis became primary osteoarthritis and secondary osteoarthritis. Scoliosis, most often a congenital condition that is diagnosed early in life, was made into an adult condition listed along with the bona fide diseases. In this way the list of diseases S. "had" grew from one to five.

Second, her conditions were made to appear *serious.* In the diagnosis of fibromyalgia, the doctor explained how she exhibited both pain amplification and referred pain: "Everything conspires to increase the pain," he told her. If this were the case, the implication was, she must be in terrible pain. (In fact, she wasn't.) In delivering the diagnoses, the doctor did not mention that osteoarthritis and scoliosis are extremely common conditions and in her case very mild. The scoliosis was so inconsequential that S. had made it through four and a half decades of her life without even being aware that the curvature of her spine was slightly awry. In neglecting to fill in this important information, the doctor created the impression that S., with her five diseases, was much worse off than most people. The apparent severity of her conditions was also underscored by the disease-management plan. In outlining this plan, for example, the doctor told S. that she "actually ha[s] serious inflammation that really needs to be controlled." Hence the need for Plaquenil, a new (for S.) and potentially dangerous drug. She must use wrist splints at night because the "right wrist is collapsing both down and in." She must start doing sit-ups and leg lifts every day because "the knees . . . are in really bad shape," a judgment that other doctors she consulted later did not share.

Third, the conditions S. "had" were *chronic*—for life. As noted above, the plan Dr. D. outlined was for disease "management," not treatment, and certainly not cure. Clearly, the conditions would be with her until death. Finally, in D.'s labeling scheme S.'s conditions were *progressive.* If she had thought things were pretty bad already, she should realize that they would most certainly grow worse. This part of the discourse— the prognosis—would not be fully fleshed out until about a week after the first appointment. But in this initial meeting the doctor introduced the theme that the future would be bleak, allowing S. to play around with it in her mind as she considered how to proceed. Use of the term *degenerative arthritis* for osteoarthritis sent a clear message about the likely course of the disease. The image of the worsening future was also used to stress the need for strong drugs. Thus, S. "needs [Plaquenil] to protect against further inflammations." She needs to take hormone replacement therapy "to prevent osteoporosis; [you] need to worry about [thinning of your] bones," he told her. All this would become much more graphic in a few more days. But as early as the first visit, the doctor began to convey to S. in strong language that she needed a serious, intensive, multipronged management program. Essentially, the doctor "gave" his new patient these conditions (except the psoriatic arthritis, which she already "had"), represented them as serious, progressive, and lifelong problems, and then presented himself as both available and almost uniquely qualified to take charge of their management.

Amelioration. All the preceding activities—the quantification, the labeling, and so on—are but preparation for the ultimate work of biomedicine: to fix the pathology, thereby improving on mother nature herself. Given the urgency of meliorating the problems, the question of what caused them becomes secondary. Dr. D., for example, showed little interest in what had produced S.'s conditions. Aside from some offhand references to their likely genetic origin and certain biological character, he ignored the issue altogether. What occupied D.'s attention was the urgency of moving on to the treatment phase. In the discourse of scientific medicine nothing could be more obvious than that the patient who *has* serious medical conditions *needs* serious medical care. In applying this logic to S., Dr. D. liberally sprinkled the word *need* around his diagnosis and management plan for her conditions. S.'s inflammation "really needs" to be controlled; the neutral alignment of the wrists "need[s] to be preserved as long as possible"; for S. it is "necessary to build muscle strength around the knees"; S. "needs to worry about [her] bones," and so on. And the massive ten-part intervention program, which the doctor introduced immediately after the five-part diagnosis, purveyed the strong implicit message that there was a serious medical need to do something fast. Not only did S. need help, she needed better, more intensive, more long-term, and more sophisticated rheumatological care than she had received from any doctor before. She needed, in short, the skills of Dr. D.

In this chapter we have seen how the doctor's deployment of the discourses and practices of biomedicine yielded a compelling new narrative about S.'s body and its ills. Dr. D.'s story worked to alter S.'s bodily identity, invading her consciousness and transforming her into a willing patient who was eager to accept the kind of treatment this doctor liked to provide. In five short hours S.'s sense of her self and her life had been radically—yes, even violently—rearranged in the name of doing good medical science and providing quality patient care. But the effects of these powerful discourses would not remain confined to the realm of cognition. In the next chapter we will see how they spilled over into the material world, turning S.'s body into a drug zone in which her new doctor could experiment freely to find "the best drugs for her conditions."

CHAPTER 2

Medicating the "Fibromyalgic"–Arthritic Body

Once attached to the patient, the new diagnostic-interpretive grid became a powerful force. In the last chapter we saw how it began to reshape S.'s mental world, infecting her bodily identity and emotional state. Now we see that the new grid had a corporeal effect as well. That five-part diagnosis became the rationale and the blueprint for massive interventions in her body. The rationale for the interventions was straightforward. If the generic problem was biological or bodily, the solution was pharmacological alteration of the body. If the specific problems in S.'s case were untreated inflammation of psoriatic arthritis and fibromyalgia-related lack of sleep, the solution had to be a stronger antiinflammatory drug and new medication to make her sleep. The treatment followed logically from the definition of the problem.

The diagnostic grid specified chemical intervention in the diseased body, but it did not indicate which medications should be applied or how they should be administered. These matters were parts of a drug discourse that supplemented the diagnostic discourse, fleshing out the last part of the story of S.'s ills (about the treatment plan) that was crafted in the initial meeting. The doctor's drug discourse amounted to a *pharmacological philosophy*, because it contained both an implicit epistemology (a theory of knowledge) and an implicit ontology (a theory of existence or being) of disease treatment. This philosophy carried the theme of objectification advanced in the diagnosis a great deal further. The doctor's discourse on drugs contained six weighty assertions: drugs are the treatment of choice; there is a best drug for each condition; the patient must be "tolerized" to these drugs; serious side effects might occur; all symptoms must be attacked simultaneously in a multifaceted treatment program; and the initial phase of treatment must be one of scientific experimentation in which the doctor-scientist uses his superior knowledge of the body and the drugs to experiment on the patient body to find the best pharmacological package for her ills. Implicit in this pharmacological philosophy was an epistemology according to which the doctor's knowledge was the only knowledge that counted and an ontology in which the patient-as-person (as opposed to the patient-as-body) did not exist. The discourse on drugs left the patient with some acute philosophical dilemmas to work out on her own.

When put into practice this discourse on drugs had notable effects on the patient's body. The first few weeks of experimentation produced extreme discomfort: huge headaches, sleepless nights, and day-in, day-out fatigue. Eventually the doctor found a combination of drugs that helped, giving the patient some welcome relief from the symptoms that had brought her to him. But these benefits were realized at significant cost: the onset of new and even more debilitating symptoms. These new ills included neurological problems such as headaches and, later, mental fogginess as well as conspicuous pain in the neck and upper back. None of these symptoms had been present at the time of the initial consultation. These new ailments compounded the patient's distress: not only did they cause discomfort, but their emergence after treatment began simply made no sense.

This diagnostic-treatment grid had another effect that may appear esoteric to the reader but provides a critical clue to the mysterious happenings of later months. This second effect was on the doctor's interpretation of the new neurological symptoms. In his tool kit of medical knowledges the doctor had a number of competing explanations that he could have drawn upon to understand these new symptoms. He chose the one that was compatible with his previous discursive constructions of this patient. Because he was convinced that the patient "had fibromyalgia," that fibromyalgia was her most serious condition, and that the antiinflammatory Indocin was the "best drug for her arthritis," he attributed the neurological symptoms to fibromyalgia, rejecting as less relevant the well-known evidence that Indocin often produces such mental disturbances. While the choice of interpretation made eminent sense in terms of the doctor's formulations of the situation, it was to have baneful consequences that surfaced in the spring and multiplied during the summer and fall.

In this chapter we examine what happened when this six-part discourse was turned into practice. The first section details the doctor's discourse on drugs and draws out its epistemological and ontological implications. The second section describes how S. was turned into an experimental subject of rheumatological science. The third, fourth, and fifth sections trace the history of the drug experiments through three phases: an initial phase in which the doctor tried the "best drugs" for the patient's conditions, a middle phase in which he backtracked and substituted weaker drugs for his preferred medications, and a final phase in which he succeeded in tolerizing the patient to some of the best drugs for her ills. In each phase we probe the effects of the drug discourse and practice on the patient body and on the doctor's interpretation of the patient's new symptoms. A final section draws on information in S.'s charts to document the marked improvement in initial symptoms and the equally marked deterioration in the newly problematic aspects of her health.

A Pharmacological Philosophy

As noted above, Dr. D. had a distinctive pharmacological philosophy that complemented and supplemented the diagnostic discourse described earlier. The pharmacological discourse was part of a larger treatment discourse and associated program. This expanded treatment plan stipulated the use of special devices (orthotic devices such as special shoes and arch supports, an orthopedic pillow), exercises to strengthen the muscles surrounding weak joints, and a behavioral modification program designed to monitor and manage all activities affecting the sites of musculoskeletal pain.

While all these changes in the patient's daily life were important, they could not solve the basic problem, which, in D.'s view, was a biochemically aberrant body. The solution could only be the use of powerful drugs to alter the biochemical functioning of that body. To this end the doctor elaborated a highly complex discourse specifying which drugs were to be used, how they were to be administered, and many other matters. This discourse on drugs, along with a related set of practices, became the centerpiece of the whole treatment program. Putting the discourse into practice became the major focus of the efforts of doctor and patient during the first three months of treatment.

The central elements of this drug discourse were sketched out during the first consultation and then gradually elaborated over the next few months as the doctor's medication plan was mapped out, the initial results discussed on the phone, and the plan modified and tried again. As the experiments progressed and the conversations multiplied, the doctor filled in many pieces of his larger philosophy of care. The term *philosophy* of care was the doctor's. But the term *pharmacological philosophy* was the patient's. What this philosophy added up to, in S.'s view, was a high-risk, drug-intensive, doctor-controlled process of medicating the patient body. She agreed to it—indeed, she actively participated in it—because the doctor promised her real relief from her symptoms, because she believed his promises, and because she saw no alternative course of action at the time. I will have more to say about that compliance in the next chapter.

A Six-Part Discourse on Drugs

The doctor's pharmacological philosophy consisted of six central elements. First, *drugs were the treatment of choice.* Since the patient's problem was a bad body, the solution was to make it better by changing its biochemical functioning. Of course, the body could not be made completely well. That was out of the question, because, as the doctor frequently reminded her, "the genetic environment can't be changed" (Diary, March 18). But, with use of the appropriate drugs, the rheumatological body could be improved upon so that the patient would both feel and function better.

If drugs were the drug of choice, lifestyle and other treatment strategies recommended in holistic approaches to medicine were deemed unworthy of serious consideration. On several occasions S. asked about these approaches, only to learn that her doctor was not an enthusiast of them. Indeed, he was quick to dismiss them, often in a tone of scorn. In answer to her question about stress, she was told crisply that the research shows that fibromyalgia is "definitely related to stress" but that there is "virtually no connection" between stress and psoriatic arthritis (Diary, March 29). A probe about stress-reduction strategies was brushed off without even a formal response. The doctor was also discouraging about diet and exercise. Massage got a thumbs-up, as long as it was not the Swedish variety (Diary, April 19). Everything the doctor said made it clear that drugs were to be the first line of defense, the essential foundation of the entire disease-management program.

Second, Dr. D. maintained that *there was a single best drug for every condition.* At least this was true for S.'s conditions, which were common ones. Though the doctor did not say how he came to this conclusion, presumably it was based on the results of scientific research and his own clinical experience. The doctor's treatment strategy was to start by giving the patient the "best-choice" drugs for her conditions. If the drugs worked and the patient suffered few or only mild side effects, that was perfect: the regime was in place and the doctor was happy. If serious side effects emerged, however, the doctor would *"tolerize the patient to the drug,*" the third element of the drug discourse. In other words, he would *change the patient to fit the drug,* not the reverse. If the patient experienced unbearable side effects, the doctor's strategy for tolerizing her to the drug was to backtrack and start over by administering the drug in smaller dosages or in weaker versions. He would let the drug "percolate through" the patient's system and then, when the time was ripe, increase the dosage or switch to the stronger version until it reached the optimal level. In using these potent drugs, the doctor's hope was that eventually (though when, one never knew) the underlying disease process would be slowed or even arrested, so that the dosage of the drug could be reduced (Diary, March 21 and 29).

When the patient's symptoms were serious and the best-choice drug took a while to build up to effective levels in the bloodstream, the doctor might try another form of patient tolerization. With this technique he would begin by administering the ideal level or form of the drug, asking the patient to live with the side effects for a few days to a few weeks with the expectation that they would eventually subside, allowing the drug, now up to optimal levels in the blood, to work its wonders. If the side effects became unmanageable, the first response would be not to drop the drug, but to introduce another drug to counteract or cover up the side effects. For example, if the drug produced headaches, the patient might be ordered to take Extra-Strength Tylenol or, if that did not work, Tylenol with codeine, a prescription drug and a narcotic, to suppress them. That solution should be tried for a good long time, generally speaking, for two to four weeks (Diary, March 27). "When 'we' walk away from a drug, it is for good": that was Dr. D.'s clearly and frequently articulated philosophy (Diary, March 13). In other words, "we" must stick with the drug of choice, using it until it is either demonstrated beyond all doubt to be ineffective or the side effects become so intolerable that the patient reports extreme misery or simply refuses to take the drug any longer.

Fourth, since the "best" drugs are often if not always the most powerful ones, the patient must understand the *potential for serious, even dangerous and, in rare circumstances, deadly side effects.* The patient must accept the possibility that she may experience some of these side effects. Clearly, this is a high-risk approach, in which both patient and doctor must remain ever vigilant lest the patient body suffer permanent damage. The patient must watch closely for side effects and let the doctor know immediately if problems crop up. The patient must also have blood work done and perhaps also other tests performed regularly, usually weekly or monthly, so that any anomalies in the biochemistry of the body, which might signal damage to internal organs, are caught early. The doctor's role is carefully to monitor the results of the blood work and to be available to answer patient phone calls about any problem. In return for the patient's cooperation in exposing her body to such toxic drugs, the doctor promised to do his utmost to make the drugs work and to make the patient symptom free, while doing "no harm in the long run" (Diary, March 27). He never explained what he meant by "harm" or "the long run."

In taking this drug-intensive approach to treatment, the doctor faced the risk of a medical malpractice suit should things go wrong. From his point of view he was taking large legal, financial, and professional risks to make his patients as near to symptom free as humanly possible. The reader might well wonder why he would risk so much for the comfort of his patients. Although one cannot be certain, from other things her doctor said, S. believed that he assumed these risks because he genuinely wanted to make his patients pain free, because he had supreme confidence in his ability to do so, and because, when everything worked as it was supposed to, he could cherish an image of himself as a larger-than-life physician, a godlike healer. Underlying the high-risk approach, then, were humanitarian impulses, a healthy dose of hubris, and appealing myths of the doctor as a medical miracle maker. Whereas patient successes supported these myths and made the doctor happy, failures were difficult to admit. Failures meant not only that the doctor had made a technical mistake but also that his larger-than-life perception of himself was unsustainable: he was not godlike but only too human. The doctor had good reasons to protect himself from seeing his mistakes.

Fifth, the doctor insisted on adopting a *multifaceted approach in which all the patient's conditions are attacked together and at the same time.* He was plainly contemptuous of the disease-by-disease and symptom-by-symptom methods of other rheumatologists. It is "not enough to simply change one drug or inject one joint," he would say scornfully, implicating his colleagues. "Everything should change together" (Diary, March 8). Or he would say impatiently, "It is stupid to just chase pain," that is, to administer painkillers *after* pain has emerged; "all the pain pathways must be closed in advance and together."

But putting such a regime in place is a tricky business that requires a great deal of hands-on work. This brings us to the sixth and final element of the discourse, the necessity of conducting *scientific experiments on the patient to find the proper pharmacological package for her ills.*

Since different people have different biochemical makeups, the way their bodies metabolize individual drugs and the way the drugs interact vary from patient to patient. Therefore, the doctor, who had established himself as the expert on the biochemistry of the body, must "walk [the patient] through various new treatments, trying each one out" (Diary, March 8). The patient, he explained, is an "N of 1": the drugs may work or not, depending on the patient's individual biochemical makeup and drug tolerance. In other words, each patient must become an experimental subject for a few weeks to several months until the doctor finds the best chemical combination for her body. In S.'s case, Dr. D. said that he would need three to six months of "aggressive treatment" to find a stable regime that worked (Diary, March 21).

An Epistemology and Ontology of Care

These six elements created a hierarchy of value in which the diseases became more important than the patient, use of the "best drugs" more important than worries about side effects, and the doctor the expert on and arbiter of both diseases and drugs. The lowest value was attached to the patient-as-person, as sentient, thinking and feeling human being. We have seen how, in the initial consultation, the work of diagnosis had severed the patient's mind and emotions from her body, placing the former beyond the scope of medical interest. The treatment process furthered this violent dismemberment of the patient by marginalizing the patient's perceptions of her body, including her sensations of painful side effects, and excluding them from consideration in the treatment process. Although S. did not fully realize it at the time, her concerns about side effects were being silenced, pushed aside by her doctor's more pressing concern about using the scientifically determined "best drugs for her conditions." Built into this pharmacological philosophy, then, was an epistemology in which the doctor's knowledge was the only knowledge that mattered and an ontology in which the patient as a thinking and feeling person did not exist.

Although Dr. D.'s approach represented the logical conclusion of the discourses of biomedicine, it was a good deal more radical than the perspectives of other doctors with whom S. had worked. For example, D.'s view on stress and psoriatic arthritis—"virtually no connection"—was different from that of S.'s previous physician, Dr. K. That doctor had acknowledged that stress probably played some role, while making it clear that stress management was beyond the scope of her practice. The idea that the *doctor* should dictate the level of risk that the *patient* would have to accept, with no input from the patient, was also extreme. Dr. K. had always discussed drug choices with S., allowing her to make an informed choice among treatment options. D. had deleted the patient's views of acceptable side effects from the process, turning her into a body without mind or sensation. Finally, the notion that there is a single best drug for every condition, and that it should be the drug of choice for every patient, was also quite radical. Other doctors with whom S. had worked believed that one could identify a best drug *for each patient*. D. had carried the objectifying logic of biomedicine to an extreme, turning the patient into a collection of diseases, each of which had an optimal medical response. The *disease* had become the object of medical attention, eliminating the person altogether.

The overall effect of these discourses on the patient was one of epistemological and ontological invalidation. Although S. did not have this language at the time, she understood that her knowledge and bodily sensations were being marginalized, and this neglect of her perceptions disturbed her immensely.[1] For example, this doctor's assertion that there is no connection between stress and psoriatic arthritis ran counter to S.'s bodily experiences, which at times showed a temporal association between stressful circumstances in her life and the onset of new swelling. S. wanted to pursue the links between stress and pain, but the doctor's curt replies to her questions made it clear that stress and other psychosocial topics had no place on his agenda. The doctor's sharp dismissal of issues that concerned the patient silenced her. As her worries were brushed off the biomedical table like so many crumbs of stale bread, she stopped mentioning them. As time went by, this sort of subtle power dynamic—this asserting of the doctor's knowledge and diminishing of the patient's—slowly ate away at the patient's confidence that her knowledge of her body counted for anything or even made any sense. This experience is what I mean by epistemic invalidation.

The drug discourses had the same invalidating effect on S.'s ontological sense of being-in-the-world. With the diseases named the sole object of medical attention, the patient's ideas and feelings ceased to exist. This was a radically disorienting experience, especially when those feelings included headaches and other perceptions of pain that stemmed from the treatment itself. (By contrast, pain associated with the named diseases were allowed a valid existence.) This new, unnamed, but very real pain had no ontological status. This process of invalidation is well illustrated by the best-drug discourse. An important corollary of this discourse was that any negative reactions to the best drugs were secondary matters, nuisances to be managed and made to go away. In countless ways, the doctor made it clear that patient complaints about side effects were not reasons to change the drug routine unless the side effects were very, very bad. This approach to treatment denied the legitimacy, even the existence, of the patient's sensation of discomfort, forcing her to exclude from her sense of being pain that was only too real a part of her lived experience. The discourses on drugs thus presented the patient with profound philosophical predicaments. S. struggled every day to find meaning in the fact that her ideas and feelings had been voided out of existence. Unable to find a way out of these philosophical prisons, she fell into a deep depression whose course is traced in a later chapter.

Tolerizing the Patient to the Drugs: S. Becomes an N of 1

As we saw earlier, the doctor had determined that S.'s bodily problems were serious ones requiring a multipronged chemical attack. The most important problems now, Dr. D. had declared, were the fibromyalgia, with its associated sleep disorder, and the inflammation of psoriatic arthritis, which affected numerous joints. The osteoarthritis and scoliosis were less worrying and did not respond to drugs in any case. They could be forgotten for now.

Working as methodically as a laboratory scientist, D. mapped out his treatment plan and how it would be modified should the initial results not match expectations derived from previous "experiments" on other patients. The correct strategy for S. was to attack the fibromyalgia first. This problem underlay all the others, the doctor said, so "we" would have to get this one under control first. (The doctor often said "we" when he was issuing orders or imposing his construction on things.) The strategy here was to introduce medication to get the patient into deep sleep and to keep her asleep throughout the night. The best drug for this purpose, the doctor said, is Elavil, an antidepressant that, when used in small quantities, induces deep sleep. If that did not work, the next-best choice would be Flexeril, a weaker drug that is chemically related to Elavil. Flexeril is a muscle relaxant that is also supposed to produce deep sleep. (More information on the medications used for S.'s conditions can be found in table 2. The text mentions only the side effects that Dr. D. told S. about in their consultations.)

The treatment of psoriatic arthritis proposed by the doctor relied on

Table 2

Medications and Their Uses and Side Effects

Medication (generic name)	Class and Uses	Common Side Effects and Other Concerns
Fibromyalgia Medications		
**Elavil (amitriptyline)	Antidepressant; in small doses promotes deep sleep	Dry mouth; constipation; blurred vision; drowsiness, dizziness; headache; nausea; unpleasant taste, and increased appetite, especially for sweets. Weight gain common.
*Flexeril (cyclobenzaprine)	Muscle relaxant; promotes deep sleep	Blurred or double vision, any change in vision; dizziness or lightheadedness; drowsiness.
Ambien (zolpidem)	Hypnotic, for short-term treatment of insomnia; induces sleep	Daytime drowsiness or dizziness; possible depression.
Arthritis Medications		
**Indocin (indomethacin)	NSAID, to reduce inflammation and pain	Headache and feeling spaced-out common. Also standard NSAID side effects of skin rash; bloated feeling or gas; diarrhea, mild nausea, or vomiting; dizziness, lightheadedness, or drowsiness; headache; mild heartburn, indigestion, or stomach pain or cramps. One of the most toxic antiinflammatories.
Clinoril (sulindac)	NSAID	Standard NSAID side effects (see Indocin).
Oruvail (ketoprofen)	NSAID	Standard NSAID side effects (see Indocin).
**Methotrexate (methotrexate sodium)	DMARD, to reduce inflammation and to retard disease progression	Black, tarry stools; bloody vomit; diarrhea; reddening of skin; sores in mouth and on lips; stomach pain; loss of appetite; nausea; likelihood of liver damage, increasing with cumulative dose of drug. Increasingly considered the drug of choice for serious arthritis.

(*continued on next page*)

Table 2 (*continued*)

Medication (generic name)	Class and Uses	Common Side Effects and Other Concerns
Arthritis Medications		
**Plaquenil (hydroxychloroquine)	DMARD, to reduce inflammation and to retard disease progression	Diarrhea; difficulty in seeing well enough to read; headache; itching; loss of appetite; nausea or vomiting; stomach cramps or pain. Less common but more serious is damage to retina of eye. Generally well tolerated.
Prednisone (oral steroid)	Corticosteroid, to reduce inflammation and suppress immuno-logical responses	Major side effects, increasing with dose and duration, include: ulcers; mental changes including psychosis and depression, infection, acne; redistribution of body fat, muscle wasting, increased hair growth, bruising; loss of calcium and fragile bones, increased risk of fracture and osteoporosis, cataracts.
Steroid Injections	Corticosteroid, to reduce inflammation	Same as Prednisone but risks are lower because joint injections are rare.
Headache Medications		
Tylenol (acetaminophen)	Painkiller, for temporary relief of minor pain	Side effects minimal.
Tylenol with codeine, Tylenol #2 (acetaminophen and codeine)	Painkiller with narcotic for moderate pain relief	Possible addiction; constipation; fecal impaction; sluggishness.

NOTE: NSAID = Nonsteroidal antiinflammatory drug; DMARD = Disease-modifying antirheumatic drug. Includes only relatively common side effects.
**Dr. D.'s "best-choice" drugs for these conditions
*Dr. D.'s next-choice drugs
SOURCES: Fries 1995; Medi-Span 1995; Starlanyl and Copeland 1996; US Pharmacopeial Convention 1996

a combination of a nonsteroidal antiinflammatory drug to reduce joint swelling and two drugs in a stronger class of disease-modifying antirheumatic drugs, which some evidence suggests might slow the process of joint destruction. In the class of antirheumatics the doctor wanted to increase the dosage of Methotrexate, which S. had been taking for four years, to the highest level recommended for a person of her size. In addition, he wanted to add a new drug in the same class, Plaquenil. Plaquenil is an antimalarial drug that has been shown to help patients with arthritis, although the mechanism by which it works is not understood. The Plaquenil would not kick in for six to eight or even twelve weeks, the doctor said, and treatment could not begin until S. had undergone a baseline retinal exam. Both drugs had potentially dangerous if rare side effects, Methotrexate on the liver and Plaquenil on the eyes. S. had tolerated fairly high doses of Methotrexate, with no apparent adverse effects. But she had refused to take Plaquenil for years, worrying about the potential for damage to her eyes. Dr. D. now dismissed those worries, noting that retinal damage could be avoided with regular use of ultraviolet-blocking sunglasses, weekly vision checks by the patient with an Amsler Grid (a printed square of vertical and horizontal lines resembling a giant Tic-Tac-Toe box), and semiannual opthamalogical exams. The use of Plaquenil was not optional; it was an essential part of a treatment package whose design was the prerogative of the doctor.

The changes in the antirheumatics could be introduced gradually over the next few weeks. What could not wait, the doctor insisted, was a switch to a stronger antiinflammatory. This was an urgent priority, for the inflammation in S.'s joints was serious and getting worse. The best drug for her, the doctor declared, was Indocin. He warned of potential side effects, including headaches and mental changes (Diary, March 8; see chapter 1 for details). But they did not worry Dr. D. If the side effects became a problem, the patient was to take megadoses of Extra-Strength Tylenol to suppress them until her body became acclimated to the drug. If she was like most patients, she could eventually be "tolerized" to it.

We now look to see how this pharmacological discourse was turned into practice. We are interested in three aspects of this practice: how effective the drugs were, what side effects or new symptoms the patient experienced, and how the doctor interpreted the new symptoms. (Whether the new problems were side effects of the drugs or new symptoms of S.'s diseases was the crux of the interpretation problem. In the discussion below I try to use the term the doctor and/or patient considered correct at the time.) Between March 8 and June 14, when a stable regime of medication was finally established, the doctor tried three different combinations of drugs to bring S.'s problems under control. He began with the "best-choice" drugs for her conditions. When they produced unbearable side effects, he backtracked, substituting weaker drugs in the same class. His hope was to establish a tolerance for the strong drugs, which in time he would reintroduce. The side effects went away, but the arthritis drug was deemed insufficiently effective. So the doctor put his patient back on the original antiinflammatory, this time in a sustained-release form that was supposed to be gentler on the user.

A crucial task during these months of experimentation was to determine what was causing a new set of problems that emerged about the time treatment began: headaches, a feeling of "spaciness," and, a few weeks later, neck and upper-back pain. Though S.'s reports on her bodily state provided input to the analysis, the interpretation was the exclusive prerogative of the doctor, who was now the expert on S.'s body. The doctor offered what he considered an appealing metaphor for their respective roles: he was the artist, she a canvas on which he would paint.

The doctor was highly creative in his approach to locating the cause of the new symptoms. Initially he proposed two possible explanations, which we can call the Indocin and fibromyalgia theories of the new symptoms, and acted on the second. Later he dropped the Indocin theory in favor of the fibromyalgia explanation. As time went by the doctor embellished the fibromyalgia theory with two additional hypotheses. The interpretation that the doctor ascertained to be correct was highly consequential, for it became the basis for decisions about what treatment would follow. The doctor's interpretive frame would be inscribed on the patient's body.

Dr. D. Starts with the "Best Drugs for Her Conditions"

On her way home from the airport after her first visit with Dr. D., S. stopped by the drugstore to fill her new prescriptions. Following D.'s orders, S. began taking Elavil, the sleep enhancer, and Indocin, the antiinflammatory, on that very night, March 8. The Indocin was the regular form of the drug, in which the dosage peaks and then subsides. Since sleep was determined to be S.'s most serious problem—and S., who had not gotten a good night's sleep for a very long time, agreed wholeheartedly with that assessment—during the first two weeks both doctor and patient concentrated on resolving the sleep disorder.

The day after she began taking the new medications S. started keeping a record of all the drugs she consumed and their effects on her body and mind. She created a private chart for a number of complicated reasons that she did not try to come to grips with at the time. Among those reasons was S.'s desire to help the doctor sort out the effects and side effects of the drugs. Another was her conviction that she was a better judge of her bodily state than her doctor. A third was her hope that a detailed log of any and all side effects would help to protect her from the risks associated with the strong drugs. In this chapter we draw on that chart for information on what medications S. took, when she took them, and with what result.

How effective was the Elavil? For the first three nights the patient took her pills two hours before bedtime and got about five hours of sleep. But the effect was not quite as anticipated. Instead of sleeping through the night she awoke at 2:00 or 3:00 A.M. and could not get back to sleep. In the afternoon she was overcome with a sickly, swooning feeling that left her no choice but to take a nap. The Elavil seemed to be putting her to sleep in the daytime while failing to keep her asleep at night. She called Seattle to report the problem. The doctor replied that Elavil rarely puts patients to sleep the next day. She should try taking the pills at bedtime instead. The swooning feeling, he insisted, was not drug related (Diary, March 11).

On the fifth day the headaches began. S. had never had headaches before. These were horrible: huge, throbbing headaches that made all activity impossible. On March 12, she noted in the chart, she had a "splitting headache." On March 13 the headache was "50 percent worse." She called the doctor again. Here is her account of what he said:

> [D.] thinks the headaches are unlikely to be related to the Elavil; his two hypotheses are (1) Indocin and (2) neck pain, leading to headaches. Says the neck pain will come more to the fore as treatment proceeds, decreasing only over time . . .
>   When "we" walk away from a drug, it is for good, that's the philosophy—so he wants to stick with the Elavil for a bit longer. He needs to know more about how the drug pharmacology interacts with my physiology. So, more experiments for the next few days. [N]ew strategy: (a) Use Tylenol with codeine to kill off the headaches. ([Possible] side effects: affects thinking, makes one nauseous, [gives one] stomach problems, constipation; is a narcotic but not addictive.) . . . Take . . . two pills four times a day. (b) Stick with the Indocin, four times a day. (c) Take one tablet of Elavil at dinnertime. (Diary, March 13)

Note how, only five days into treatment, the patient has already turned herself into an object of her doctor's experiments, so that his "need to know" becomes the driving force behind the continued drug work: "He needs to know more . . . So, more experiments for the next few days." The hierarchy of precedence established by the drug discourse—doctor over drugs, drugs over side effects—has taken firm root in the patient's mind. The doctor's "need to know" is evidently more important than the patient's need to gain relief from the new symptoms. Indeed, her need for deliverance from the headaches is deemed so trivial by Dr. D and, in turn, S. that it gets no articulation whatsoever.

The March 13 entry is important also because it contains the first word about neck pain, which the doctor cites as a possible explanation for the headaches. He seems to have known that his treatment would exacerbate any neck pain—"the neck pain will come more to the fore as treatment proceeds"—yet he had failed to mention this drawback to his program of care in the initial consultation. S. learned of this cost, which would vex her to no end over the next year, only *after* the treatment that fostered it had begun.

This diary entry also needs to be marked, because it establishes a pattern of interpretation of side effects and drug practice that was to persist for the full eight months that S. remained in Dr. D.'s care. The doctor *recognized* that Indocin might be the cause of the headaches—indeed, that was his first theory—but he *acted on* the assumption that they were related to neck pain and sleep difficulties associated with the fibromyalgia. He gave the fibromyalgia theory preferential attention, I believe, because it followed so logically from the diagnostic discourse. In the diagnosis the doctor had determined that S. had fibromyalgia and that this was her most serious and fundamental problem. If this problem underlay most of the symptoms she exhibited at the first appointment, it only made sense that it was now also causing the new problems.

The interpretive emphasis given to fibromyalgia also followed from the doctor's pharmacological philosophy. The drug discourse had made Indocin the drug of choice for the inflammation in S.'s joints. It was important not to drop that "best-choice" drug unless it was absolutely necessary—and it was not yet time for that. "When we walk away from a drug, it is for good," he said, reminding her of his ("our") philosophy and putting less-than-subtle pressure on her not to demand that he drop the drug too soon. Put more pointedly, the doctor's conviction that Indocin was the best drug for S.'s arthritis subtly discouraged him from pursuing the Indocin theory of headaches, for were that drug indicted, he would have to use a second-best drug for the joint swelling. The fibromyalgia theory was more appealing, for it allowed him both to keep his patient on his preferred arthritis drug and to attribute the new symptoms to his specialty disease, which he had already determined was S.'s major problem. In short, the fibromyalgia theory of the neurological symptoms rose to the top because of its discursive rationality—its tight fit with already established discourses of the patient body.

Despite the massive dose of Tylenol with codeine that S. was taking, her headaches did not go away. The Tylenol seemed to help on some days, but it was worthless on others. On the night of March 17, S. went to bed at 10:00 P.M. and awoke at 12:30, 2:30, 4:30, and 6:30 A.M. On March 18 she wrote on her chart: "Splitting headache all day, ringing in ears, dry heaves. *Huge* bags under eyes." She called Seattle once again. Below is her record of that conversation. Note how once again S. accepts the discourse of the scientific experiment, in which the doctor-scientist makes the decision to backtrack, even when the patient is the one suffering from the headaches:

> Called doc about horrible headaches. Luckily he decided it was time to backtrack . . . Most of the problems are probably due to the fibromyalgia; certainly the headaches are, he thinks. Wants to know mechanisms underlying the symptoms, so can decide how best to treat . . . Thinks headaches [are] due to fibromyalgia; if any drug, then certainly Indocin, not Elavil . . . Basic problem is most likely upper back pain. [This causes] no sleep [which] leads to headaches. (Diary, March 18)

By now fibromyalgia had emerged as the leading explanation for S.'s problems, including her headaches. Yet in perhaps a silent admission that Indocin might also be implicated, the doctor took her off the drug, putting her on a weaker antiinflammatory instead. Here is the new regime, as described in the same diary entry:

> New regime: Clinoril . . . No neurological side effects, well tolerated. [A] few side effects, mostly in kidneys. Stomach, potential for ulcers. Tylenol with codeine—take 1,1,1,2 until headaches settle down. [For sleep, switch to] Flexeril, [which is] like Elavil, but less potent, fewer side effects. Take two hours before going to bed. (Diary, March 18)

Dr. D. Backtracks for Two Weeks

S. went off Elavil and Indocin on March 18, switching to the weaker drugs, Flexeril and Clinoril. The headaches promptly went away and stayed away—at least as long as this new regime remained in place. Now the worries centered on how effective these second-choice drugs would be in producing the desired effects. S.'s diary tracks the changes, jumbling up her doctor's views with her own:

> Results of new experiment . . . inconclusive . . . Clinoril is in Indol group, which is most effective. Different people metabolize these drugs differently, though. Want to continue this one.
> Flexeril—try moving this to bedtime, in hopes that the 12:30 wakeup will not happen. Maybe wait til I tolerate it, i.e., get metabolically acclimatized, then maybe down-dose this. Usually within weeks the drugged feeling goes away. The not-so-secret strategy is to move from Flexeril to Elavil and then eventually reduce the dosage of Elavil . . . Stop Tylenol with codeine—this may be contributing to the drugged feeling. Switch to Tylenol Extra-Strength . . . for pain control . . . Call tomorrow . . . to report on sleep under new . . . timing routine. (Diary, March 21)

But sleep refused to come easily. S. struggled to make it through the sleepless nights and the days of exhaustion that invariably followed, while her doctor did his very best to come up with a drug package that would work for this biochemically aberrant new patient. Faced with a patient who could not get to sleep, he added a second sleep medication. Unlike Elavil and Flexeril, Ambien was a serious sleeping pill, a narcotic that was supposed to knock her out.

> I must be biochemically bizarre. No matter what, I cannot sleep. Last night took a Flexeril at bedtime, was wide awake til about 1:30, then dozed off a few times before giving up . . . Naturally, feel wretched today.
> Doc thinks this is weird too. What's bizarre is this business of waking at 1:30 or 2:30 and never quite going back to sleep again . . . Also weird is that the drugs I've tried . . . do not kick in at the right interval, or else [do] not knock me out enough. So. He's going to try to induce sleep, then use Flexeril to keep me asleep . . . Ambien is a sleeping pill . . . Must take just before bed . . . Call doc . . . on Monday. (Diary, March 22)

But the Ambien worked too well. It put her to sleep not only at night but during the day as well. When the doctor halved the dosage, the patient got no sleep at all.

S. was miserable from all the experiments. She was barely able to carry on a life and fulfill her university duties; creative thinking and writing were out of the question. As the ordeal stretched on and on, with no end in sight, her consternation about the drugs' effects on her cognitive functioning grew ever deeper. She was a scholar and a teacher; her mind was her life and livelihood. She could live without some of her joints, but a clear head was absolutely essential. She registered these worries with her doctor, but he refused to take them seriously:

> [Told D. I feel] like I [am] in a torture chamber, with nothing ever working and the side effects always making it impossible to function, let alone work. The reply: . . . "things have just begun!" (Diary, March 27)
>
> [Mentioned] mental alertness as criterion for judging the success of a drug. [The reply:] "yes, of course." I . . . wanted to register that it was very high priority for me . . . [H]e just wanted to include it along with all the others. At least I made my point. (Diary, March 29)

At S.'s second appointment, on March 29, the doctor announced that he was not satisfied with the results of the Clinoril experiment. The inflammation in her joints had not gone down. The doctor wanted to put her back on Indocin, using a low-dose, sustained-release form of the drug to avoid a recurrence of headaches (Diary, March 29). Here again the doctor quietly conceded that Indocin might have produced the headaches the first time it was used, although fibromyalgia had supplanted it as the leading explanatory mechanism. Yet despite his suspicion of a connection, the doctor put the patient back on the drug, trying to trick her body into accepting it through tolerization techniques.

S. Is Tolerized to Some of the "Best Drugs for Her Conditions"

On April 4 Dr. D. put S. back on Indocin, this time in a low-dose, sustained-release form. Because the doctor now had so much valuable (and laboriously gathered) experimental data on the effects of Flexeril and Ambien, he did not switch back to Elavil but kept her on the two newer drugs, whose workings he was coming to understand. While waiting for the Indocin to reduce the joint swelling, he continued to concentrate on the sleep problem, which had not yet been resolved. After a few more days of adjusting the dosages and timing of the sleep medications, a phenomenal thing happened: S. got almost six hours of sleep. She was thrilled.

Yet all was not well on the antiinflammatory front. On the very first day that S. began taking Indocin again, a new neurological symptom emerged: she felt spacey and faint. She reported these strange sensations to the doctor that very day, April 5. But the doctor did not want to hear about possible side effects from the Indocin. Now he asked her to stay on the drug, adding that the sustained-release version was not supposed to produce problems. He very much hoped that the Indocin would work, since it was the perfect drug for her. To make sure that problems did not emerge, he introduced it cautiously, starting her at one tablet of 75 mg. a day. S.'s description of her doctor's high hopes for Indocin brings out the strong pressure he placed on her to accept the drug without complaints:

> The hope is that I will fall in the class of patients for whom Indocin works as an antiinflammatory, that is, that it shuts off at least part of the inflammation. If Indocin doesn't work, it's unclear which of the eighteen NSAIDS [nonsteroidal antiinflammatory drugs] to use to reduce the inflammation. The hope is that, if it works, I will be able to go on a second dose of two times that (150 mg.) for five days before my next visit. (Diary, April 5)

But the spaciness persisted. S. reported it to the doctor again on April 7. He tried to reason out what could be causing the faintness. Rather than connect the neurological problem to Indocin, a theory he had already rejected, he tied it to S.'s fibromyalgia. Based on his experience with that disease, the doctor suggested that her spaciness might be related to the microenvironment of work. Here is S.'s record of the conversation:

> [It] was funny, [I] started the Indocin last Thursday. Thursday and Friday I had a strange spacey feeling, especially Thursday when I went to school [to teach]. Saturday and Sunday no such feeling at all. Then today, when I went back to school, it returned and stayed all day. Felt faint, had to rest head on wall to keep from fainting.
> So, the doctor suggested it had to do with the microenvironment of work! Right—[my university] makes me sick! More technically, [D. explained], the fibromyalgia is very environment sensitive. It could be [that] very slight adjustments in my chair, posture, [or] degree of tension, [are] making the fibromyalgia worse . . . (Diary, April 7)

S. was intrigued by the microenvironment idea, adding: "That is amazing. Especially because it is probably true." A week later she mulled over the idea some more. It seemed to fit her life so neatly that she accepted it as the truth:

> So interesting . . . his hypothesis about microenvironment at work producing the feeling of spaciness. That is a side effect often associated with fibromyalgia. He offered that notion on a Monday night. The next day, Tuesday, I worked at home and had no spacey feeling at all! Today I had a very intense morning of teaching and feel very, very tired, as well as a little light-headed. Now I have to figure out what is going on at work to produce these feelings. (Diary, April 15)

On April 15 the doctor doubled the dosage of Indocin to 150 mg. a day. The effect on the joint swelling was immediate: by the next day the pain in almost every joint of S.'s body had subsided. But no sooner did she enjoy relief from the joint pain than another debilitating symptom appeared.

In late April the headaches returned with a vengeance. They arrived in full force on April 17, two days after the dose of Indocin was doubled. They vanished on the fourth day, but then returned to stay on the sixth day of the sustained-release Indocin regime. By now, however, Indocin had dropped out of the interpretive picture altogether, with the fibromyalgia-related neck pain and sleep problems, which in turn were affected by the environment, bearing full responsibility for the headaches:

> Well, unfortunately, the bliss of restful nights and clear-headed days has come to an end, at least temporarily. Saturday, Sunday, and Monday I woke with low-grade headaches; they went away by mid-afternoon with a few hits of Tylenol. Today [Tuesday] it was a middle-grade headache. And it did not go away. So I had to call [D.], though I really did not want to bother him.
>
> He thinks it's either: poor sleep causing neck pain causing the headaches; or neck pain ([from] fibromyalgia and osteoarthritis) causing poor sleep causing the headaches. I agree, it could be either. Probably not the Indocin, because Indocin headaches usually appear soon after increasing the dosage. What to do? For now, switch to the Tylenol with codeine, six tablets today and tomorrow. Dr. D. will call me [tomorrow]. (Diary, April 23)

From the end of April on, S. struggled with on-again off-again problems of headache, poor sleep, fatigue, and yet another new symptom, upper-back and neck pain. The doctor tried everything he could think of to make things right: he upped and downed the dosage of sleep medications, boosted the painkiller, and suggested changes in the configuration of the orthopedic pillow she had begun using at his insistence. S. felt certain that the orthopedic pillow, with its uncomfortable neck roll, and the changes in sleep posture the doctor had commanded her to make, were actually contributing to the neck pain that he ascribed to her fibromyalgia. Her chart is filled with her struggles to sleep with that pillow and the countless times she cut open the casing to remove, replace, or otherwise adjust the fiber filling. The chart also suggests a temporal connection between use of the pillow and emergence of the neck pain. On April 23 it indicates that S. started sleeping with the pillow nightly, and on April 24 she began experiencing neck, shoulder, and upper back pain daily. S. suggested the pillow hypothesis to her doctor. But D. "nixed the idea, [explaining that] the pillow does not exacerbate [the pain], [it] only makes the pain more obvious" (Diary, April 30). Once again S. was silenced, her interpretations of her care ridiculed and rejected. These experiments and hunts for explanation produced little but frustration for the patient and probably the doctor as well. On April 30, for example, S. writes: "Weekend experiment—increasing Flexeril from 15 to 20 mg— was a complete failure. I got an hour or two more of sleep [five hours instead of four] . . . but felt completely drugged, headachey, and unrested all three days. So, more bad news. [Dr. D.] wants me to . . . "

This greater focus on the fibromyalgic neck pain gave the doctor a chance to elaborate his view of microenvironmental causes into grander ideas about the ergonomics of postmodern life. Here is S.'s account of this enlarged interpretation:

The mechanisms underlying the neck pain are not tension or tensed muscles, but too much of the wrong kind of movement; they are mechanical. This is an interesting concept I had not encountered before. The environment of postmodern life truly contributes to these problems: desk and library work (especially craning neck over desk), sedentary lifestyles, working without breaks, talking for long times on the phone, reading or watching TV while lying on one's back—all these promote bad body positions. In people who already have underlying problems, the ergonomics of postmodern life can make things much worse. (Diary, April 30)

This expanded version of the fibromyalgia theory of S.'s new symptoms seemed to fit her situation perfectly: her life was filled with such "postmodern" activities, which were probably making her pain worse. The approach to these problems was for the patient to observe closely her daily activities, looking for body postures that might be exacerbating the neck pain that was contributing to her sleeplessness and headaches. Activities magnifying the pain were to be performed differently or eliminated from her life. Dr. D. encouraged this hypervigilance with talk of patient empowerment: "Being able to identify the environmental stressors, or sources of increased pain, is an important part of the process [of] . . . tak[ing] charge of one's life again" (Diary, April 30). But S. was very discouraged. As if it were not bad enough to have all these physical ailments, now her doctor was telling her that her lifestyle and chosen occupation were making her conditions worse.

In late April a new, even stranger hypothesis came to the fore: exercise is causing the headaches. Since she began feeling a little better, S. had been swimming almost daily. She had even begun to do neck-ranging exercises in the water, thinking that the stretching would improve the range of motion of that now troublesome neck. By this time S. had gotten into the interpretive act, using information on her chart to analyze her daily activities for clues about what was going wrong. With all the new emphasis the doctor was placing on neck pain, she began to wonder if maybe the swimming and added neck exercises were not making things worse. Despite her worries about letting a doctor into this sacrosanct part of her life—S. had a special relationship with water that went back to her childhood summers spent by a Maine lake—she wanted desperately to get better. According to the doctor's ideas about treatment, self-monitoring and self-management were the keys to improving her fibromyalgia. So she swallowed her worries and suggested the idea to her doctor. What he told her contradicted everything she had always known to be true about her health. Yet these perverse new ideas seemed to be supported in her own life:

> Turns out that swimming is not particularly good for arthritis—too much strain on the neck. I was really feeling that last night while swimming—all that turning of the neck to breathe . . . Also, the neck-ranging exercises . . . [that] my New York physical therapist recommended are bad. (!) (Osteo) arthritis [which I have in my neck] usually results from . . . excessive force on a normal joint, or normal force applied to an abnormal joint . . . [Either] tends to make the arthritis worse. So, it seems that rest is better than exercise! This is really baffling; everything I've always known to be "true" turns out to be wrong. D. says that 50 percent of the time, going to a physical therapist makes his patients worse! . . . So, no more neck exercises! (Diary, April 24)

Since swimming was now identified as part of the problem, it too was included on the list of proscribed activities. On April 30, after yet another experiment with the sleep medications led to more headaches and sleeplessness, S. was ordered to cut back the Flexeril, take a full dose of Tylenol with codeine, and "cut out all swimming" (Diary, April 30). The ban on swimming appeared to bring immediate results: the headaches went away and stayed away—for three days. But then they returned, for no apparent reason. And her neck pain grew worse. Like so many other hypotheses the doctor had offered, this one received inconsistent support—on some days it worked, on others it didn't. Yet despite the mixed results, the ban on swimming remained in effect on the theory that it was best to eliminate all possible sources of the new symptoms to make them go away. Once the symptoms had disappeared, the activities could be reintroduced gradually and in a graded fashion so that the symptoms would not recur.

S. was utterly despondent at the thought of giving up her swimming. (This story is told in a later chapter.) But she toughed it out and came to accept the doctor's interpretation as her own. After all, she believed that she had fibromyalgia and that the doctor was an expert in managing it. Also, some of the ideas associated with the fibromyalgia theory—especially the microenvironment and exercise hypotheses—turned out to gain some, if erratic, support from her life. By now very much "inside" the discourses of biomedicine with her doctor, S. did not blame him for her new ills or challenge his interpretations of the symptoms. Quite the contrary, she was happy that he was so thorough in analyzing her problems and thankful that he was frank and gentle in breaking the bad news to her.

Dramatic Improvement and Dramatic Decline: Bodily Results

Drawing on data from the patient's charts, we now step back to examine the overall record of improvement—and decline—in S's bodily conditions over the first three months of treatment. We then ask why S. did not challenge her doctor's practices and find the answers in the drug discourses and practices themselves.

Old Problems Partly Solved, New Ones Created

Throughout May and early June, the Flexeril-Ambien-Indocin SR regime was stabilized, and S.'s two major problems, the inflammation of psoriatic arthritis and the fibromyalgia-related sleep dysfunction, were brought largely under control. The Indocin seems to have been a dream drug, inducing a rapid reduction in the swelling of all but three of S.'s joints. The doctor injected these joints with corticosteroids, and the swelling and pain in them disappeared. The increased dosage of Methotrexate and the new antirheumatic, Plaquenil, introduced in mid-April, undoubtedly contributed to the overall improvement in S.'s joints and produced no evident ill effects. From all appearances, the treatment for the arthritis was highly successful.

S.'s fibromyalgic sleep disorder was also alleviated to some extent. With Ambien to put her to sleep and Flexeril to keep her there, she often managed to get six hours of sleep or so. Although she never felt truly rested, six hours a night was more than she had been getting before. Data from her daily charts show that during April, May, and early June, one night in three was disturbed by very poor sleep, and two days in five were marred by serious or incapacitating fatigue. S. was functioning at little more than half-capacity, but being able to count on six hours of sleep two nights out of three gave her a measure of predictability she had not had before. And, despite the diagnosis of fibromyalgia, S. continued to enjoy respite from the "pain all over" that characterizes the disease. Her chart shows not one day of whole-body pain during the spring.

By mid-June, then, S. was successfully tolerized to some of the best drugs for her conditions. She was on the very best drugs for psoriatic arthritis and two next-best drugs for the sleep disorder. She was to remain on this regime, which had taken so long to work out, for the next five months.

These gains were not achieved without a cost, however. The major cost was a complex of painful new symptoms whose causes remained poorly understood. During April, May, and early June, S. experienced on-again, off-again the mental spaciness, which occurred one day out of seven. This symptom was a little worrying, but it could be tolerated. More serious were the intense headaches, which seemed to arrive out of nowhere one out of every four days. The third new symptom—neck and upper-back pain—emerged in full force in late April. It grew far worse in May, when S. suffered neck and/or upper-back pain two days out of three. Overall, during the eleven weeks of treatment in the spring, S. endured pain in that region almost one day of every two. From the patient's point of view, these new symptoms were worse than her original complaints. Over the years she had learned to cope with the joint swelling and poor sleep, managing a busy career and active personal life. But now the neck and upper-back pain kept her from engaging in her favorite forms of recreation. And the headaches kept her from doing anything at all.

Discourse and Dissent: Why There Was No Patient Protest

Yet despite the emergence of these new symptoms, S. did not challenge her doctor's interpretation or treatment of her bodily situation. Why not? The first and foremost reason was utter exhaustion. In good part because of the drug experiments, throughout the spring this patient was on the verge of physical and emotional collapse almost all the time. She had to focus her scarce energies on making it through the day. With her physical, emotional, and mental capabilities depleted, she simply did not have any resources left that would have enabled her to step outside her daily struggles for survival to gain a larger perspective on the situation.

Although sheer exhaustion is enough to explain why S. did not challenge her doctor, like much in this story, the issue is more complicated than at first it appears to be. In this case there are two other things the reader needs to know to understand why S. could not imagine that her doctor might have made a mistake. First, she was immeasurably happy—ecstatic would not be too strong a word—to have some relief from her initial complaints, which had been with her for years. As the drug discourse had indicated, the "best drugs" worked. The patient attributed the improvements to her doctor's intimate knowledge of the rheumatological body, the correctness of his drug-intensive approach to treatment, and the extraordinary personal efforts he had devoted to working with her, day after day, week after week, to make her better. S. followed her doctor in putting him on a pedestal and in believing that the effects of his practices always matched his intentions. She could think of no earthly reason that he might intentionally cause her harm. To the contrary, she believed that he was doing everything humanly possible to help her; if things had taken a turn for the worse, it was certainly through no fault of his.

A second reason that S. did not actively question her doctor's management of her case is that the diagnostic discourse had sunk in. Moreover, the diagnostic beliefs had interacted with the drug practices in convoluted ways that left her in a Kafkaesque maze of confusion. More specifically, S. now believed she "had fibromyalgia" and was persuaded, in part by evidence from her own body, that the doctor's fibromyalgia theory of the headaches and neck pain was at least partly correct. After all, he had told her early on that, as treatment proceeded, pain in her neck would come to the fore. Although he never explained why that should happen, and this puzzle remained a source of anger and confusion for S., it had happened just as he had predicted. How could she fault him if her body was simply manifesting the symptoms his theory had predicted? Furthermore, the attribution of the two major new symptoms to fibromyalgia, a perplexing new disease in which the doctor was a rare specialist, worked to make her all the more dependent on him for help. Since these new symptoms were now an incontestable part of her bodily condition, and he was a specialist in the disease of which they were part, he was one of the few rheumatologists anywhere who could help her understand and treat them. And the fact that he was the one whose treatment had precipitated the new symptoms meant that he had more detailed knowledge of their specific causes than anyone, anywhere. If anyone could help her, it had to be him. Paradoxically, then, the further S.'s treatment progressed and the worse the new symptoms grew, the more dependent she became on this particular doctor to make them right. How could she allow herself to distrust someone who, alone in the world, seemed to hold the keys to her health?

This account of the doctor's discourse on drugs and its effects during the spring raises troubling questions. Politically, why was the patient so compliant? Why didn't she resist the doctor's intrusions into her life or simply stop going to him, a step that would have saved her considerable time and money? Intellectually, why was the patient so credulous of her doctor's theories, when the evidence from her body lent them only partial support? Psychologically, S. seems to have lost the ability to differentiate her own interests from those of her doctor. How did this frightening loss of self occur? These questions are critically important, because what happened in the spring, when the regime of medication was worked out and the structure of the doctor-patient relationship negotiated, laid the groundwork for everything that was to follow during the summer and fall.

In the next four chapters I review the developments of these crucial months again and again, sifting through different aspects of the doctor-patient relationship for clues about why things turned out the way they did. By pulling back successive curtains veiling the medical encounter, we will see how the seemingly innocuous idea that the patient "had fibromyalgia," once inserted into that relationship and worked and reworked in specific conversations, produced effects that were ultimately so harmful. We begin with the power of persuasive talk to produce behavioral and intellectual acquiescence.

CHAPTER 3 **Producing the Good Patient**

To Dr. D.'s delight S. turned out to be a very good patient. She listened carefully to everything he said, taking copious notes at every appointment. She accepted his diagnoses of her conditions and readily adopted his changing interpretations of her new symptoms. She followed his treatment orders to the letter, changing this drug and that, this dose and that, all with scarcely a word of protest. She worked hard to make the best of an often bad situation and covered her discouragement with a brave smile. Moreover, she became actively involved in her own treatment, eagerly searching out information on her conditions and asking informed questions. Carefully observing her own life, she offered observations and hypotheses that fit into and filled out the doctor's interpretive framework. On top of all that, S. was an engaging person (he told her that one day), fun to talk to and fun to see. This is the kind of patient that doctors dream of.

This chapter explains how S. came to be such a good patient. By "good patient" I mean what Dr. D. meant: a patient who remained in treatment (that is, who *was* a patient), followed the doctor's orders (was "compliant"), and trusted her doctor's judgment, abilities, and promises to make her better ("had a good attitude").[1] Whether S. would be a good patient was always an open question. It was in doubt because, as we have seen, after treatment began she experienced a rash of new symptoms. How was it that S. not only held on and followed orders, but did so in such an upbeat, trustful way?

S.'s medical diary reveals that her positive response to her doctor was in good part coaxed into being by the doctor himself. In the last two chapters we saw how the discourses and practices of biomedicine secured a powerful grip on S.'s body and mind. In this chapter we look at the work done by the *rhetorics* of biomedicine, disclosing how the doctor's active attempts to persuade his patient to believe his story, follow his orders, and trust in him had the effect of turning a skeptical patient into an adoring one. In discussing the doctor's persuasive skills I speak of rhetorical *tactics.* By calling these verbal maneuvers tactical I mean to signal that, although the process remained unconscious, the rhetorics were formulated and deployed to produce specific effects. That the doctor's words could be unconsciously chosen for particular persuasive purposes is not surprising. The process had to be unconscious, because his biomedical mind-set did not allow him to see his work as anything but pure science. And the connection between specific verbal practices and specific effects is simply the product of years of clinical experience in which the doctor had faced problems of patient creation again and again. Over time he had worked out conversational gambits that would transform various unhelpful attitudes into helpful ones, with the effect of converting cautious or doubtful or resistant patients into good ones.

The doctor's rhetorics worked so well because they were based on the discourses, the powerful and well-known "truths," of biomedicine, which were then embellished for persuasive effect. The listener not attuned to the conversational use of rhetoric would think she was hearing "the truth," when in fact the truth had been subtly stretched. The doctor's claims were not false, they were just exaggerated for effect. The reader should keep in mind that Dr. D. was following accepted practice here. As noted in the Problematique, doctors must sometimes resort to such language to get recalcitrant patients to comply with their orders. S. was nothing if not recalcitrant, at least initially.

In S.'s case we can identify three phases of good-patient construction, or three sets of rhetorical maneuvers, each addressed to a different patient problem. In the first two weeks of treatment, when the patient remained skeptical of her doctor's ability to help her, he painted a potent mix of frightening and hope-inspiring images to keep her in treatment. Then, when the patient appeared on the verge of dropping the drug treatment, the doctor brought out heavy linguistic guns to overpower her resistance. Finally, when the medications began to work, he marked and encouraged his patient's new attitude of trust with declarations of patient benefit and physician victory over entrenched bodily foes. These rhetorical maneuvers produced remarkable effects. Within six weeks the patient's initial skepticism had been transformed into cautious hope and faith in her doctor. The doubtful and resistant patient had been transmogrified into the compliant patient. By the end of three months S. was a happy trooper who not only followed orders with a smile, but worshiped her doctor as a generous human being who had given her a new lease on life.

Such rhetorical blandishments and assaults might have persuaded other patients that the doctor was deceptive if not dangerous. And indeed, Dr. D. reported that many patients had dropped out of his treatment program. But with this patient the doctor's rhetorical flourishes found a receptive audience. To understand why S. was so responsive to his enticements and threats, we need to look at the habits, beliefs, and desires she brought with her from three domains of her life: her lifelong training in the cultures of science and gender, her social location as a scholar, and her decade-long experience with rheumatological medicine.

S.'s interpersonal manner was a product of a long process of gender training in which girls are socialized to please, especially in interactions with boys and men. That education in gender had left its mark on her conversational style, which tended to avoid direct conflict and confrontation. Although I do not pursue gender issues in this chapter, the reader should keep in mind that S. may have had a particularly strong dose of socialization into pleasantness. Hadn't the famous Cornell neurologist commented on how pleasant she was?

Raised in a middle-class family, S. also shared her culture's, and especially her class's, great respect for scientific knowledge and professional expertise, especially as applied to the human body. Indeed, her social location as a knowledge producer gave her a particular affinity to knowledge-based expertise that rendered her perhaps more susceptible to scientific claims and more eager to see the application of scientific methods to her own body than other patients might be. Her image of "the knowing doctor"—the singularly knowledgeable specialist who would teach her all there was to know about her body—was one of the core beliefs that kept her in treatment through the difficult weeks before the drugs began to work.

S.'s vulnerability to her doctor's rhetorical pressures was also shaped by her individual biography, in particular, her history of rheumatological ills and care. That history, like the histories of so many chronic patients, had left her with a growing number of bodily problems that caused real difficulties in her daily life but had gone unacknowledged and unattended to by medical science. These difficulties included poor sleep, bent toes, and more. The persistence of these vexing problems created in her a deep yearning to find a doctor who could name and mend her ills. S.'s medical biography also included years of experience with standard rheumatological medicine, which offered quick-fix solutions to the most serious symptoms, paying no attention to the larger, less clearly defined complex of maladies of which her joint problems were but a part. This experience left her with an aching desire for a caregiver who would take the time to help her understand everything that was wrong. Dr. D., with his time-intensive, hands-on, all-encompassing approach to rheumatological medicine, replaced that longing with hope. And indeed, the image of "the caring doctor"—the compassionate and generous human being who personally attended to her every problem—became the second core belief that sustained her during those first few weeks. To be sure, these images of the knowing and caring doctor reflected the reality: Dr. D. was more thorough, he took more time, and he cared more about his patients than any doctor S. had ever known. But in her bewilderment S. saw only truth, missing the possibility that the science behind it might be flawed. In her neediness she saw only care, overlooking the dark underside of control.

Although physician rhetorics, coupled with patient susceptibility, form the heart of the story of constructing the good patient, the reader should keep in mind that the rhetorics built on other discursive and material practices that we examined in earlier chapters. For example, the discourses of medicalization deployed in the initial consultation cognitively and emotionally prepared the patient to be receptive to the rhetorics of compliance that followed in later conversations. Some material practices had similar effects. The way in which the doctor structured the initial consultation, for instance, forced the patient to make a huge up-front investment in the process, virtually ensuring that she would come back at least a few times to make all the time and money she had spent worth it. In S.'s case, five hours plus $1,000, mostly of her own money, vastly increased her commitment to making Dr. D.'s approach work.

This chapter focuses on the conversational negotiations and contests, the sparring and back-and-forths that played themselves out over the first three months of the doctor-patient interaction, turning the almost-bad patient into an incomparably good one. The first two sections map out the rhetorical gambits the doctor deployed to overcome patient skepticism and tamp down patient subversion, thereby solving the problems of keeping the patient in treatment and gaining her compliance. The third section traces the evolution of a private patient discourse, in which images of the doctor as an exceptionally knowledgeable and compassionate physician become the guiding thoughts that made her willing to place her faith and future in her doctor's hands. The final section examines how, once the treatment began to work, the doctor rhetorically solved her "attitude problem," turning patient doubt into adulation. This last section also explains how both doctor and patient could believe the patient was in such good shape when the evidence from her body was mixed at best. The answer lies in the distorting discourse in which they were both trapped.

Overcoming Patient Skepticism

As we saw in the last chapter, Dr. D.'s first major task was to find a viable regimen of medication to correct his new patient's problems. This turned out to be a difficult and time-consuming process. During her first few weeks as an "N of 1," the patient complained often about the new symptoms she was experiencing and expressed skepticism that the doctor could ever do what he promised. Dr. D. faced the daunting task of convincing his new patient to believe in him and to stay the course when the bodily evidence gave her every reason to drop out.

To this task the doctor brought the formidable verbal skills that he had used to such good effect in the initial consultation. To counter the patient's skepticism, he painted frightful scenarios of a future of worsening illness, offered tantalizing promises of a symptom-free and drug-free future under his care, and conveyed heroic images of himself as the brave healer who dared to defy managed medicine and go it alone, all for the good of his patients. Were they fully effective, these verbal maneuvers would have produced the perfect patient—one who feared the decay of her body, worshiped her doctor, and dared to hope for something better as a lifelong patient of Dr. D.

Scary Scenarios

As noted earlier, S. began taking the drugs prescribed by her new doctor on March 8. Three times over the next ten days she called him to report "awful, swooning feelings," "massive, splitting headaches," and "horrible headaches" that she could not abide (Diary, March 11, 13, and 18). The doctor responded not by changing the medications, but by underscoring the urgent need for S. to get serious medical treatment, a point he had introduced in the March 8 appointment. She was in terrible shape, he told her, and would get progressively worse unless drastic corrective measures were taken now. In other words, all the drug work and associated suffering were necessary not simply to ease a current condition but, more important, to ensure that her bodily ills did not worsen in the not-so-distant future.

The centerpiece of this line of argument was the formal prognosis, the second part of the larger story the doctor had crafted about her ills. Wondering whether all the agony was really necessary, in the March 18 phone conversation S. asked about her prospects for the future, something the doctor had only hinted at before. The doctor took this opportunity to lay out his formal prognosis for her. He began with the generic outlook for the conditions S. "had," then turned to her specific case. In pressing his points, he made artful use of the rhetorics of reification, in which a known past is projected into the future, making an unknowable future seem knowable and known. Here is what he said, as reconstructed in S.'s medical diary on the basis of detailed notes she took during the conversation:

> Got into discussion of long-term strategy. [The] goal is to treat (not cure, dummy) the underlying problem . . . So, what are the prospects for treatment? (1) Psoriatic arthritis: Cannot change its natural history, scant evidence that can . . . Are a few cases of sustained remission, but only a few. (2) Osteoarthritis: Cannot change course of. Cartilage degradation is biochemical process that cannot intervene in. But can change things that impact on it. Can improve the mechanics . . . Can make quality of life better . . . (3) Fibromyalgia: Is curable, though rarely, and may come back. Eminently treatable. Comprehensive approach to mechanisms . . . (4) Thoracic scoliosis: Won't change, is mechanical problem . . . What are we aiming at? Up to and including symptom-free condition. Estimate six months of aggressive program to see benefits. (Diary, March 18)

The doctor proceeded to elaborate on what might happen if "aggressive treatment" was not undertaken immediately:

> [The] problem is that pain grows and magnifies, and new deformations lead to new manifestations of osteoarthritis. [We] want to stop this process in its tracks. Want long-term protocol that does that. Five percent get arthritis mutilans, [in which] all joints are destroyed. Thanks [S. says to herself]. Psoriatic arthritis is weird in that pain is not parallel to joint erosion or destruction. Someone with psoriatic arthritis might feel fine but actually, inside, their bones are eroding away. (Diary, March 18)

The doctor was outlining some scary scenarios for the future: her pain will "grow and magnify"; her bones will develop "new deformations" until eventually "all joints are destroyed." Indeed, S.'s bones might be "eroding away" at that very minute, even though she felt fine!

So far the doctor had been describing the general prognosis for patients with S.'s conditions. Now he addressed the question of S.'s own probable future:

Psoriatic arthritis takes a multiplicity of pathways. Based on my history, it seems that my arthritis is following the "rheumatoid pattern" seen in 30 to 70 percent of patients. This is progressive, erosive, deforming. [There is] no way to predict [the] progression of [the] disease. [But] I won't crumble away. (Thanks!) Even if every five years a couple of joints are eroded, that is not so terrible.! (Diary, March 18)

Although the prognosis for psoriatic arthritis is hard to call, the doctor presented some essentially meaningless numbers—a 30 to 70 percent probability of progressive disease, reflecting, no doubt, the mixed results of the scientific literature—to make an indeterminate conclusion seem more determinate. The doctor cautioned that the future of S.'s disease could not be known, but then proceeded immediately to "assure" her that her bones wouldn't crumble away. In other words, what he *believed* was not that he could not know her future but that he *knew* her future, and what he knew was that her disease was erosive. She wouldn't turn into crumbles because the erosion would occur slowly—over decades rather than years or months. In this shift of emphasis, achieved so quickly and effortlessly, the future of the disease, which is actually uncertain because it is subject to many unidentified factors, has been rendered certain. The rhetorics of reification have done their work.

Hearing that his patient was upset by his dreary prediction for her life, the doctor added in soft, kindly tones that he liked to be "frank, not brutal" (Diary, March 18). This little phrase, which the doctor offered every time the patient grew noticeably distressed, worked to amplify the reality of what was distressing her by presenting the doctor as the candid ("frank") teller of the unfortunate truths of her body. The phrase also worked to absolve the doctor from responsibility for what he was reporting or its effects on the patient: he was merely reporting the truth; he had no hand in its creation. The second part of the phrase—"not brutal"—called attention to the doctor's deep consideration for his patient's feelings. By accentuating his supposed concern for his patient's emotions, these words deflected attention away from any selfish interests the doctor himself might have in telling the story he has told. The doctor cared only about his patients, the phrase said; he had no thoughts for himself. This little phrase, used in moments of emotional vulnerability, had deeply distorting effects on the patient's understanding of what was going on. It was one of the most potent expressions Dr. D. kept in his big doctor's bag of linguistic tools.

S. did not want to believe that her arthritis was progressive, but she could not deny that it had grown worse in recent years. Her sarcastic "thanks," in reaction to the doctor's reassurance that she would not "crumble away," suggests that she was not quite able to reject the fearsome "rheumatoid verdict," even though she could not fully accept it either. She put the matter on hold until more information came in.

Heavenly Promises

After outlining for S. this rather too-graphic picture of a future marked by progressive erosion of her joints and deformation of her body, the doctor switched gears to offer some words of comfort and hope. No matter if your musculoskeletal system is falling apart, he said, what counts is how you feel and function. (Such words might be comforting to patients whose bodily decline could not be stopped.) And I will help you feel and function better. Just trust me. I am not worried about a thing!

> Doc knew I was totally depressed by this talk of progressive disease . . .
> Trying to make me feel better, he said that the critical measures of how
> one is doing [are] how much pain one is in and how one is functioning.
> What is going on under the skin, in the musculoskeletal system, does not
> really matter. He is "not worried about anything" (that's so I don't get
> depressed that the first ten days have made me feel no better and much
> worse). (Diary, March 18)

Why should S. accept Dr. D. as the savior of her body? Because he could promise her heaven. Exploiting the rhetorics of scientific domination over nature, he stressed his ability to conquer her illnesses and make her, if not disease free, then at least symptom free. "What are we aiming at? Up to and including [a] symptom-free condition . . . in six months" (Diary, March 18). Dr. D. made these promises again and again in response to S.'s never-ending doubts and queries about where she was headed and why she should tolerate all the suffering. S. filed this report of the doctor's extravagant assurances about the future:

> Just saw [Dr. D.]. He does not accept the idea of limits—says there are none.
> [I] could be doing the marathon next year, once my shoes are properly
> fitted. That is quite comforting. Aim is to narrow the range of variation
> in the symptoms. And ultimate aim is to be symptom free [and] to get rid
> of all the medication. (Diary, March 29)

The doctor could not change the underlying conditions, which, he emphasized repeatedly, were genetic or biological and "would always be there lying in wait to emerge." But, he promised, he could make her symptom free and drug free. For a chronic rheumatological patient such as S., accustomed to the idea of lifelong joint pain and dependence on medication, such promises sounded like miracles. They seemed too good to be true.

S. did not fully believe the promises, especially the pledge to make her drug free. She asked the doctor how he would know when it was time to reduce the dosage of the drugs. His answer was hedged and cautious, fueling her doubts. He replied that such a decision depended on the results of a clinical examination and the amount of time the patient had been on the drug. And oh, by the way, he added, only drugs that do not need to remain at a constant level to be effective could be reduced and eventually eliminated. And which ones were those? S. decided not to pursue this line of inquiry. She remained skeptical, commenting to herself that his reply was "a reasonable answer" (Diary, March 29). In other words, it did not inspire much hope. To her, the promises were dubious at best.

Heroic Images

Too-good-to-be-true promises were not the only reason S. was given to accept Dr. D. as her savior. The other reason was his own less-than-quiet heroism. Making brilliant use of the rhetorics of the heroic scientist, S.'s doctor portrayed himself as uniquely qualified, motivated, and institutionally well placed to provide her with extra-quality care. What was brilliant about this rhetorical project was its rootedness in institutional fact, the aw-shucks humility with which it was carried out, and its emphasis on patient benefit with corresponding de-emphasis on gains the doctor himself might reap from striking this maverick pose.

Dr. D. conveyed the idea that he was better than other doctors repeatedly, if indirectly, by noting that S. had been undertreated in the past. Although careful not to criticize them directly, a step that would have violated professional norms, D. made it clear in indirect ways that he had nothing but disdain for the work of S.'s previous physicians. For example, he often said that the short-term rounds of the cortisone-based drug, Prednisone, which she had taken to control flares in the past, "just indicate that the baseline treatment is failing" (Diary, March 8). Or he would say, "[Your] toes should have been treated much earlier. Silent synovitis [inflammation of the joint lining] has been at work for a long time" (Diary, March 8). And on many occasions Dr. D. found opportunity to heap scorn on his colleagues in rheumatology generally for their collective failure to diagnose fibromyalgia, his specialty.

Dr. D. also represented himself as institutionally well placed to treat S.'s conditions. He was an outspoken critic of managed care, which, he emphasized on many occasions, puts profits before quality of patient care. The doctor stressed how he himself refused to join any managed-care plan, presenting a heroic image of himself as someone who had taken great professional and financial risks to buck the system to guarantee top-quality patient care. S. knew from her private investigations at his medical center that he had indeed taken professional risks in maintaining a rigid anti-HMO stance. She remained unconvinced about the financial risks, however. Her information on her doctor's financial situation was sketchy, but she knew that much of the cost of his long appointments and drug- and test-intensive treatments was displaced onto his patients, for his charges were far above the "standard and customary" fees most health insurance plans, including her own, were willing to cover. She also had reason to believe that her doctor had a financial interest in the orthopedic pillow he pushed, although she never checked that out.[2] The suspicion was based on the doctor's remark that he had personally developed the pillow, as well as on the gossip of patients who believed that his wife was nominal owner of the pillow company.

If one side of the doctor's discourse on managed care was the heroic doctor who refused to join the crowd and lower his standards, the other side was the pitiful chronically ill patient who has no place in the new world of managed care. S.'s discussion of the sharp limits placed on the use of tests at her primary care facility in California inspired in Dr. D. a long disquisition on the deleterious effects of managed care on patients with chronic rheumatological conditions. D. was adamant that managed care had no interest in treating patients like S. Here is how he put it to her:

> Managed care wants one of three things to happen to chronic-condition patients: get better, get much worse and go into [a] nursing home (which managed care does not have to pay for), or die! (Diary, March 11)

Nobody else will treat you, he darkly implied, so you have no choice but to come to me. S. did not comment on this remark in her diary, but it sank in. It left an impression because she knew from her experience with her first West Coast doctor that the aim of managed rheumatology was to get rid of the symptoms and get the patient on her way—in the most expeditious fashion possible. It took but one visit to Dr. D. to see that his approach was infinitely more thorough. In a world of managed care, Dr. D. was a welcome exception to the rule of fifteen-minute appointments. His comment underscored that hard truth.

Thwarting Patient Subversion

The first ten days of treatment were bad for S., but the next ten were worse. None of the drug regimens worked, and the headaches and exhaustion were so debilitating she could hardly function. One night in late March she announced on the phone a "subversive thought": dropping the sleep medications altogether. From the change in his voice, S. could sense that the doctor was growing alarmed. Her mind raced ahead to figure out what he was thinking. Perhaps he saw this as a serious insurrection. He might even lose the patient. Something had to be done to bring her around. What he did was to pull out some heavy discursive and rhetorical guns. With these verbal maneuvers he effectively threatened the patient with serious physical deterioration if she did not shape up and do as he said, charged her with responsibility for the failure of the drugs to work, and trivialized her suffering, describing it as nothing compared to what was to come.

Although not consciously deployed for this purpose, the doctor's conversational tactics worked to silence the patient's complaints and suppress her rebellion. This exercise of medical authority was effective in part because it was covered up by the language of scientific sensibility and patient power. Dr. D. was extremely adept at these concealments. Never once did he raise his voice or speak in a threatening tone. To the contrary, he consistently spoke in a soft, calm voice, maintained a measured tone, and peppered his conversation with the impressive-sounding terms of medical science. The effect was to make everything he said appear reasonable, objective, logical, scientific. A second camouflaging practice was to conversationally invert the actual hierarchy of power and authority. Even as the doctor exerted his medical authority to the utmost, he verbally downplayed his power, using the collective "we" rather than "I" as the subject of important sentences, describing critical treatment decisions as belonging to the patient rather than the doctor, and, on one occasion, depicting himself in mock-humble terms as "your humble servant." Although the doctor was more transparent than he perhaps realized (the "humble servant" gambit was particularly unsubtle), his tactics were remarkably effective in restraining complaints and snuffing out patient subversion.

Threats

S.'s talk of subversion produced an immediate reaction. Within seconds the doctor launched into a long lecture on "getting on the same track philosophically." By this, it soon became clear, he meant getting the patient on the doctor's philosophical wavelength. The doctor's philosophy on that night centered on the terrible condition of S.'s health and the certainty that she would "progress into serious deterioration" in a mere five years if she did not heed his medical advice. The rhetorics of reification had returned with a vengeance. S. describes the conversation this way:

> Long conversation last night about getting on the same track philosophically. He is worried that if I don't do something serious about this condition now, we will be dealing with very serious problems in five years, in his words, that [my conditions] would "progress into serious deterioration." Why this fear? Because fibromyalgia, left alone, is virtually always progressive. And because my synovitis is currently very bad and getting worse. (Diary, March 27)

Here the doctor underlined, in blood red, the points he had sought to get across earlier in the medical labeling phase of the initial consultation and the prognosis pronounced over the phone ten days later. Although the message was delivered in the cool, analytic language of medical science, it was effectively a threat: if you don't do what I say, the doctor warned, you will "progress into serious deterioration." To emphasize the progressive nature of S.'s ills, the doctor stooped to presenting as unproblematic truth an opinion that few who have published on the subject accept: that fibromyalgia tends to get worse. There is no evidence for this assertion in the literature, although S. did not discover that for a very long time.[3] The representation of her arthritis as progressive was less a lie than an exaggeration of the scientific facts—speculation dressed up as prognostication. Although S. did not want to believe these words and knew deep down that the doctor could not possibly know her future with such certainty, the phrase "progress into serious deterioration" pierced her heart like a knife. Try as she might, she could not get it out of her thoughts.

Trivializations

S. begged to be allowed to drop the drugs, because they were making her miserable. How did the doctor respond to this plea? Reaching into his bag of linguistic tricks, he pulled out the rhetorics of scientific precedence, according to which nothing must be allowed to interfere with the doing of science. As merely the objects of science, the patient and her concerns were trivial matters and deserved to be treated as such. Speaking with characteristic bluntness, D. told S. that her suffering had just begun. Given the severity of her conditions and all the work he had left to do to bring them under control, three weeks was a minuscule amount of time. In other words, she had nothing to complain about, so she should stop complaining:

> Said I felt like I was in a torture chamber . . . The reply: a few days or
> few weeks is an infinitesimal time in the grand scheme of things, given the
> conditions I have and the amount of drug work left to be done to bring
> them all under some kind of control. So, things have just begun! (Diary,
> March 27)

This silencing tactic worked. S. got the message: "things have just begun."

Accusations

A third verbal move the doctor made was to say, in essence, if the drugs are not working it is not because the treatment is flawed, it is because the patient has an abnormal body, a bad attitude, or both. Here he was making clever use of the rhetorics of biomedical infallibility, which make the object of medical attention, not medicine itself, responsible for any problems that arise. In advancing this line of argument, the doctor introduced explicitly the idea of "the bad patient," which S. quite evidently was. His hope was that he might turn her into "the good patient," changing her attitude so that the drugs would have a more favorable climate in which to work.

The first step here was to portray S.'s responses to the drugs as outside the normal range of reactions. The doctor introduced this idea of "normal" and "abnormal" reactions early on to explain why his treatments of choice did not work right away. He did not have to spell it out in black and white, for this was elementary stuff, the everyday, commonsense knowledge of medical science: drugs work well on normal patients; everyone else is abnormal. Then when problems with the treatment arose, the fault lay not with the treatment program, but with the deviant body of the patient. Note how rapidly S. picked up this discourse on normality and abnormality and applied it to her own "abnormal" body:

> I must be biochemically bizarre. No matter what, I cannot sleep . . . Doc
> thinks this is weird . . . What's bizarre is this business of waking at 1:30

or 2:30 and never quite going back to sleep again . . . Really think there
is something weird going on here. Even this doctor agrees that I am way
outside the norm in terms of response to these drugs. (Diary, March 22)

More objectionable than her uncooperative body, however, was S.'s
unhelpful attitude. It was her skeptical outlook, the doctor told her, that
was the basic problem. But S. stubbornly refused to abandon her doubts
until she had material proof that the drugs would work:

> The problems [according to D.] are: I am skeptical that he/we can ever
> find anything to ease the sleep problem; and my expectations (for treat-
> ment, alleviation of conditions) are too high. I said I was willing to suspend
> judgment for quite a long time on the first point, but I have to remain skep-
> tical until I have physical evidence that some sleep medication will actually
> work for me. This is only natural. (Diary, March 27)

The doctor also complained that S. was "forcing him" to alter his regimen sooner than he would like. Again, if the treatment was not working, it was her fault, not his. She was being too aggressive, she was having too much sway over his medical decisions. This too was an attitude
problem. In this case S. took the blame on herself, calling herself "an impossible case," a "bad patient" who needs to be made good:

> Really have to stop being so hard on this doctor. [He says] I'm forcing
> him to make many more changes much faster than he would like, and
> then throwing the consequences back at him. It's not fair. I really need
> to be the humble patient. I really am an impossible case.
>   After three days of one sleep regimen . . . I begged for a change, so
> he halved the dosages. The result was no sleep at all. So now I have to
> go back to the three-day routine and stick it out, trying to make it work.
> [The doctor says] I should be staying on a routine for two to four weeks
> if the side effects are tolerable. This is the rule of thumb. I am bad: I
> am forcing him to make changes that he really does not want to make.
> (Diary, March 27)

As for the patient's suggestion that she might go off the sleep medications, the doctor said that though he couldn't prevent her from doing
that, it was a stupid idea since it would just delay discovery of a pharmacological solution—the only kind that would work—to what was a
fixed, biological problem:

> My idea of going off the sleep medication—well, he said he couldn't and
> wouldn't oppose it. It just doesn't prove anything. If I get sleep that night,
> [there] will be no way to tell why. And the underlying sleep disturbance
> will be there, lying in wait, until some regimen is found to deal with it.
> (Diary, March 27)

D.'s response was very clever, for it downplayed the doctor's authority, making the patient appear to be in control of the decision. At the same time, it framed the matter in such a way that only one decision—continuing the drug experiments—appeared sensible. Any other decision would "prove nothing." The doctor's tactics worked, for S. abandoned her insurrectionary plan and remained on the sleep medications.

S. Develops a Private Discourse

During the first few weeks of treatment the doctor was fairly successful in bringing his new patient around. Most important, she remained in treatment, even though the drugs had not resolved the sleep problem and, overall, had made her feel worse rather than better. Why did she hold on? Certainly the doctor's verbal incitements, blandishments, and assaults had left their mark on her thinking. Some of his views—that he was a special doctor, that she was a difficult patient, that a few weeks of suffering was nothing given the severity of her conditions—sank in and left a deep impression. There were others, including the prognosis and the threat of serious deterioration, that she regarded as dubious but could not quite shake off. Still others, in particular the sky-is-the-limit promises, she rejected as too implausible to be given any credence. The doctor's imprint was real, but his words came to be enveloped by a larger understanding that grew out of S.'s own experience of the world.

For deeper insight into why S. decided to hold on despite the enervating new symptoms, we need to peer inside her private mental world, a universe of thought and feeling that remained sealed off from the doctor. There, we find, she was evolving a private discourse that reflected her own history of need and desire and provided an overarching framework of meaning within which she came to understand her relationship with Dr. D. Enfolding many of the views conveyed by her doctor, this pattern of meaning was structured around two central images: "the caring doctor" and "the knowing doctor." These were the guiding images that sustained S.'s hope and kept her in treatment during that first difficult month and beyond.

"The Knowing Doctor"

From the day of the first consultation, S. was convinced that Dr. D. was not an ordinary doctor, but a singular expert on the rheumatological body. How she got this idea is not clear, but she was certainly impressed by his examination-room lectures and frequent use of technical terms with which she was not familiar. Moreover, as she gradually came to understand, Dr. D. was a specialist on fibromyalgia. Since few rheumatologists knew much about this emergent condition, she figured, he must be on the cutting edge of rheumatological science. She was also impressed by his thoroughness and attention to the most minute detail. If he was concerned with all these things, she figured, he must know a great deal about what was causing her conditions and what could be done to alleviate them.

As time went by and the doctor's hypotheses about her new symptoms gained confirmation from her own life, S. became all the more convinced of her doctor's scientific prowess, if not infallibility. When the hypotheses failed to explain something or received inconsistent support, she followed the doctor in believing that the problem lay not in the original proposition but in the existence of other, complicating factors that had yet to be identified. There was nothing foolish about this; to the contrary, doctor and patient were simply following the logic of clinical science, in which hypotheses are developed, tested against behavioral data, and then rejected only when the evidence is overwhelmingly negative. The search for ever more causal factors could even be described as sophisticated science, for it eschewed simple, monocausal explanations in favor of a complex, multifactorial model of the patient's symptoms.

S. was so certain that her doctor knew everything there was to know about rheumatology that she was not even deterred by her own evidence, acquired from a computer search, that he had published only a handful of articles, none of them on her medical conditions. (There may have been others that were not caught by the Medline search.) She politely inquired into his research activities one day and was told that he had "tons of clinical data but no time . . . to analyze them" (Diary, March 27). "Clinical work just never ends," he said with a sigh. Never mind, she reasoned to herself, he is too busy making patients better to bother with research and publishing. Much better that he have broad, clinically based knowledge of the real experiences of flesh-and-blood patients than a lot of narrow scientific publications.

From the beginning S. constructed her new doctor as the professor and herself as the student of rheumatology. His knowledge was a resource that she could draw upon and eventually master in improving her bodily condition. Indeed, one of her original aims in keeping the medical diary was to record all the wonderful things she learned from talking to

Dr. D. With irrepressible enthusiasm, she writes: "I love to talk to [D.] because I learn so much each time I do" (Diary, April 24). Or "I really like talking to him, in part because I learn so much that is useful" (Diary, May 2).

Other patients might have been less interested in, or less impressed by, D.'s fount of knowledge about their bodies. But S. had a special affinity to knowledge. As a scholar herself, she had perhaps an overly large dose of respect for knowledge-based expertise and an overly active interest in acquiring some herself. From the first consultation, she was thrilled to find someone who gave her long disquisitions on rheumatology. And he was so willing to teach, with his endless discussions of dynamics and mechanics, all liberally peppered with technical terms. S. loved those terms and did outside research to learn what each one meant. For S., interacting with D. came to be something of a game, something fun. It was a new intellectual challenge—her favorite kind—to see how much she could learn about her physical problems. Indeed, a casual reader of her medical diary might come away with the impression that S. was more interested in mastering the science of rheumatology than in treating her own bodily ills. More than the doctor's presumed knowledge, it was this element of intellectual sport, as well as S.'s sense that there was a special bond between them based on the sharing of knowledge, that kept her in the relationship with her doctor.

"The Caring Doctor"

It was not only her doctor's wealth of knowledge that convinced S. that she had found a very special doctor. It was also his attitude of caring, of taking personal responsibility for making her better, that drew S. to him and kept her coming back even when his drugs were causing her so much pain. Many aspects of Dr. D.'s approach to patient care led S. to believe that he was an exceptionally caring physician. He paid great attention to the most minute details of her life; it seemed that no problem was too small for him to minister to. He was almost always available to talk by phone, if necessary spending half an hour or more on long-distance calls explaining the rationales for his treatments and alleviating her worries about side effects. And he was willing to walk her through literally dozens of different drug regimens, trying each one out until they found one that worked. If this behavioral evidence was not enough, the doctor frequently claimed personal responsibility for making her better. All this personal attention made a profound impression on S.

This view of the caring doctor emerged as early as March 13, only five days after the initial consultation, when S. noted to herself: "This guy is amazing—he takes it as his personal responsibility to make me feel better. I've never had a doctor who cared" (Diary, March 13). The feeling grew stronger as time went by, producing some eccentric, even comical readings of the doctor's actions. In the following passage S. describes her doctor as "a generous human being" when he agrees to reduce the dosage of his headache-inducing drugs so that S. can go on a professional trip. Other patients might have seen this gesture as the only reasonable thing the doctor could do under the circumstances.

> What is the bargain? I will stay on this [hard-to-tolerate] regime for several more days until our meeting Friday. If things are not workable, he will suggest a change so that I can go on my trip . . . This really is a generous human being. (Diary, March 27)

The doctor's frequent discussions of the special difficulties faced by patients with chronic rheumatological conditions deepened S.'s sense that her new physician possessed a profound understanding of her problems. She saw herself in his stories of how patients with chronic conditions feel "so out of control, like victims." And she was comforted by his view that such patients need to become active participants in their own care (Diary, March 29). When the doctor spoke of the misery of patients forced on an endless search for a doctor to help them, S. felt that she had finally found someone who deeply understood and empathized with her plight:

> I really can't believe in my heart that things will truly get better. I don't dare believe that. In most cases, [the doctor says,] the longer a condition has been in existence, the longer it takes to feel improvement. Seems lots of patients are like me: the fibromyalgia becomes entrenched and becomes a body-habit. I like that, I know it's true! And you become very miserable, only once in a great while coming out of your misery to try out a new doctor, who in turn fails to help you, sending you back into your miserable state. Boy, can I relate to that scenario. (Diary, April 7)

On one occasion S. asked her doctor point-blank why he cared so much about his patients. His answer—"otherwise, what's the point of being in medicine?"—only confirmed her view that she had found a special caregiver (Diary, April 19).

By the end of March S. had come to link her changing understandings of her life and body directly to her view of Dr. D. as compassionate and capable. That is, she *allowed* him to invade her mind and alter her views of her life and future precisely because she considered him a deeply caring and knowledgeable person. If he knows so much, means to do well, and cares so much about his patients, she reasoned, he could not possibly make a mistake or do me any harm. It was this kind of logic, which S. formulated very explicitly, that made her willing to trust him, to subordinate her own concerns about the new symptoms, and to put her faith and future in his hands:

> Really wish I could tape these amazing conversations. So bizarre to have someone—a total stranger—come into your life so suddenly and then re-arrange everything you had ever thought or planned for yourself. I mean, so bizarre. But this is a fine person, one who is compassionate and caring and capable in the extreme, or so it seems. (Diary, March 27)

In early April, a friend began to stoke doubts in S's mind about whether her doctor was doing the right thing in her case. (S's husband was not especially interested in the details of her treatments, so she discussed them with close friends instead. I explain why in the next chapter.) The new symptoms persisted, fueling her concerns. Such doubts might have led other patients to drop the doctor at that point. But S. was not willing to take that step. Although he had not yet fulfilled his major promises, by now he had made some other improvements in her life that were far from trivial. For example, he had advised her on what kind of shoes would be good for her arthritic toes and personally hand crafted metatarsal arch supports for her feet. Although her toes had been in poor shape for years, no other doctor had ever helped her in this way. (And such information is never published in patient self-help books, of which S. had read many.) Dr. D. had enabled her to walk again without discomfort, a benefit of immeasurable value. He also helped S. with her sleep problem. For many years S. had had trouble getting restful, restorative sleep. Dr. D. recognized the seriousness and entrenched nature of her sleep difficulties. Even if he had not fixed them, he was the first doctor to take seriously this major problem in her life. All these things weighed heavily in S.'s decision to stay in treatment.

In early April S. elaborated the "caring" discourse into a "good things" talk that elevated her doctor into a "rare and generous human being." In the following passage she lists all the "good things" the doctor has done for her:

> Have to remember the incredibly rare and good things he offers: First, he has taken seriously and named my sleep disorder, and is trying to amelio-rate the situation. For this I am eternally grateful; even if he does not succeed, he tried. Second, he is actually trying as hard as anyone humanly

could to find a way to reduce the inflammation from psoriatic arthritis . . . Third, his strategy of raising the baseline level of medication in order to avoid rounds of Prednisone . . . is really good: he is looking to the future, and the long-term future, not just the present and pain relief today. Fourth, because his approach is a massive chemical attack, it forces me, the patient, to go out and educate herself on these meds . . . Fifth, unlike any doctor I've ever gone to . . . [D.] has the patience to walk me through all the steps required to find a package of medications that will help treat my various ills. Since some of these ills are longstanding indeed and have gone undiagnosed and untreated, this is a gift of unmeasurable magnitude for which I will be eternally grateful. (Diary, April 6)

It was this idea that "he cares," developed into a larger understanding of "the good things he has given me," that helped assuage the patient's worries and tide her over the last crucial week before some solution to the sleep problem was finally found. Although to the reader S. may seem a bit too suggestible, a shade too grateful, any judgment of her reactions needs to take into account her long years of private suffering, the novelty of D.'s personal touch, and the hope he sparked in her heart.

Encouragements and Victory Proclamations: The Good Patient Is Finally Produced

At the end of the first week of April a minor miracle occurred: the sleep medications began to work. This change in S.'s bodily state cemented the transformation of the skeptical patient into a grateful one. S. had already been rhetorically seduced and pressured into compliance with her doctor's orders, but she continued to have an "attitude problem," refusing fully to trust his promises. After seeing the results on this most difficult front, however, her opinion of her doctor began to change. But the doctor did not leave S.'s full conversion into a good patient to chance. He was quick to jump on these promising developments, praising her new hopeful and trusting outlook. A few weeks later, when the arthritis medications began to work too, he declared victory over the arthritis and fibromyalgic tender points, presenting himself as a hero, a medical miracle worker who did everything he had set out to do, and more. It worked: by the time she left the West Coast in June, the cautiously skeptical patient had become an adoring one. To understand why, we need to appreciate the real improvements in her body, the rhetorics the doctor deployed, and the peculiar rheumatological discourse in which both of them were ensnared.

S. Begins to Sleep and Is Told Her Attitude Has Improved

After four weeks of torturous experimentation, in early April S. and her doctor found a combination of sleep medications that worked. On April 5, S. got her first good night's sleep. On April 7 she wrote: "For the first time in years and years and years, I have actually felt almost person-like; I can imagine what that might feel like." This change in sleep brightened her attitude toward her doctor, whom she credited with producing the sleep. Now it was not only a few "good things" he had given her, but the "gift of sleep"—a most valuable present indeed. Another was "the gift of optimism—striking how my general mood has improved since the day I began getting a decent night's sleep" (Diary, April 12).

This change in outlook was quickly picked up by Dr. D. Indulging in the rhetorics of patient benefit, he openly praised her new, more hopeful attitude:

> Re: my attitude, [Dr. D. says] it certainly has improved. Seems that a month ago when we started this process I had little hope that any improvement could be achieved, thought it couldn't. Said it was okay if the condition just didn't get worse. (Diary, April 7)

Just a few weeks earlier Dr. D. had complained that her bad attitude was partly responsible for the delay in bodily improvement. Finally her outlook had begun to brighten, and her doctor wanted to mark and encourage the progress.

Dr. D. Declares Victory and S. Becomes a Happy Patient

But sleep was just the first problem the doctor had set out to solve. After sleep there were still the inflammation of arthritis and the tender points of fibromyalgia. By the time of S.'s third visit to Dr. D., he was ready to mobilize the rhetorics of domination over nature and announce the first victory over those foes. Remember that the doctor, not the patient, was collecting the objective, quantified data that, according to the discourse of biomedicine, were required to assess whether and how much the patient's conditions had improved. In an appointment in mid-April, the doctor proudly proclaimed his first certifiable success in reducing the fibromyalgia and arthritis. He began by announcing the results of the most recent blood work: her sedimentation rate, a measure of inflammation, had dropped from fifty in mid-March to thirty-five in mid-April, tantalizingly close to the normal range of zero to twenty. The clinical examination produced more good news:

Doctor's visit today . . . Some good news for a change: two fewer tender points ([down] from 18 to 16); among the still-tender points are many that involve just "mild pain;" the number of "active [arthritic] joints," based on clinical examination, has fallen from 21 to 13: almost in half. That is quite extraordinary. (Diary, April 19)

Note how, although these were the doctor's rather than S.'s measures of her bodily state, and she had never felt the tender points or perceived them as a problem—except when her doctor pinched her—S. was very impressed by D.'s early success in treating her problems.

As we have seen, S. had begun to think of the improvements in her life as "gifts" the doctor had given her. She shared these ideas with the doctor during the April 19 appointment. Dr. D., pleased that his patient was coming around, told her that she looked "illuminated" that day. He praised her new attitude of acceptance, hinting that it was almost religiously inspired. Beaming, because both her body and her attitude had improved, S. left the doctor's office a very happy patient: "Doctor's visit today . . . Was very rewarding and made me feel good . . . Really hope I can talk to him again soon. He's a feelgood doctor" (Diary, April 19).

This same dynamic—in which Dr. D., based on his objective measures of her well-being, tells S. that she is better and S. then begins to feel better—played itself out at the next two appointments:

Fourth doctor visit. Seems there has been "global improvement," though, if you had asked me, I would say things are pretty much the same. My wrists are both acting up and my neck has been quite painful, some days all day long. This despite the fact that I have been really favoring my neck by not swimming . . . Anyway, the doctor was very happy about things, so I am happy too.

Number of inflamed joints has fallen from 13 to 5. Dactilitis [another one of those scientific terms] has dropped from 4 to 2. Basically, I felt little pain from the toe joints he was pinching; actually there was a little pain, but it was slight. The psoriasis [psoriatic arthritis] is much better too.

Funny how, because the doctor thinks I'm doing so well, I feel that way too. I didn't think I was doing particularly well until he suggested so. Said that, objectively, I'm doing really well. And, according to his perception, I'm doing well subjectively too. Maybe so; I think that seeing him makes me light-hearted and happy, so I'm probably acting happier on days I see him than others. Basically, he's right, though. Today I got an inkling of what it might feel like to actually feel pain-free, like a "normal," healthy person. It felt so, well, amazingly wonderful. (Diary, May 17)

Note how, in this passage, S. was initially skeptical, for her impression of her physical state was the opposite of her doctor's. Although she was not fully convinced that she had experienced global improvement, she was susceptible to her doctor's judgments: "Funny how, because the doctor thinks I'm doing so well, I feel that way too." And because the doctor said she was doing beautifully on a subjective level as well, her emotional state perked up too. Just to make sure that she felt better, he injected the three joints that remained painful with corticosteroids, which almost always do the trick.

At the last appointment before S.'s departure for the East Coast, the doctor reported that her sedimentation rate had fallen to thirty, just ten points above normal. The physical exam also yielded pleasant surprises: "Mostly good news: number of inflamed joints has fallen from 22 to 13 to 3. Tender points have decreased [from 18] to 6 . . . " (Diary, June 14). At that appointment the doctor reinjected one of the joints that had not responded the first time. This injection took, leaving S. in a state of near-perfect health, at least by her doctor's measures. This dramatic improvement in the second of her two initial medical problems turned the cautiously trusting patient into a worshipful one. Her faith in Dr. D. was so great that she would not dream of seeing another doctor, even when she was on the other side of the country for five months.

A Distorting Discourse That Counts Some Symptoms but Not Others

S.'s sky-high belief in her doctor's skills reflected the actual improvement in her physical conditions as well as her doctor's rhetorical enhancement of those improvements. Yet the impression of dramatic recovery also depended on a rather peculiar discourse that counted some things but not others. This is the same discourse of rheumatological medicine that we encountered in the initial consultation, only by now it had been materialized on the patient body. Three components of this rheumatological discourse worked to distort S.'s perceptions of the changes in her body.

First, the doctor had "objective" measures of the condition of S.'s joints, but he had no good gauge of her second problem, the amount and quality of sleep she was getting. For this the doctor had to rely on the patient's reports, which were by definition "subjective." Because there was no scientific measure of sleep, this aspect of the patient's health did not count in the overall assessment of how she was doing. As we have seen, in this domain the improvement was real but inconsistent; even after the sleep medications began to work, S. slept very poorly one night out of three. The notion that the doctor had done everything he had set out to do and more depended on leaving sleep out of the picture.

Second, the view that the doctor had made the tender points of fibromyalgia vanish rested on a most peculiar discourse according to which something the patient does not perceive on her own is turned into a real, nameable bodily symptom ("this is the 'pain all over' you feel," he told her), when a doctor's pinching produces sensations of pain. This discourse enables the doctor first to manufacture the symptoms and then to eliminate them, all with only the most minimal of patient participation.

Third and finally, the notion that the doctor had produced dramatic improvement also depended on ignoring all the new symptoms that emerged after treatment began. These new symptoms—headache, fogginess, upper-back and neck pain—were not what the doctor had set out to fix; they belonged to a different category of bodily phenomena. These costs of the improvements that counted were steep, but they simply carried no weight in the evaluation of how the patient was doing.

Like her doctor, S. was trapped in this distorting mode of understanding. Her bodily improvements were real, but the discourse, rhetorically amplified by the doctor, created some improvements where to her there were none and discounted some new symptoms and hard-to-measure old ones that to her were only too real. In effect, these rheumatological understandings enabled her doctor to claim credit for the positive changes that "counted," while the patient had to assume responsibility for the symptoms that remained. During the spring months S. came to accept this discourse as a good representation of her bodily reality: the rhetorics of biomedical infallibility had done their work. She accorded her doctor credit for the improvements he had made, while forgiving him for progress that was only partial and taking all the other symptoms upon herself as the "price" *she* had to pay for the gains *he* had made. That is why S. believed that her doctor was a genius when the evidence from her body was mixed at best.

In this chapter we have seen how S. was transformed from a skeptical and subversive patient into a model patient, the kind who makes physicians feel that their efforts are not in vain. I have highlighted the central role of physician rhetorics in this process, showing how the doctor actively created a good patient through the use of verbal tactics that began with soft enticements but, when it became necessary, turned to hard-edged accusations and threats. At the beginning of the chapter I suggested that the patient's cultural training in gender made her especially vulnerable to the rhetorical appeals of biomedicine. In the next part of the book I expand on this theme, showing how gendered expectations and behaviors colored everything that transpired in the medical encounter. Although biomedicine is a powerful apparatus of cognitive and social control, it alone could not have done the damage that was to be done to the patient's body and mind. It was the combination of biomedicine and gender that was so deadly.

Part Three | Doing Gender

CHAPTER 4   A Most Pleasant Patient

A fundamental issue in S.'s relationship with her doctor was that of power: Who would define her conditions and decide how they would be treated? In this contest the doctor enjoyed decided cognitive advantage. As we have seen, the discourses of biomedicine had severed the patient's mind from her body and defined the doctor as the expert on her body. The doctor was also advantaged institutionally: the interaction took place on his turf, he controlled the relevant scientific knowledge, and he possessed the formal qualifications required to order diagnostic tests and treatment protocols. Moreover, his personal power as a representative of institutionalized medicine was buttressed by the cultural authority of science and scientific medicine in American society at large. Given this imbalance of power in the biomedical relationship, the operational question was not so much who would control the process—obviously, the doctor would—as it was how much room there would be for the patient to resist aspects of the process she did not like and to insert her own understandings into the doctor-defined process.

S. was caught in the classic patient bind: she had the bodily conditions that her doctor was an expert in treating. How could she gain more control over the medical process when she was dependent on his medical expertise to help her with some real (and some not-so-real) physical problems? She wanted and needed his medical help but actively disliked the prospect of having to turn control of her body and important parts of her life over to a doctor. And this doctor was a particularly controlling one: he had offered a package deal in which the patient was to accept three to six months of "aggressive treatment"—including massive pharmacological intervention, considerable discomfort and danger, and intrusions into many aspects of her life—and in exchange he promised to produce real bodily improvement while doing no harm in the long run.

The hierarchy of science was overlaid with the hierarchy of gender, further narrowing the modes of resistance available to S. Research on women's psychology has shown how, in a society in which achievement in the public domain has long been a male prerogative, the fundamental self of many women is relational, based on intimate relations with others, especially men.[1] This is especially so for mainstream—that is, white, middle-class, heterosexual—women, a category to which S. belonged. This research suggests that, in a society that does not want to hear what girls have to say, in adolescence many girls pick up the discourses of "femininity" that teach them to form pleasant exterior selves while silencing inner voices that are critical or angry, attitudes considered unappealing in girls.[2] Socialized to adapt their social selves to others' needs and to cultivate an "ethic of care" in which they care for others' well-being more than for their own, these girls may become deeply confused about where their self leaves off and the selves of others begin. The blurring of boundaries reduces their ability to recognize abuse and leaves them at psychological risk of depression when they discover that they have no self.[3] Although this line of research has not been extended to the psychology of patienthood, we will see that these are the very psychosocial dynamics that unfolded in S.'s relationship with her doctor. Yet S.'s case is more complicated, for in her the psychodynamics of *femininity* were overlaid by the psychodynamics of *feminism*.

S. had a complex and contradictory gender identity that merged an iconoclastic feminist self that she had fashioned in college with a more compliant feminine self that had been created for her during childhood and adolescence. Coming of age in the late 1960s and early 1970s, she was swept up in the promise of the women's movement, with its discourses of opportunity, justice, and equality between the genders. The foundational text of the women's health movement, *Our Bodies, Ourselves* became her personal Bible on matters of sexuality and the body, both central to identity construction in her baby-boom generation.[4] Inspired by the autobiography of French feminist Simone de Beauvoir, during her junior and senior years at Wellesley College she decided to decline the conventional role of mother and to construct a different life based on work in the wider society.[5] In graduate school at Columbia University and then in a high-powered research job in New York City, she fashioned a gender identity based on feminist ideals. She married, but neither she nor her husband saw her as a "wife"; if anything, her unconventional marriage encouraged her self-image as an iconoclast who actively defied the rules of the social order. S.'s feminism gave her important skills and resources. It made her ever alert to the existence of gender and other forms of power, and it gave her potent tools with which to analyze their workings. It also emboldened her to "speak truth to power" on many occasions when most would keep quiet. But her ability to tap those skills was situation specific. In most domains of her personal and professional life, S. was able not only to poke fun at the inequalities of the world but also to challenge them. The medical domain was different. Underscoring the exceptionally intense authoritarianism of biomedicine, here S.'s stick-up-for-herself identity could not gain expression. As guides to action in medical settings, she often fell back on the rules of another gender identity, that of femininity.

Long before S. could create herself as feminist, she had already been created as female, imprinted with the cultural rules of gender subordination. While S. understood that her pleasantness was culturally constructed, at the time of the encounter with Dr. D. she did not yet see the contradictions between her femininity and her feminism. She did not yet understand how the cult of feminine pleasantness consigned her to silence the very self to which her feminism had sought to give voice. Trapped in the cultural routines her feminism opposed, she could not foresee how her lifelong gender training in pleasantness would become a liability, in the end wounding her psychologically and guaranteeing a failure of communication with her doctor that would impose further costs on her physical health. What was this femininity, and what did it teach her?

Growing up in a small New England town in the 1950s and 1960s, S. had a sterling training in femininity.[6] Her parents were white, well-educated, and solidly middle-class, placing them in that burgeoning postwar middle class that could not only aspire to, but readily achieve, the culture's ideals. Their goals for their five daughters were the 1950s goals for middle-class girls: college, marriage, and motherhood. The fourth of the five girls, S. got an early start in her education by closely observing her older sisters, from whom she learned the ingredients and the rewards of being a "good girl." Her understanding of being a good girl is neatly captured in the final stanzas of her fifth-grade poem, "What Teeth are Made For":[7]

> Teeth are made for good appearance,
>   Candy and cake make an interference.
> Visit your dentist every year twice,
>   Then you'll get a smile that's sweet and nice.

Of course, S. had a "bad-girl" side as well. But the good-girl side tended to predominate, because it was so richly rewarded. Unlike many academic women, who were "brainy" but not especially popular as adolescents, S. had been in the "in crowd" her whole young life. A résumé of her childhood and adolescent accomplishments would show not only good marks in school but also an outstanding record of success in the institutions of femininity. She had been a Brownie Scout, a curved bar–rank Girl Scout, a junior varsity and varsity cheerleader, a high school beauty-queen candidate, and a Kappa Kappa Gamma sorority girl during her freshman and sophomore years at Bucknell University, where she spent two years before transferring to Wellesley. And she always had boyfriends—lots of them. S. had played by the rules and won again and again. What were those rules?

The rules of gender that S. had internalized and lived by can be boiled down to six fundamentals. These codes of male-female behavior applied not to all relationships with men, but to a small number of relationships that were intimate, sexually or otherwise, and of relatively long duration. The fundamentals are these: (1) Men have power. (2) A woman's happiness and well-being depend on her ability to form intimate relationships with men. (3) The way for a woman to create and maintain these all-important relationships is to make herself pleasing and pleasant. (4) Open conflict and disagreement threaten a relationship and must be avoided at all costs. (5) When the woman's views or goals differ from those of the man, the woman must subordinate her opinions and objectives, silence herself, and publicly accept the man's authority. (6) Although a woman cannot challenge male authority openly, she can contest his decisions and pursue her goals indirectly by quietly working "behind the scenes," either on her own or in alliances with other women, manipulating him and/or the environment to promote her interests. Although such silent forms of resistance cannot be expected to unseat or even destabilize male authority, they make women feel they have "done something" to right the wrongs in their lives.

Twenty-five years after she had abandoned femininity for feminism (or so she thought), S. unconsciously applied this very same set of gender codes to her relationship with Dr. D. From the very beginning it was clear that this relationship fell into the category of intimate relationships with men, for by the end of the first appointment the doctor had made massive interventions in her life by redefining her bodily reality and outlining a program for deep intrusions into her body and her life. This new medical relationship was not only intimate, it was also threatening, for the doctor wanted to use dangerous drugs to bring her newly identified conditions under control. To S. the stakes appeared very, very high. They were high because she now "had" five chronic rheumatological illnesses, this doctor presented himself as uniquely capable of treating them, and his treatment program carried the risk of life-threatening side effects. Doubly silenced by biomedicine and gender, S. fought for her health and her life with the only weapons she had: sweet compliance and silent rebellion. Drawing on the gender codes she had been taught in childhood and used again and again throughout life, she hid her real thoughts (rule five) and put on a happy face of compliance (rule three), while working out her doubts and anger in the private spaces of her writing and friendships with other women (rule six). S. fought tooth and nail like a girl—and she lost. (She would win a victory of sorts in the long run, but that story comes much later.)

This chapter relates the gendered tactics that S. used in her attempts to guarantee a good medical outcome and to protect herself against harm. Chapter 5 sets out the silent resistances she waged, while chapter 6 charts the devastating psychological price she paid for challenging her doctor through indirection. This chapter begins with feminist maneuvers, which largely failed, moves on to feminine ploys, which mostly worked, and concludes with the costs of both. S. began defensively, deploying her feminism in ways she thought might make her doctor feel vaguely insecure. Her hope was to discourage him from falling back on sexist routines, which he was reputed to follow with other women patients. Although she succeeded in keeping flagrant sexism out of the examining room, her doctor foiled her attempts to leverage her social scientific knowledge about the body into some power, authority, or even voice in the deliberations on her care. When these feminist tactics failed, S. unconsciously fell back on the feminine routines she had learned as a girl. Working on the assumption that good medical care depended on a warm doctor-patient relationship, and that a warm relationship required making herself likable, S. set about making herself pleasing in every way she could. With her doctor as target, she staged an impressive patient-promotion campaign designed to seduce him into liking her through winsome dress, conversational charm, and the open expression of affect. S. succeeded in making her doctor like her, but her project of creating a lovable outer self hurt her inwardly. To appear so agreeable she had to silence her critical self, actively suppressing her worries about many of her doctor's practices. Though some of the whims and whimsies S. indulged in are quite funny and the stories she told herself quite fantastic, her efforts to get help in this way were ultimately tragic. Not only did they divert much-needed energy away from the task of fixing her body; they were also destined to fail. For by taking herself out of the relationship with her doctor, S. ensured that their communications would break down. And the costs of that breakdown, in terms of her physical and emotional health, would prove very high.

A Feminist Front

S.'s experience in New York had made her wary of male doctors and their often imperious ways of treating female patients. Her friend Anna had warned her that Dr. D. was a particularly controlling sort, micromanaging his patients' lives and haranguing them about things they could not control. With perhaps a touch of middle-class conceit—Anna had a working-class background—S. felt confident that she could work out a balance of power with Dr. D. that was less hierarchical than what Anna had described. Two aspects of the situation appeared promising. First, S. was considerably older than D. and thus, she figured, wiser about the ways of the world. Second, S. was an established professional person in her own right. She saw her doctor as a colleague, someone who, like her, was an expert in a particular field of knowledge. He had an M.D., she a Ph.D.: to her that made them equals. With these advantages of age and position, she believed, she could negotiate her way to power, or at least to a balance of power that gave her some say in her treatment. Her tool of choice was her feminism, which she had used to good effect many times before.

Feminism as Protective Armor: Keeping the Bully at Bay

To ensure that her doctor did not bully her the way he had bullied Anna, S. deployed her feminism as a protective armor to ward off overtly sexist treatment. Without consciously planning it in advance, in the first minutes of the initial consultation S. began working to "throw patriarchy off guard" by introducing her personal and professional life in frankly feminist terms. She described her unconventional family life—a bicoastal marriage, no children—as happy and satisfying, undoubtedly unnerving her doctor, who, she learned later, was a conservative family man. In telling him about her research on China's one-child-per-family population policy she framed her intellectual interests as "gender politics," elaborating with frightful stories of parents allowing their baby girls to die because they had wanted a son. This off-putting, subtly threatening phrase, "gender politics," was perhaps meant to keep such politics, at least male-dominated ones, out of the examining room. The feminist bravado must have made an impression, for S.'s description of herself came through in the typed report on the appointment that the doctor placed in her file. The first full paragraph of that report begins thus: "The patient is a 46-year-old married female, without children who works as an Associate Professor of Anthropology for the past 1 1/2 years at UCI. She spends her summers in New York from where she came, where she had worked as a specialist in Chinese affairs and gender politics and attended graduate school at Columbia University" (Dr. D. Report, March 8, 1996).

Throughout the spring months S. continued to deploy her feminism in small and large ways to destabilize conventional gender codes. Though far from a conscious strategy, these little ploys were meant to keep her doctor off guard, to make him feel vaguely insecure so that he would not fall back on comfortable sexist conventions. For example, S. refused to use makeup, knowing that this made him mildly uncomfortable. Perhaps to make sure that he got the point, she once joked about her "bare face." Because S. saw herself as her doctor's intellectual match, it irked her that she was expected to call him "Dr. D." while he called her by her first name. For a long time she refused to use that form of address, simply directing a question or comment to him without referring to him by any name.

These tactics seem to have worked to keep the bully out of the examining room. In contrast to the domineering manner Anna had described, and to the scornful ways in which he sometimes treated nurses and assistants, Dr. D. never once addressed S. in an intimidating manner. To the contrary, in his interactions with S. the doctor adopted a laid-back interpersonal style. He spoke self-confidently but softly and left conversational spaces in which S. could say at least some of what was on her mind. Although it is impossible to know how much influence S.'s flaunting of her feminism had on the doctor's interpersonal style, his relatively nonthreatening manner should probably be seen as a minor victory for her. If it was a victory, though, it was a Pyrrhic one, for it lulled S. into a false sense of security, a feeling that she was safe in this relationship with her doctor. A sense of vulnerability and preparedness against imminent danger would have been more helpful.

Feminism as Tool of Empowerment: The Failed Syllabus Initiative

S. also tried to use her feminism and professional accomplishments in more aggressive ways. The goals here were to challenge the objectifying discourses of biomedicine that had made her into a body without a mind and to gain cognitive authority for herself in the deliberations on her diagnosis and treatment. One tactic she adopted was to insert little reminders of her professional identity into conversations with her doctor. She did this because, after the initial get-acquainted conversation, the doctor never asked about her work, which occupied about 90 percent of her life. S. did not like being treated like a mindless body and felt that the biomedical discourse the doctor was using violated the reality of her life. Another bolder tactic was to define herself as an expert in a subject of interest to her doctor. Her hope here was that her specialized knowledge would become a source of power for her in the doctor-patient interaction. She tried this strategy once—in the syllabus incident described below—only to see it fall flat on its face.

One day in mid-May Dr. D. shared with S. his interest in "fat fibromyalgics" (Diary, May 17). He hoped some day to do research on women's body images and their relation to fibromyalgic disease. S. was thrilled to hear this, because her own research interests included the cultures of beauty and the body in contemporary American life. Issues of thinness and the diseases of femininity were very much part of this intellectual program. S. started thinking about how much fun it would be to do collaborative research with her doctor: she would bring her insights as an anthropologist and gender specialist, he his expertise on disease and the body, and together they would do cutting-edge anthropological-biomedical research on this issue. She had already come up with the perfect title for the grant proposal: "Fatness and Fibromyalgia: Body Image and Body Practice in the Etiology of a Rheumatological Condition."

Of course S. could not broach this possibility directly, for to her doctor she was just a patient, a rheumatological body to be treated, not a person with a mind, let alone intellectual interests equal to his own. The first step, then, was to show him that she was an expert in something of interest to him. So at the next appointment, S. brought her doctor a copy of the syllabus for her course, "The Woman and the Body," which dealt with body image and body politics in theoretically sophisticated ways. In making this rather bold move—after all, doctors are supposed to be the givers of information, patients the receivers—S. had two hidden agendas. First, she wanted to show him that there were sizable social science and humanities literatures on body image, a subject he had expressed interest in, and that she had mastered them. Should he so desire, she would be more than happy to introduce him to this work. Her second agenda was less innocent still. The syllabus had a strong feminist content. In asking her doctor to pay attention to it, she was testing him to see how he would react. S. had already decided that her doctor sorely needed an education in feminism. Even if he did not fully "get it," at the very least, she figured, a dose of feminist psychology and sociology would help him to understand his patients better and hopefully induce him to treat them more sympathetically. With these subversive thoughts in mind, S. waited for his reaction.

She had expected at least a politely enthusiastic response, with perhaps comments on how interesting the course sounded. At the next appointment, however, the doctor said nothing about the syllabus. How had he forgotten such an important matter, S. wondered to herself? S. screwed up her courage and asked him if he had "had a chance" to look at her syllabus. He said, yes, he had spent about ten minutes going over it. What was his reaction? After a long pause, he asked, "Why are the reading assignments so short?" And that was all he said. He had refused to say anything about the content of the course. The message could not be clearer: there is only one knowledge expert here, and it is the medical doctor. And an education in feminism? Not a chance! The doctor had cleverly deflected this move, once again defining his patient's knowledge as irrelevant and maintaining his own position as master of the doctor-patient relationship.

Feminine Seductions: Sweet Compliance

Although S.'s feminist moves had helped protect her against the insults of blatant sexism, none of them had succeeded in giving her power, authority, or even a voice in the negotiations over her medical care. Feminist measures failing to meet her needs, S. largely abandoned them and fell back on feminine tactics rooted in a feminine identity she had acquired in childhood. Unconsciously following gender routines internalized early in life, she construed the problem as one of relationship. Her basic assumption was that, if she could create an intimate and trusting relationship with her doctor, he would personally attend to her medical needs and protect her from harm. The first prerequisite for having such a relationship—personal attraction—was readily met. But that was just the beginning. If S. were to create the perfect relationship with her doctor, she must devote every effort to making herself likable. To S., likable meant pleasant. So she set about making herself pleasing in every domain of behavior she controlled—appearance, conversation, and sentimentality. Together these efforts added up to a multipronged patient-promotion campaign designed to win over her doctor and, in this way, guarantee delivery of good rheumatological care.

Fond Feelings

If S. wanted to build a close relationship with her doctor, she must have been attracted to him personally. And so she was. The chemistry between them was charged. But the attraction ran deeper than that. Although Dr. D. guarded the secrets of his life with great care, through the slow accumulation of tiny facts—he had shoulder-length hair in college, his medical bag was a "very 1970s" faded denim, he believed in patient advocacy—S. came to see her doctor as a soul mate who shared her 1960s and 1970s values of changing the world for the better. She saw in him a sweetness, an innocent idealism, and she was powerfully drawn to these qualities she sensed in him because she had not given up that idealism herself. She describes these complicated feelings of tenderness and bonding in an entry made in a computer file intended for her eyes alone:

> You know, there is something incredibly sweet, innocent, idealistic about this guy. There is a small vulnerable place, and I want so badly to move into it. I'm not sure exactly why. It's as though the world has not yet gotten to him, that he still believes he can do good in the world. I truly hope he continues to think this for a long, long time. I feel I need to reach out to people like that, to remember why I am doing what I am doing, to engage with them and do it together. Does this make any sense? (Transition file, May 20)

S.'s feelings about her doctor were so deep and personal that she consciously decided to stop telling anyone, even her husband, about their conversations, and to confine her reflections on the relationship to her writing:

> Keep thinking about my conversations with [D.], which are so special to me. Think I will keep them totally private . . . I'm seeing them as so special as to be something I do not even want to share with anyone. (Diary, April 27)

Thus it was that S. built a wall of silence around her relationship with her doctor, so that no one—not even her closest relatives—could see what was going on behind it. And the more intimate the relationship grew— that is, the more intense the feelings S. invested in it—the more reluctant she became to tell anyone about it.

Why S. would shift her emotional attentions from her husband of four-teen years to a doctor who was a complete stranger might baffle read-ers unfamiliar with the social dynamics of chronic illness. With chronic illness, family members live year after year with someone who routinely needs help with daily chores, often complains, sometimes gets moody, and generally can be something of a pill to live with. Over time close relatives of the chronically ill become emotionally drained and begin to tune out. This same dynamic had played itself out in S.'s relationship with her husband. Although he cared deeply about his wife's well-being, he tended to interpret new messages about her physical problems as "more of the same." His reaction to S.'s dramatic announcement at din-ner one night that she had a new chronic illness and had found a prom-ising physician to treat it was something like "Oh no, not this again." He had grown tired of hearing about new diagnoses and self-important specialists. After this conversation, S. felt that she could not get emo-tional support from her husband to deal with the trauma of the fibromyal-gia. And so she stopped talking to him about it. This left her husband totally in the dark. One morning, when they were having breakfast to-gether on the patio, S. became so upset about her worsening symptoms that she started sobbing uncontrollably. Her husband, at a loss to un-derstand what was happening, asked with great concern, "*What's wrong, dear?*" He simply had no idea how devastated she was. The only person in the world she felt she could go to for real help was her doctor. And Dr. D. was not only a rare specialist in her conditions, he seemed to per-sonally care about how she was doing. It was in this situation of social isolation, so common in chronic illness, that S. invested so much emo-tional energy in her doctor.

Sartorial Seductions

The most visible arena of S.'s patient-promotion campaign was that of appearance. On her trips to Seattle, she chose to dress herself not in the drab, shapeless attire of the female professor, but in fetching Barbie-doll outfits that showed off her girlish figure. In donning short, waist-nipping jackets and above-the-knee pleated skirts, all in bright but tasteful col-ors, S. constructed a little-girl image that not only pleased the male eye but also left the male ego intact. Although at the time she thought of her-self only as "looking good," in fact the wardrobe she displayed for her doctor sartorially infantilized her, inverting the age hierarchy to his ad-vantage and preserving the doctor's authority in the relationship. By showing off the patient's figure, the outfits also subtly sexualized her (the message was understated: no bare breasts or thighs here), presenting her as an object of desire in a context in which expressions of overt sexuality were totally taboo. Even as she asserted her feminism, then, S. played her femininity to the hilt, spinning a tangled and sticky web of contradictory meanings that must have left her doctor utterly confused. Her aim was to visually and, as we shall see shortly, conversationally and emotionally seduce him into liking her in hopes that, once trapped in her web, he would take extra-special care of her rheumatological needs.

One can only pity the poor doctor who thought he was playing the game of medicine when his patient had spiced things up by adding the game of gender. Judging from his own rather lackluster presentation of masculinity, and from his other patients, who were mostly older, overweight women who probably (though who knows?) had scant interest in either femininity or feminism, the doctor apparently had little experience in the sport of sexuality. Indeed, as if to test and then confirm her doctor's lack of sexual savvy, one day when she was lying on the examining table having her joints inspected, S. laughed out loud at the thought of being simultaneously an object and a subject of medical scrutiny. She said, teasingly, "You're going to regret ever taking me on as a patient." "Oh, no," the doctor replied earnestly, "I never regret any of my patients." From this S. concluded that her doctor was a pushover.

Conversational Compliance and Charm

The second element of S.'s patient-promotion campaign was conversational niceness, a term embracing both compliance and charm. S.'s interactional style was to be obliging to a fault. Not once did a hint of the anguish or anger one might expect from someone in so much pain creep into her voice. Previous chapters have documented how "nice" S. was even in the darkest days of the drug experiments. Here I bring some of these examples back into focus to suggest that they were not isolated instances, but part of a larger if unconscious project of conversational compliance aimed at winning her doctor's favor.

S.'s communicational compliances worked in different ways to endear her to the object of her affections. Some of her responses functioned to validate the doctor's ideas, making him feel smart and appreciated. For example, on hearing her doctor's microenvironmental theory of fibromyalgic pain, S. enthusiastically endorsed it, offering supporting evidence from her own life. Other conversational tactics worked to subordinate

S.'s concerns or perceptions to her doctor's, reinforcing the doctor-patient hierarchy. For instance, when the doctor's drug regimens did not work as hoped, S. always asked the doctor what to do next rather than offering her thoughts on what might be done. A third set of patient responses authorized the doctor's exercise of conversational power. For example, when the doctor complained that the patient was "forcing him" to alter the drug regimen too soon, rather than defending herself, S. accepted the criticism, telling herself that she was a "bad patient." A fourth type of interaction removed the threat of patient resistance by presenting the patient as unfailingly cooperative, uncomplaining, and non-threatening to the point of self-abnegation. The most striking example of this occurred when S. wanted to abandon the sleep medications. Instead of simply dropping the drugs, she announced in advance that she was contemplating "subversion," giving her doctor a chance to intervene to stop her before it was too late. In using such linguistic tactics S. sought to place herself in a class of special patients who could always be counted on to shore up the doctor's professional ego, preserve his authority and power, and never complain or challenge him, no matter what.

Had S. confined her conversation to acquiescences, she would have had to suffer a good number of dull conversations. To entertain herself and her doctor, and no doubt also to give herself an extra edge, she indulged her love of satire and spoof, seasoning their conversations with lessons, illustrations, and jokes from her own life. Once, wanting to explain to a rather incredulous doctor how gender worked in American culture, she found herself singing the Brownie Scout song to him: "I've got something in my pocket that belongs across my face . . . I'll take it out and put it on, it's a great big Brownie smile!" S. could describe the cult of female pleasantness and sing its anthems, but she could not see how it trapped her in its deceptions and indirections. Yet while S. remained caught in the cult of femininity, she was adept at making that culture serve her ends. From the small smiles on his face and the warmth in his voice, the doctor seemed charmed by her wit and her wiles.

Sincere Sweet Talk

A third element of S.'s bid for attention was the open expression of positive affect. While she kept much of her anger and distress to herself, when she was happy with her doctor's medical care she made a point of telling him so. This was not flattery but the expression of genuinely and deeply felt sentiment. The reader may perhaps think it warped that S. adored and idolized someone whose behavior was systematically snuffing out her life spirit. And warped it was. But the worshipful feelings followed a psychological logic: S. almost *had* to think she adored her doctor to justify letting him intrude so deeply in her life. She *had* to put him on a pedestal to justify letting him treat her as a lesser being, a body with no mind. Whatever the inner dynamics, on a conscious level the feelings were real and deep.

The most uninhibited expression of positive affect can be found in an extraordinary letter S. wrote to her doctor in mid-April. We have seen that, in early April, when the medicines started to work, S.'s spirits soared. So too did her approval rating of her doctor. She wanted to mark her inner progress and share her new feelings of gratitude with him. She tried to convey these feelings to him in an appointment on April 19, but it proved embarrassing to say these things face to face. And in the appointment, time constraints made it impossible for her to say everything she wanted to say, which was as much "I am in charge of my body" as "thank you for your help." She decided to put her thoughts and feelings into a letter, the vehicle she always used to say important things. Because the letter S. wrote was constructed with such care and because it conveys so well the complexities of her approach to and understandings of her relationship with her doctor, I include it here in its entirety. Just below in this section I will focus on the feelings imparted by the letter. Treatment of other elements of the communication is left for a later section.

20 April 1996

Dear Dr. [D.],

My words of gratitude, offered in some haste and not a little embarrassment yesterday, were too fleeting fully to convey the feelings I wanted to share with you. I thought it might be useful to put those words on paper to make them more real and permanent, and part of your no doubt ample collection of patient appreciations.

In the six weeks since I have been working with you, I have gone through many different phases of emotional engagement. After our first meeting I was extremely depressed that my list of conditions had quintupled, from the psoriatic arthritis I knew I had, to include the primary and secondary osteoarthritis, fibromyalgia, and scoliosis that I did not know I had. After a while I became angry that you had delivered a needlessly distressing diagnosis; after all, scoliosis and osteoarthritis are very common conditions, hardly requiring treatment, thus, I was thinking, not meriting mention. Why had this new doctor tried to make me feel so bad? As if the quintupling of conditions weren't enough, he offered a very poor prognosis: if untreated, in a mere five years I would likely "progress into serious deterioration."

I had always managed the psoriatic arthritis well, or so I thought, by trivializing it: I figured, my sisters had bad eyes, I just had bad skin and an uncooperative musculoskeletal system. Also, my older sister, who also has psoriatic arthritis, had miraculously gone into remission in her mid-30s; of course that will happen to me too, I rationalized, then put it out of mind.

Your "dismal diagnosis and poor prognosis," which I have dubbed DD&PP, forced me to rethink that dismissive portrayal of my bodily realities. In trying to deal with this blow to my identity and expectations for the future, I have talked to many friends and family members and read widely in areas such as stress management and natural healing.

The outcome is a new stage of engagement, one of great gratitude to you for giving me the gift of a DD&PP. Why is it a gift? First, because your medical managerial regime entails the application of serious drugs, it has forced me to educate myself about these medications and the diseases that would lead you to prescribe them. This knowledge has been wonderfully empowering, making me feel less dependent and more in control of my own bodily well-being. It has also made me take responsibility for my own health: after all, it is my body and my life that are involved here. I realize that I need to take my health care into my own hands to make sure that all resources available are drawn upon in managing my admittedly serious conditions.

Second, it provides me a welcome opportunity to make a number of major life changes I have been contemplating, yet always putting off, for years. These changes—in life goals, social connections, and many other areas—should contribute to a healthier, less stressed way of living that will, if not directly influence the course of the disease, at least provide a fertile emotional and whole-body climate in which the medications you prescribe do their work.

Finally, your gloomy medical forecast presents me with a challenge: to prove you wrong! Of course, it is not a fair contest, because I will have your medical assistance in proving you wrong. But I plan to go beyond the medicine and do some life work; hopefully my interventions will enhance the effects of your medicines.

The second gift I have been given is, well, you. In my fifteen years as a (reluctant) consumer of rheumatological medicine, I have never encountered a doctor who deeply cares about his patients as you evidently do. As early as our first meeting, despite the bad news you delivered, I became convinced that your aim is to make your patients better, rather than simply help them get by, the unstated but actual goal of all the other doctors I have seen. Some of the questions on your protocol gave you away as a caring doctor. It was not just that you asked questions many times more detailed (and numerous!) than those any other doctor has ever asked; it is also some of the specific questions you asked that revealed an unusual person inside the white coat. In particular, the question about hooking one's bra in the back suggested to me a rare respect for women's human dignity, to say nothing of an intimate knowledge of the lived microrealities of their lives. I also especially liked your comment about depression: you said you would not deal with that directly, but that depressed outlooks are often by-products of serious physical conditions, and that treating those conditions often helps alleviate the depression. That observation really rang true for me: over the last six years—exactly the time frame in which the arthritis has become serious—I have been intensely depressed, a sharp departure from the generally sunny outlook of my younger days.

I am, to put it simply, just thrilled to have you as a collaborator in working to improve my health. Please do not think that, in using the notion of collaboration, I harbor secret intentions of trying to usurp your medical authority. Far from it! It is precisely that authority, more specifically, all that clinical experience and biomedical knowledge, that I look forward to drawing on as time goes by. This special combination—of plentiful personal commitment, clinical experience, and biomedical knowledge—makes you a rare kind of doctor indeed.

I already have ample evidence of the potential benefits this blend of expertises and attitudes can offer: my ability to sleep, absent for twelve years, has returned. My ability to walk, in jeopardy for twelve months, has been restored. In the case of the sleep, it was your willingness to walk me through different combinations of drugs, and to deal with the unhappiness stemming from the mixes that did not work, that finally produced a success. You have already done more for me in a month than any other doctor has done in a decade.

As you struggle to resist the HMO-ization of American health care—an attitude for which I have profound respect—I hope you can take heart from, and find courage in, the feelings of deep gratitude patients like me have for you and your very special kind of medicine.

With the warmest best wishes,

S.

In this letter S. sought to draw her doctor closer to her by sharing with him the very private and intense feelings he had provoked in her. She begins by noting her own embarrassment about being so frank, making it "okay" for him to be embarrassed as well and clearing the way for greater openness about feelings in the future. Although S. was not able to express negative emotions toward her doctor when she felt them, she takes the opportunity now to describe the history of her depression and anger at him, highlighting how they had given way to the positive emotion of gratitude.

Writing straight from the heart and in astonishingly direct language, S. proceeds to tell her doctor exactly what she likes about his approach to her medical care. She appreciates his caring attitude; his plentiful commitment, experience, and knowledge; and the fundamental improvements he has made in her abilities to sleep and to walk. Note how she interprets his earlier question about hooking her bra in the back or front as evidence of "a rare respect for women's human dignity." Other patients—indeed, the doctor himself—might give it a less feminist cast. While we have noted the doctor's mastery of rhetoric, we should not leave this letter without observing that S. was not averse to the use of rhetorical flourish herself. She ends this paragraph with such a splash, writing: "You have already done more for me in a month than any other doctor has done in a decade." Rhetoric notwithstanding, the emotions expressed here are heartfelt. S. truly adored her doctor and wrote a patient "love letter" to tell him so.

It was so important to S. that the letter be taken in the spirit intended that she followed up on its reception very closely. Oddly, though, the doctor said nothing about it, not even a simple "Thanks for your letter." As days turned into weeks, S. grew worried that she had overstepped her bounds or been too personal in expressing her feelings of gratitude. In the following diary entry S. stews about whether she has committed a serious faux pas:

Wonder if he got my letter. If so, is it not strange that he did not mention it to me? Maybe it was embarrassing to him. Maybe at our next meeting I will ask him if he got it, and if he minds if I write letters once in a while. For me, if not for him, this is a pretty intense experience, invoking very powerful feelings. He of course has to protect himself against feeling those feelings, and he does so, appropriately, by drawing a sharp line between his professional and personal life. (Diary, April 27)

In an appointment with her doctor three weeks later, S. finally found an opening in which to inquire into these delicate matters. Here is her diary description of the conversation:

Had [a] chance to talk to doctor about . . . setting boundaries between what is personal and what is public or shared information. He had pointed out that it was important to maintain a doctor-patient relationship in the clinical room, to ensure that doctorly functions like injecting the patient['s fingers] can be effectively performed. (Guess it is hard to inject someone if you empathize with his/her feelings too much.) I wondered if this was an unintentional hint that I was overstepping those boundaries, or had somehow done so in the past. So I took the opportunity to inquire about that, focusing my question on the letter I had sent. I . . . said I had worried after I sent the letter that I might have overstepped some bounds, been too personal. He said, no, he appreciated everything I had said, especially the part about gratitude, and that it is rare for someone to express appreciation. So, I said, would he please let me know if in the future I overstepped that boundary, because I want him to feel safe with me. He promised he would let me know, and said he found the boundaries I had set totally fine, that I was an engaging person, and so on. So it seems my worries were not justified. That is totally cool. (Diary, May 17)

S.'s painfully candid "patient love letter" and the diary entries recording how closely she followed up on its aftermath lay bare the huge amounts of psychic energy she devoted to the work of nurturing and strategically managing that all-important doctor-patient relationship. Clearly, in her mind the essential task had little to do with monitoring her bodily treatment or outcomes. Rather, her job was to construct a relationship with her doctor based on feelings of mutual affection and trust. Her relational reasoning was that, if they truly liked and felt safe with each other, he would protect her from medical harm. Another element of that reasoning was that, if she could position herself as a special patient who stood out from the rest, she could ensure the delivery of extra-quality health care. This is why, when she picked up a pen to write to her doctor, she chose not to drop him a thank you card, but to craft an elaborate once-in-a-lifetime kind of letter that her doctor could never forget.

Her bid for attention and affection appears to have worked, for the doctor said that he "appreciated" her words of gratitude, that such expressions of praise are "rare," that the boundaries she set were "totally fine," and that she was an "engaging person." S. was immeasurably happy to learn that her derring-do had paid off: "So it seems my worries were not justified," she writes with evident relief. "That is totally cool."

Yet while the letter served S.'s relational ends, it is important to note the unbalanced character of the relationship she so painstakingly constructed. What is striking about the diary entries is the one-sided "ethic of care" they betray: S. is deeply solicitous of her doctor's comfort level in the relationship, but neglectful of her own comfort and safety. She asks the doctor to tell her if she ever "oversteps her bounds" because "I want him to feel safe with me." When the doctor injects some delicate joints, she worries about his sense of professional competence and how it might be eroded if she says anything that causes him to empathize with her pain. She even toys with the idea of asking the doctor's permission to write him letters because she wants to protect him from embarrassment! Evidently, S. is more concerned about her doctor's feeling of safety in the relationship than she is about her own sense of security or her ability to tell him what is in her heart. This dynamic would be almost amusing if its effects were not so damaging. For in slighting her own safety in the relationship, S. leaves herself exposed and vulnerable to any dangers that may be present in her doctor's approach to her care. In overlooking her own needs, she takes one party out of the relationship, guaranteeing a failure of communication. And in prioritizing the social relationship over the bodily treatment, she takes an indirect route to healing that rests on a host of relational assumptions that might not apply in the medical encounter.

Silencing the Critical Self

S. succeeded in creating a warm and intimate relationship with her doctor, but her project of fashioning a sweetly compliant outer self imposed inner costs. To make herself agreeable in every interaction she had to suppress her concerns about her doctor's more questionable practices. She had to silence her critical self, sometimes to the point of self-abnegation. S. stifled her worries not out of a desire to deceive her doctor but out of a deep-seated fear that if she allowed him to see her doubt and anger he would stop liking her and stop devoting special attention to her bodily needs. In her mind, good medical care was contingent on a close doctor-patient relationship, and a close relationship demanded the absence of open conflict. The only way she knew to eliminate conflict was to mute her own concerns. The ever-agreeable self she presented to her doctor was an inauthentic self, but S. was not aware of that at the time. The whole process of silencing the doubtful inner self and projecting a pleasant outer self—for these were two sides of the same coin—occurred unconsciously, as she enacted the routines of feminine acquiescence she had taken in at a tender age.

The pressure on S. to silence her inner self was particularly strong because it came not only from the rules of feminine docility but also from the codes of scientific medicine. The reader will remember how biomedicine severed the patient's mind from her body, making the doctor the sole expert on the body. The discourse of biomedicine the doctor was applying not only did not invite patient participation in the diagnosis, prognosis, and treatment, it also excluded that participation by definition. Subjected to two powerful silencing mechanisms, S. had no real choice but to keep her thoughts to herself.

The Energy Required to Suppress Inner Doubts

S. may have appeared passively compliant on the outside, but on the inside she was devoting massive amounts of energy, both cognitive and emotional, to suppressing actively her critical faculties. Throughout the spring she constantly had to quash her worries about everything from her doctor's qualifications to his definition of her problems and treatment of her ills. The first three chapters were brimful of examples. Here I review a few of the most important instances, adding detail to suggest how much effort was required to be inauthentic.

S. harbored on-again-off-again doubts about the diagnosis of fibromyalgia but believed her doctor would ridicule her and refuse to treat her if she rejected his diagnosis of his specialty disease. So she buried these concerns by convincing herself that the diagnosis was helpful in one way—it had named her "sleep disorder"—and that it was innocuous in any case. (How wrong she was about that!) S. thought the prognosis of "progression into serious deterioration" was a gross exaggeration of the probable curve of her illness. But she stilled her concerns about her doctor's intentions by reinterpreting the prognosis for him in more qualified and probabilistic terms. She was alarmed that he refused to pay attention when she said that preserving her cognitive functioning was of utmost importance. But she swallowed her worries, consoling herself with the thought that "at least I made my point." She did not believe the doctor's promises to make her drug and symptom free, but she contained her worries about his motivations by telling herself that a little hyperbole did not matter and that it had no bearing on his professional integrity. S.'s biggest fear was that she was losing control over her body and life to an utter stranger. But she stifled this fear too by telling herself that her doctor was an exceptionally knowing and caring person who was doing everything humanly possible to help her.

Mental Acrobatics behind the Conviction of Self-Control

The kinds of mental contortions through which S. put herself to rationalize away her worries about losing control are well illustrated by the April letter quoted above. The two greatest sources of her mental anguish had been the doctor's diagnosis of a second major rheumatological disorder and his prognosis of "progression into serious deterioration." Though mere words, they exerted tremendous power over her by redefining her life as one dominated by disability and disease. To get out from under their power while retaining her doctor's help, in the April letter S. reinterpreted the role of the diagnosis and prognosis in her treatment. No longer would they be labels he pinned onto her in a disempowering act; to the contrary, they would become tools of empowerment for her. How did she perform this mental somersault?

In her letter S. made herself the active agent of her care by accepting her doctor's "dismal diagnosis and poor prognosis"—which she irreverently dubbed a DD&PP—not as a true representation of her reality, but as a gift she decided to accept. It was a gift because it empowered her to take charge of her own health and life: it forced her to educate herself and take responsibility for her own health; it gave her an opportunity to make other long-put-off changes in her life; and it presented her with the challenge of proving her doctor wrong. To underscore the point, she announced boldly the type of doctor-patient relationship she planned to have: it would be one of collaboration in which she drew on the resources provided by her doctor to improve her health. While respecting his medical authority, she would take her health care into her own hands. And to make sure her brazen, take-charge proclamations did not injure his pride, she threw in a slew of compliments, discussed above, for good measure.

S. was tickled pink with her letter and the new formulations it had worked out. These understandings gave her ways to continue receiving her doctor's help while leaving her ultimately in charge of her body and life. As if in unconscious acknowledgment that a satisfactory relationship had finally been established, a week after she mailed it she "decided to start playing the patient role and calling him ['Dr. D.']" (Diary, May 2).

These convoluted formulations served S.'s cognitive needs well. As solutions to her real problem of loss of power to her doctor, however, they were sadly pathetic. S. thought she was in control, but her control was all in her head; it was fantasy rather than fact. The letter was an exercise in deluding the self, which only delayed her realization that her doctor's brand of medicine offered, at most, microempowerments, faux empowerments within a larger context of disempowerment by the discourses and practices of biomedicine.

S.'s project of securing her doctor's help by silencing her critical inner self and creating a falsely pleasant outer self is understandable in light of the codes of gender and biomedicine in our society. But it was also tragic, because it was destined to fail. By taking that angry self out of the doctor-patient relationship, S. virtually guaranteed that their communication about her body would go awry. And the costs of this failed communication—both physical and psychological—would be steep. Had she been able to present her critical self or to tell her doctor what she really thought, the medical relationship might have taken a different turn or ended much earlier, giving S. a chance to find a less controlling physician to help with her ills. S.'s project was also tragic because it involved such a huge dissipation of energy and imagination. Had her vigor and ingenuity been harnessed instead to the task of healing her physical self, S.'s bodily and emotional health might have improved instead of deteriorating at an alarming rate.

So far we have seen only the sweetly seductive side of the girl games S. was playing. But there was a roughly rebellious side as well. In the next chapter we look at the resistances and rebellions against medical authority that S. staged during the spring. What was unusual about these revolts was that they were all mounted in secret, so that her doctor never even knew they took place.

CHAPTER 5

Silent Rebellion and Rage

Although S. had made herself ever pleasant on the outside, on the inside she was filled with an unspeakable rage. She was angry because she desperately needed her doctor's help, but that help was delivered in a fundamentally violent way and she had to silence her concerns about that violence to receive it. Her anger about biomedicine was fed by a deeper anger about having a chronic illness that she had done nothing to deserve. Yet she could not share these feelings with her doctor, because she was deeply fearful that doing so would imperil the warm, trusting relationship on which she felt her care depended. So she fought the injustices of her world "like a girl": in private.

Twice silenced in the public space of the doctor-patient relationship, S. created private spaces in which her anger and rebelliousness could be expressed. The most important of these spaces were her writing and her friendships with other patients. By maintaining a diary and a daily chart, S. found ways to resist the discourses of objectification and quantification and to record the "subjective" truths of her life. In her friendships with other patients she found a safe space in which to air doubts, stage defiances, and nurse her rage. During the spring S.'s writing and friendships provided emotional sustenance and deepened her understanding of her plight. In the long run, these modes of resistance would provide crucial resources that enabled her to pull herself back from the brink of madness. Though lived in anguish and confusion, these months of nonspeaking supplied rich opportunities for the psychological and political growth that allowed her to find her voice in the end. In the short run, however, these silent resistances and rebellions hurt S.'s cause more than they helped it. For they were limited forms of resistance that precluded genuine communication between patient and doctor and left the doctor's practices intact. And the anger, finding no outlet, ate away at S.'s spirit, producing symptoms of psychological distress that will be traced in a later chapter.

Although S.'s silent mode of resistance followed codes of femininity learned in childhood—in particular, that open challenges to male authority are taboo—her feminist identity was not totally submerged. To the contrary, much of the *content* of the critiques S. and her friends developed was explicitly feminist, striking themes similar to those highlighted by the women's health movement in its early condemnations of the authoritarianism of male doctors.[1] Although one gender identity remained dominant, the two coexisted, jostling around inside S. in an uneasy tension.

This chapter takes us into those hiding places where S. waged her secret battles against biomedicine. In the first section we peer into her personal records and computer files, looking for resistances that never got waged. In the second section we eavesdrop on her conversations with friends, looking for rebellions that never got staged. While S.'s political options were constrained by her gender training, the reader should remember that her abilities to recognize and resist the dangers inherent in her doctor's brand of biomedicine were also compromised by the material realities of pain. In part because of her prior conditions, and in part because of the drug experiments the doctor was conducting on her body, throughout the spring her physical, emotional, and mental capacities were stretched almost beyond the limits of human endurance. These material realities of pain made it difficult for her to gain a larger perspective on her situation or to mount an effective resistance to her doctor's encroachments on her life.

Writing as Resistance

S. was silenced in the public space of the doctor-patient interaction, but there were other, more private spaces in which she could speak her thoughts and feelings. The most important of these spaces was her writing. From the day of the first appointment S. began keeping two records of her "adventure" with Dr. D., a medical diary and a daily chart. These records served diverse, sometimes contradictory ends. It was here, in the private space of her writing, that S. dared to articulate the tender feelings she had toward her doctor. It was here that she negotiated truces between the warring parts of herself, the part that hurt and achingly wanted his care and the part that sensed danger and urged wariness and caution.

Although the diary and chart had many embedded meanings, both served important oppositional functions. They were resistant modes of expression, because they recorded parts of S.'s bodily reality that she knew intuitively to be true but that had been excluded by her doctor's discourses as irrelevant to her care. Without being fully conscious of it,

S. felt deep down that her doctor's approach was too narrow, and she wrote her own history of her case to fill the gaps left by his. Through her writing, she challenged her doctor's discourses of objectification by restoring the wholeness he had shattered when he split her body from her mind and emotions and by recovering her own authority to know and to speak about her body. This authority had been denied when her doctor made himself the expert on her body. In her writing S. also defied her doctor's erasure of her bodily history. She recovered her own history by retaining the original computerized file of her health, simply adding new chapters to it to cover the experience with Dr. D.

That the diary and the chart were oppositional forms of expression is evident from the fact that S. had never maintained such meticulous records before. In the past S. had not felt the need to keep detailed accounts of her health care, because she had virtually complete trust in her doctors. Although she wanted badly to believe in Dr. D., in her heart of hearts she never fully trusted him, because his drug-intensive approach was self-evidently dangerous and his safeguards were not fail-safe. S. also sensed in Dr. D. a subtle element of compulsion—you do what I say because I am the expert—that she had never sensed in a medical relationship before. In keeping these private records S. sought to protect herself from harm by documenting everything that happened. It was as though, through the sheer accumulation of mind-numbing detail, she could somehow save herself should something ever go wrong.

The Diary

For several years S. had been keeping a medical diary to chart the ups and downs of various joints and the changing regimens of medication applied to control the pain and swelling in them. The entries were spare, because the point of the exercise was simply to record information that might be medically useful in the future. A typical entry might read: second finger of right hand swollen, Methotrexate increased to five pills a week. There was no thought of recording her feelings about her conditions, their treatment, or anything else.

That changed when S. began to see Dr. D. The first and most obvious change was a lengthening of the typical entry: it took S. two and a half single-spaced pages to record all the diagnoses and treatments he outlined at the initial consultation alone. In the first three months the diary grew to almost twenty-five pages; by mid-November, when her relationship with Dr. D. came to an end, the diary had expanded to fifty single-spaced pages.

The content of the diary entries also changed. Sensing that the doctor would massively alter her life—remember, the first entry began, "I think my life will never be the same"—S. started to record in great detail everything of consequence that transpired between them. She did this because she was a compulsive recorder of the facts of her life and because the experience provoked intense feelings of hope and fear that she could contain only by writing them down. New meanings were added to the diary as time went by. When S.'s emotions began to include shock and despair as well as hope and fear, she used the diary to untangle those complicated and contradictory feelings. When the relationship with her doctor needed to be worked on, she used the diary to plot strategy. When S. became confused by paradoxical developments in her bodily state, she used the diary to clarify her understandings of what was going wrong. When the side effects of the drugs (or the "symptoms of fibromyalgia," as her doctor called them) grew harrowing, she wrote that down too. Without intending to, S. produced a record of everything that went wrong and all the things her doctor—and she herself—did to produce those troubling outcomes.

The Chart

On the day of her first appointment with Dr. D., S. also started to keep a daily chart of her bodily conditions. Although she had created mini-charts of selected aspects of her health before, this is the first time S. had maintained a comprehensive chart on her well-being. The "S.G. Well-Being Chart"—an ironic name, given what was to happen—would also have a much longer life span than that enjoyed by any of the special-purpose charts of the past.

Initially S. created a rough "drug chart" to keep track of the medications she was taking, as well as their effects, side effects, and interactions. She was worried about the drug experiments the doctor planned to put her through and concerned that he could not monitor the drugs' effects as well as she herself could. A few weeks into treatment S. revamped the chart to provide spaces for many more items. Her doctor displayed great interest in his drugs and their effectiveness, but he had announced that other aspects of her physical well-being that were important to S. had no place in his medical regimen. So S. decided to maintain her own records of the things that counted to *her*. She reformatted the chart, typed it up on her computer, and printed out multiple copies so that the records could be maintained into the indefinite future.

Reproduced in figure 1, the chart provides spaces for recording a large

Date:
Page:

	Monday	Tuesday	Wednesday	Thursday	Friday	Saturday	Sunday
Meds (night before)							
Meds (same day)							
Other Factors Affecting W-B							
Sleep Timing and Pattern (night before)							
How Feel (drugged, other side-effects)							
How Function (0–5)							
Pain-Free Index: Specific pain (0–5)							
General Pain (0–5)							
Exercise							
Mood (0–5)							

Figure 1. S.G. Well-Being Chart

amount of information on health and health care. The horizontal layout makes it easy to see changes that occur from day to day during a given week. Weeks can be aggregated into months and months into seasons, so that the whole course of disease and its treatment can be charted over long periods of time. Without thinking of it this way at the time—she was just "doing what comes naturally"—S. was using science both to assist her doctor's science and to challenge it.

The specific items included in the chart reflect both the doctor's narrow yet "objective" views about the proper focus of medical attention (arthritis and fibromyalgia) and the things impacting it (the drugs) as well as S.'s larger "subjective" views of the forces underlying her health and the dimensions of her health and well-being worth noting. These items, listed in the left-hand column, merit close scrutiny.

The first three items cover inputs into health: sleep medications, "other meds" (those for arthritis and pain relief), and "other factors affecting well-being." "Other factors" was a category S. employed to cover any unusual activities, stressful circumstances, or interpersonal developments that might affect how she felt.

The next five items deal with the effects of these factors on S.'s physical health and mental capacities. These include four items measuring bodily well-being: the timing and pattern (or quality) of her sleep; side effects from the medications; "specific pain" associated with the arthritis; and "general pain" associated with the fibromyalgia. The category of general pain included headaches as well as muscle pain in her neck and upper back, both symptoms associated with fibromyalgia. S.'s inclusion of this item—which she later relabeled "neck, back, headache" and even later relabeled "fibromyalgia"—signals her growing conviction that she had the condition. The fifth item, "ability to function," S. included to assess how well and for how long she was able to perform her research, writing, teaching, and other professional activities. The doctor expressed interest in the four bodily measures but he never once asked S. about her professional work. Yet her ability to work was of paramount concern to S. herself.

The last two items on the chart are elements of S.'s well-being that she considered critically important but that her doctor evidently did not, since he virtually never inquired about them. One of these was aerobic exercise, something that had been a central component of S.'s life and sense of well-being since childhood. The doctor asked about swimming, her favorite form of exercise, only after she had brought it up and then only to proscribe it. The other was "mood." In including this item, S. wanted a place to note whether she was feeling depressed and pessimistic, which was only too common at the time she created the chart, or happy and optimistic, a state she wanted keenly to recover. Mood was important not only in its own right but also because depression seemed to have an independent and deleterious effect on her physical well-being. To chart changes in her emotional state over time, S. needed to describe her mood not only in words but also as numbers, which could be manipulated to obtain averages and trends. For this purpose she developed a scale that allowed her to rank her outlook on any given day from 0 to 5, with 0 meaning something like clinical-level depression, 3 indicating neither happiness nor sadness, and 5 signaling elation, feeling on top of the world.

The chart construction carried political significance of which S. was only partly aware at the time. As we saw in chapter 1, S.'s doctor had reduced her bodily reality to a set of "objective" numbers, which he recorded privately in her file and used to determine how and how fast her health was improving. (In Dr. D.'s accounting system S.'s health only improved; it never got worse.) Without particularly thinking of it this way, in creating her own chart S. was giving the "subjective" parts of her life—especially her mental capacities, exercise, and emotions—equal weight, at least in her own accounting scheme, by turning them into numbers as well. S. was fighting her doctor's numbers with her own; she was using quantification to resist quantification.

No sooner had she created it than the chart became an active participant in the medical process. From the beginning S. drew on it regularly in reporting to her doctor the effects and side effects of the drugs. In no time at all, the discourse of the chart—what it said about how she felt—became an important part of S.'s reality. That is, how she felt according to the chart became crucial in how she really felt. For example, including an item for fibromyalgia made S.'s "fibromyalgia" all the more real to her by keeping her focused on aches and pains that she might otherwise have brushed aside as unworthy of note. The daily ritual of filling in the form made the symptoms cluster in her mind, gradually solidifying her belief that she had the disease her doctor said she had. And the more she believed she had fibromyalgia, the more she suffered from its physical symptoms. Ironically, in using her chart to track her "fibromyalgia," S. succeeded in enhancing her doctor's power over her life. Clearly, the chart could work to support, as well as oppose, biomedical power.

Later in the spring, after the doctor had introduced his microenvironmental hypothesis of S.'s new symptoms, the charts became the basis for S.'s research into the activities in her life that were exacerbating her pain. Although the doctor maintained firm control in the public space of the doctor-patient relationship, because they reflected her own reality and priorities, these charts allowed S. to retain some control over her life and treatment throughout the spring and summer. In the fall the charts would enable S. to reclaim control over her life. By providing quantified evidence of how much her physical and mental health had declined, the charts literally saved her life. But here we are getting ahead of ourselves.

Friendships as Spaces for (Silent) Rebellion

A second space in which S. felt free to air her doubts and anger was provided by relationships with her sisters and a few close women friends.

Unfortunately, most of these confidants lived thousands of miles away in places as remote from southern California as Georgia and Maine. But through telephone and e-mail conversations, S.'s sisters and friends were able to provide enough emotional sustenance to keep her from drowning in a sea of despair.

For discussion of critical medical matters, however, S. turned to her friendships with fellow patients, who shared her experiences of disease, depression, and disempowerment. For years S. had actively sought out others who suffered from similar rheumatological conditions. After S. began seeing Dr. D., two of these friendships—with Dana and Anna—became crucial sources of life support for her. Through phone conversations, e-mail messages, and occasional in-person visits, S. and her friends created a positive, nurturing environment in which together they could name their doubts, scope out their doctors' faults, and invent alternative treatment strategies that went beyond the narrow scientistic techniques of their medical practitioners.

This second form of silent rebellion against medical manipulation had both its strengths and its limitations. By providing a safe space for airing big doubts and trying out little defiances, these friendships contributed significantly to S.'s understanding of her plight. Yet the anger that these conversations sparked did not spill over into the public space of the doctor-patient relationship. Silenced by the codes of science and gender, S. took her anger only to the point of "mind rehearsals," in which she told herself again and again that her doctor's treatment of her case needed to be challenged.[2] Yet so fearful was she of jeopardizing that all-important relationship that she never dared to bring those challenges out into the open. S. was left with a silent, inexpressible rage, while her doctor, not knowing what was going on in these private spaces of her life, continued to manage her case in the way he had determined was correct. He thought she was happy with his care—indeed, had she not said so in every imaginable way?—when she was seething with a rage that she could hardly admit to herself.

Big Doubts

In early April S. spent an intense afternoon with Dana, a friend who had a full-blown case of fibromyalgia, with all of the characteristic symptoms. Comparing notes, they realized that S.'s doctor was full of hot air: S. could not "have fibromyalgia," since she did not have "pain all over," the main symptom of the disease. His diagnosis was simply wrong. Moreover, they decided, the prognosis that had caused S. such anguish was overblown at best, since no one can predict the future.

S. grew angry at her doctor. Why had he said these things of such dubious truth? She and Dana began to speculate on the sinister motives that might have led him to exaggerate the truth and cause her so much psychic pain. They came up with two: to increase her feelings of dependence on him, and thus keep her in treatment, and to justify his use of dangerous drugs. Here is S.'s account of that conversation:

> Had such an amazing talk with [Dana] . . . [I] . . . realize[d] that this doctor doesn't know what he is talking about when he says my conditions are progressive. Doctors don't know anything [for certain about individual patients]; at most, they know statistical averages, they can *never* say what will happen in an individual case. What he *should* have said is that, based on the last six years, it *looks* like the psoriatic arthritis is progressive. There is no telling what it will be like in the next six years.
>
> I really don't know what basis he has for saying he anticipates "serious deterioration" in five years if I don't do anything now. I really doubt that. So what business does he have telling me things are so bad? I really think it is a deliberate strategy of his to make his patients feel bad—worse than they are, if they're not too badly off—so they will feel dependent on him. He says they go through "catharsis." But that is crap. What I have gone through is three weeks of horrible depression. That is not catharsis. And since one's mental state is a major factor in how the condition does, I would say he has made me worse, not better. That needs to be talked about.
>
> [Dana] is also extremely skeptical about the "diagnosis" of fibromyalgia. *She* has fibromyalgia, and seriously. She is in constant pain . . . [and] cannot even wear a light jacket, it feels so heavy and painful on her shoulders. God. I don't even feel any pain . . . So why is he telling me I have fibromyalgia? Maybe a very mild case, one that causes passive rather than active pain. And I know for sure I have a sleep disorder. But I feel like he's trying to make it out as worse than it really is. *Why?* Why make me feel worse than I am??? To justify putting me on such strong medicine? (Diary, April 3)

We have already met another friend, Anna, who was also a patient of Dr. D. Like S., Anna lived in Southern California, and flew up to Seattle every other month to see him. In talking to Anna, S. discovered that she was not alone in feeling disempowered by D.'s style of practicing medicine. Here is S.'s record of that conversation:

> Saw Anna again yesterday. She talked of nothing but her weight problem and how [Dr. D.] is constantly badgering her about it and how awful she feels that she cannot, just cannot, overcome it. He needs to use positive

reinforcement. Anna says she cries after every time she sees him! That is just terrible. He needs to learn—and use—some feminist psychology. Making his patients feel bad is not helping them get better . . .

Anna had two very good explanations for why he gives his patients such dismal diagnoses: "reality check" for the patients, and "ego enhancement" for the doctor. (If the patient gets better, the doctor can claim credit, if she does not, it is not his fault, the disease is too entrenched to be manageable.)

Many of his patients complain of his micro-managing their lives. Anna tells the story of his strongly insisting that she stay on Methotrexate, even though the side effects on her stomach were just horrible—constant pain, upset, and so on. She is caught between a gastroenterologist . . . and the rheumatologist . . . She feels very disempowered by this; we need to change that.

[O]ne time [D.] shared with Anna a hypothesis about why women in "powerful positions in business" stay heavy—to . . . protect themselves from men . . . Anna and I think this is basically wrongheaded: the pressure to be thin is so strong in our culture that virtually all women would give anything to be thin. (Diary, April 12)

Putting their experiences together, Anna and S. concluded that not only was Dr. D. no feminist; his youth notwithstanding, he was nothing but an old-fashioned sexist. Here, then, was a third reason for his needlessly dismal diagnosis and prognosis: he was a perpetrator of a sexist system of scientific medicine in which male doctors take advantage of women's socialization into habits of dependence and obedience to place them in subordinate positions in a hierarchy in which male physicians hold power. Here is how Anna and S. formulated the matter:

Weird how this doc is so old-fashioned about doctor-patient relationships: he insists on embodying the authoritarian model, when today many doctors are following "partnership" models in their relations with patients. Why? What generation does he belong to, anyway? Can he do this because the vast majority of his patients are women with chronic diseases who feel lousy about themselves? (Diary, April 12)

Small Defiances

These friendships also provided space for the active defiance of medical authority. In early June, after a particularly harrowing day, S. sent a distress e-mail to Dana, asking for her thoughts about how to cope with new limitations the doctor had placed on her life. Dana called her the next day, and they talked for two hours.

Knowing how well S. had managed her conditions before she had started seeing Dr. D., Dana expressed strong skepticism about whether this new doctor was handling her case correctly. Dana, who had two years of experience with biomedicine's approach to fibromyalgia, was a master at stoking doubt and dissent. She asked probing questions that challenged D.'s overall management of S.'s case. Dana's queries also encouraged S. to disobey some of her doctor's orders and to try new strategies that lay outside the domain of conventional medicine. S. was easily convinced, because Dana's perceptions matched her own:

> [Dana] asked how it was that I am now feeling so much fibromyalgic pain when I have been doing so well for so many years? What has happened in the last few months? I was doing so well with the swimming—why, [Dana wondered,] did I stop??? These are very good questions. I have begun to suspect that this neck-roll pillow [the doctor badgered me to use] is actually *giving me neck pain!* I've had neck pain for several days in a row, for no obvious reason. Last night I used the pillow upside down and, voilà, no neck pain. What a finding! (Diary, June 1)

Dana also questioned some of the doctor's medications, pointing out that Tylenol with codeine, which D. kept prescribing for S.'s pain, did nothing for her. S. had already begun to suspect the same thing. The next day she reduced the dosage from twelve tablets to none—and felt no pain at all (Diary, June 1). Dana also urged her friend to defy her doctor's interdiction on swimming. S. needed little encouragement on that front:

> [S]he urged me to get exercise, regardless of what the doctor says. She has a number of friends with fibromyalgia who feel so much better when they exercise, even when they have active pain. And I have little active pain (except the neck). So today I went swimming again—it was so lovely. I used the mask and snorkel and did just eight double laps. So far I feel nothing untoward, though I did have to take a half-hour rest immediately afterward. (Diary, June 1)

Finally, Dana urged S. to go beyond conventional treatment and try alternative means of pain reduction, such as massage and meditation, which the patient herself controls.

Inexpressible Rage

Emboldened by these talks with her friends, S. determined to turn her anger into action. But deeply fearful of unsettling or, worse yet, destroying that carefully crafted relationship, she did not dare to openly challenge her doctor. Using her diary to build up courage, she resolved again and again to confront her doctor. Indeed, the passages just quoted contain several examples of such resolutions. Realizing that the doctor has made her worse rather than better, S. wrote with determination: "That needs to be talked about" (Diary, April 3). Seeing Anna caught between two doctors with opposing agendas, S. wrote bravely, "we need to change that" (Diary, April 12). Again and again she mentally rehearsed how she would challenge her doctor:

> The point is, to use this guy for the good things he offers . . . But I will have to negotiate a new relationship that makes me less of a dependent. (Diary, April 3)

> At my next appointment I really want to challenge this doctor for giving me so many meaningless diagnoses and seemingly deliberately trying to provoke an emotional reaction of depression. Also, the idea that this stuff is progressive—it only *looks* that way, no evidence can scientifically say that it is. (Diary, April 6)

But no matter how many times she rehearsed how she would rise up and confront her doctor, S. could never bring herself to do it. The boldest action she was able to take was resolving to prove her doctor's prediction wrong by doing everything in her power to get better within his time frame of five years. In the following diary passage she decides that this is what she will do with her anger:

> So, my task is to utilize the tremendous resources he has to offer to *prove him wrong* about the progressive character of the fibromyalgia and psoriatic arthritis. This will be my goal for the next five years, the period during which he predicted "serious deterioration." I will prove him wrong, using his methods and some of my own. (Diary, April 6, emphasis added)

Working up her courage, S. announced this decision to her doctor in the late April letter. But the pitiful truth of the matter is that her challenges existed in words only. She broadly hinted to her doctor that she did not accept his prognosis, but her behavioral solution to the problem did not require him to retract it or to change his treatment program in any way. Unable to speak her anger, S. could advance only a feeble challenge that left her doctor's program intact and placed the onus of making a change on herself.

Given her location in the hierarchies of science and gender, S. had little choice but to "fight like a girl." On the positive side, her methods of resisting through writing and rebelling through conniving with friends enabled the accumulation of resources that allowed her to escape with her life in the end. Over the long run, the silences provided psychological spaces for political growth that nurtured S.'s capacity eventually to speak out with authority and self-confidence. On the negative side, however, these modes of challenging biomedical power failed to protect S. in the crucial early months of treatment, when the understandings and drug regimens that were to prove so harmful were being worked out and put into place. And because the revolts were all staged in private, their message that something was terribly wrong did not get through to the doctor. Shown only his patient's sweet outer self, he could not see the angry inner self that boiled beneath the surface. Doctor-patient communications suffered accordingly.

These political and communicational costs of S.'s "girl games" are already high, but there were psychological costs as well. Forced to hide her true feelings behind a falsely pleasant exterior, S. fell into a deep depression that eroded her will to fight at all.

CHAPTER 6   **A Depression Worse than the Disease**

We have seen how, in the initial consultation, the doctor spoke in powerful scientific language that split his patient into two parts, objective and subjective, and declared the objective part the sole domain of medical interest. Yet for the patient, the affective component of the medical encounter was fundamental to the lived experience of her illness. For her the emotional repercussions of the doctor's interventions came to be more serious—and debilitating—than the bodily ills that had brought her to him in the first place. This chapter tells the painful story of how the doctor's discourses of biomedicine, filtered through the patient's psychology of gender, precipitated yet another disease—depression—which manifested itself both mentally and physically.

The chapter begins by describing how, from the patient's point of view, the doctor effectively *produced* her depression by diagnosing five chronic diseases, including a second major condition, and giving her a prognosis of worsening pain and deformity. Although her physical condition had not yet changed, the mere idea that she had a second serious lifelong illness eroded her sense of pride in her body and shattered her image of a happy future, producing feelings of sadness and diminished self-esteem. S. could not directly contest the diagnosis and prognosis, because the language of science had defined the doctor as the expert on her body. She tried to place her depression on the medical agenda, but the doctor rebuffed her efforts. He refused to acknowledge that depression might be a by-product of his practice and told her to accept as "cathartic" his dark view of her future. As if to rub salt into her psychological wounds, he talked of disability and death, implying that these were in store for her soon. Faced with a bleak diagnosis and prognosis, and with pointed reminders of her impending death, S. fell into a deep depression that, try as she might, she could not shake.

The next section traces how the doctor's diagnosis of fibromyalgia became a self-fulfilling prophecy, giving S. a complex of new symptoms that she had not had before. Interpreting these as manifestations of his specialty disease, the doctor instituted a treatment program of close monitoring and restriction of the patient's activities. Whereas the diagnosis and prognosis had produced only the *fear* of loss, the doctor's ban on her favorite activity led to a *real* loss of a major part of her life. Her depression deepened, becoming a pervasive melancholy that gnawed at her, sapping her energy and will to persevere.

The final section documents S.'s descent into despair as she sought out the biomedical literature to find comforting news, only to discover that her newly diagnosed condition would last fifteen years or more. Despite the energies she poured into the task, she was unable to vanquish the monster. By mid-June, when S. left the West Coast to spend five months back east, she was barely managing to hold everything together.

While the doctor's biomedical discourses and practices fostered feelings of loss and low self-esteem, the psychological makeup that S. bore as the mark of her femininity left her particularly vulnerable to "biomedical depression." As we have seen, S.'s relational reasoning led her to silence her critical inner self and to create a falsely agreeable social self to maintain the intimate relationship on which her care and safety depended. But this relationship-first approach to care exacerbated her feelings of loss, for she had voided her true feelings so that she could get help. S.'s relational strategy also eroded her self-esteem, for she had betrayed her self to please another. S. felt the pain of self-betrayal all the more keenly, for she had given up her feminist values—those of standing up for herself and speaking her anger—and embraced feminine routines of sweet compliance and silent rebellion that, on an intellectual level, she deeply deplored. And finally, all the energy S. expended to silence her concerns and suppress her rage depleted her stores of physical and psychological strength. This loss of stamina no doubt contributed to the physical symptoms of depression that emerged in the spring and grew markedly worse in the summer and fall: apathy, insomnia, and loss of appetite and weight. Trying to get help the only way she knew how, S. ended up deepening her psychic and physical wounds.

S.'s feminine strategies for getting help had a second major psychological consequence whose manifestations have been documented in previous chapters but not yet explained. This consequence was a blurring of boundaries between self and other and a resulting confusion about the corporeal reality of the self. We have seen how, in an effort to make her doctor like her, S. followed an ethic of care in which she was more attentive to her doctor's needs than to her own. As she made his needs and happiness the focus of her attention, she lost touch with her own needs, leaving herself exposed and vulnerable, with no one to protect her from harm. As the boundaries between her self and her doctor's self blurred, she came to take his views of her body as her own. This psychological dynamic helps to explain how S. came to believe that she had fibromyalgia despite the absence of all-over pain and how she accepted her doctor's assessment of "global improvement" when the evidence from her body said otherwise. These examples of S.'s disowning her own knowledge provide evidence of a profound confusion about the reality of her body. Incapable of distinguishing her perceptions from her doctor's, and unprotected from harm, she was unable to see the abusiveness of her doctor's approach to medical care. Even as he abused his institutional and discursive power by tolerizing her to drugs of proven toxicity and then using threats and accusations to coerce her compliance, she wrote in her diary that he was a generous human being and told him in a letter that she was thrilled to have him as a doctor. This case certainly tests the limits of the feminine ethic of care. When the patient's concern about making her doctor happy comes *at the expense of her own bodily and mental health,* the self-destructive potential of the ethic becomes painfully clear.

Bleak News: Depression Descends

Since her early forties S. had suffered from bouts of depression about the pain caused by her arthritis and the occasional limitations the disease placed on her life. The depression came and went with major flares of the disease. In the spring of 1996 she was also fighting a tenacious unhappiness about her work life. Her transitions to a new job, a new institution, and a new field—to say nothing of a new location three thousand miles from home—had been anything but smooth. The job stresses had been costly to her emotional health, leaving her weakened and vulnerable to new sources of psychic distress. Her husband, who was also struggling with a new bicoastal life (which in his case involved two homes to maintain, new jobs in several cities, and incessant travel) was under incredible stress as well. He had little energy left over to help S. deal with her problems. As if all these life strains were not enough, S.'s doctor became a major source of new distress. Soon after she started seeing Dr. D., S. fell into a deep, unremitting depression about her health. The feelings of despondency grew directly out of two aspects of the doctor's treatment of her case: the diagnosis of a second serious disease and the prognosis of progressive physical deterioration.

The Diagnosis

As we saw in chapter 1, S. emerged from the initial consultation shocked and despondent. The doctor had told her she had five chronic rheumatological problems, when she had thought she had only one. While three of them were relatively tractable, the fibromyalgia was not. From the doctor's point of view she had two serious conditions, and the new one was more worrying than the old, since it had become "entrenched," a "body habit."

S. was devastated to learn that she was twice as ill as she had thought. She had struggled for years to maintain a sense of her bodily identity as "normal," despite the existence of an occasionally debilitating joint condition. Most of the time she had succeeded in convincing herself that she was "basically healthy." As hinted in her April letter, she had considered her arthritis a minor inconvenience—little different from the inconvenience of, say, poor eyesight—not a major impediment to a happy life. This comforting image was now torn to shreds. The diagnosis of a second serious illness placed "normalcy" out of reach, pushing her over a psychological cliff. Although her physical condition had not changed a whit, the mere *idea* that she was so sick, that she would never again be "normal," cast a black pall over her spirits.

The doctor had talked about depression at that first meeting, but he had not acknowledged that his diagnoses or treatments could *create* depression where there had been none or *reactivate* a preexisting tendency to feel hopeless. He said only that depression was secondary to the physical ailments; once the ills were under control, the depression would disappear. In other words, talk of depression did not belong in the doctor-patient interaction. In effect, S.'s practitioner had produced a new, disease-related depression and then denied that it was producible, negating S.'s experience of her emotions.

The Prognosis

The prognosis came in a phone conversation ten days later. And it was bleak: she would "progress into serious deterioration" unless drastic steps were taken immediately. S. was terribly upset by this dismal view of her future. Her older sister, who also had psoriatic arthritis, had experienced a remarkable remission in her mid-thirties which had already lasted for twenty years. Because of her sister's happy history, S. had always imagined that her arthritis too would go into long-term remission. The doctor's violent words—violent because of their stark, terrifying message, delivered with no qualification at all—ripped into that comforting thought. S. could barely keep from crying while she was on the phone; the second she hung up the receiver she collapsed into hysterical tears. What distressed her was not the fear of her body in pain; it was the thought of her life shriveled and shrunk. S. had always imagined herself living a long and productive life. She would continue her writing and research work into her seventies, retire into a life of letters and quiet pleasures in her eighties, and die of old age in her early nineties. The doctor's talk of a deteriorating body ruptured that happy image, forcing her to see her life and dreams as sharply limited by her illness. This thought was so devastating that she could not bear to consider all its implications, even to herself. Her diary includes a one-line paragraph simply recording this fearful new truth: "Seems like I have to accept the idea of real limits" (Diary, March 27).

The prognosis might not have been so desolating had S. had some physical or emotional resources that would help her cope with it. But weeks of largely unsuccessful drug experiments had left her body drained and exhausted, her soul devoid of hope that her physical problems could ever be eased. Coming on top of this, the prognosis pushed her to the edge of emotional collapse:

> Well, this news Dr. [D.] has given me has really set back my progress toward getting out of this state of eternal depression. It's bad enough to be told that you have not one, but [five], serious conditions, but when you add to that, feeling lousy absolutely every single day from all the drugs he is experimenting with, it's really pushed me back to the brink, if not over. I really feel like someone told me I had a fatal disease. (Transition file, March 26)

Retirement, Disability, and Death: More Doctor-Talk

As if to make the prognosis more real, the doctor soon began to talk about her retirement. That was the last thing on S.'s mind. In a major career move, she had just moved to California to take a new job. From her point of view she was at the beginning of her life's work, not the end:

> Somehow we got onto the subject of what I want to do, and he suggested that I was planning to retire. Retire! Ha! I said, I haven't even *begun* to do the things I want to do. And I repeated that, for emphasis. I simply couldn't believe he was talking about retiring . . . I've just started my life work! (Diary, March 27)

Interspersed with the talk of retirement was an occasional mention of disability, aging, and dying. One day the patient got a mini-lecture on disability. Arthritis is among the most disabling conditions that exists, the doctor said, yet U.S. law does not treat it as a disability, so his patients cannot get government support. The implication seemed to be that disability was in S.'s future, perhaps right around the corner. The doctor frequently brought up the subject of death, arguing that life is really just a process of dying, and that the sooner one gets used to that idea the better off one is. Once when S. worried aloud about the loss of more joints, the doctor said it didn't matter, because she had only a few decades left to live anyway and other joints could tide her over until the end. Again and again the doctor used images of aging and dying to describe the prospects for her life.

S. found these images disheartening, to say the least. She did not want to believe all the talk about progressive illness and disability and retirement, but the doctor's words slowly wormed their way into her consciousness. She commented on this in an early diary entry: "So bizarre to have someone—a total stranger—come into your life so suddenly and then rearrange everything you had ever thought or planned for yourself. I mean, so bizarre" (Diary, March 27). Note how S. is unable to separate her doctor's views from her own, so that whatever he says becomes her truth. She notes how "bizarre" it is to have a lifetime of thoughts and plans suddenly pushed aside, but she does not or cannot stop the invasion of her mind. It is perhaps not surprising that she does not resist the invasion, for the replacement of her thoughts with her doctor's was encouraged by the discourses of biomedicine, which made the physician the expert on the patient body. The mental takeover was also promoted by the guidelines of gender she was following, which called for her to silence herself and take his truth as her own.

Although the doctor had placed depression outside the range of topics he would deal with, during her second office visit S. told him that she had become very depressed since hearing his gloomy prognosis. She knew the subject was not fully legitimate, but she considered the downturn in her outlook a major consequence of his treatment style and a fundamental aspect of her (un)well-being. She thought it was important to apprise the doctor of what was happening. But he remained deaf to her pleas for help. More than that, he declared her emotional reactions part of her problem, in effect blaming her for her psychic pain. The only way out, he told her, was to stop fighting the prognosis. Fighting the truth—that is, his truth, the biomedical truth—would only slow her progress and make things worse. She must accept the prognosis and make it part of her identity. Doing so would lead to "catharsis" and a new, more realistic sense of the self and its possibilities. This new sense of self as ill, in turn, would improve her ability to manage her diseases. S. could not quite see how this would happen, but she considered the idea reasonable enough to warrant more effort:

> Oh, and the big thing. I said I had been much more depressed since [the] last visit, especially since [the] phone call in which he told me like it is. [D. said] this is supposed to lead to "catharsis," a euphemism if ever I heard one. It leads to nothing but deep depression. But the idea is one is supposed to make the chronic condition part of one's identity . . . and then go on from there, framing a life with the condition as part of it. Fair enough. (Diary, March 29)

Try as she might, S. could not make "being a fibromyalgic" or "being a chronically and progressively ill person" part of her identity without falling into a sea of sadness. The feelings of grief became chronic, unshakable. For S. the struggles to overcome the depression became a big part of her problem, as big as, if not bigger than, the battles with the body.

The Restrictions Become Real: Depression Deepens

During the first month of treatment S.'s worries about the restrictions on her life were theoretical only: the doctor's vision of a fibromyalgic-arthritic body growing more and more decrepit conjured up fears of future loss of function and fun. Then, six weeks into treatment, to her horror her worst fears came true. In late April, when S. began suffering from severe headaches, her doctor located the cause in the one activity in her life that had always brought her pleasure: swimming.

A Ban on Swimming, a Diminishment of Life

As we saw earlier, in early April, when S. began to sleep more and feel better, she started swimming again. Indeed, she felt so good that she swam every day. For a myriad of reasons swimming was a special, even sacred part of her life: it evoked memories of a happy childhood spent on a Maine lake, it produced feelings of health and well-being, it made her body strong, and many more.

It is a painful irony, then, that it was S. herself who first raised the possibility that swimming might be causing her renewed headaches by exacerbating the neck pain. This idea had first occurred to S. as she and her doctor were looking for support from her life for his fibromyalgic interpretation of the headaches (for details see chapter 2). During that conversation, however, S. kept this unpleasant thought to herself, later noting in her diary: "Hmmm . . . wonder if . . . all the swimming . . . is contributing to this [set of problems]." As if to ward off the possibility that her swimming might be restricted, she added: "It is the one thing I look forward to every single day" (Diary, April 23).

Trying to be a helpful patient, the next day S. proposed this hypothesis to her doctor. He considered it very plausible, indeed, so plausible that he urged her to stop swimming for a while to see if the headaches went away. Thus it was that swimming came to be subject to medical proscription. S. struggled hard to swallow the thought that something that had always been an unmitigated good for her should now be tossed out of her life, and by a medical doctor, no less:

> [Dr. D.] thinks [the swimming hypothesis is] quite plausible. So I have to cool it for a little while on the swimming. So ironic, that you can make things worse while working so hard to make them better . . . [D.] says he usually doesn't "allow" his patients to swim, but since I was already swimming when I started to see him, he didn't say anything!!! Boy, having a doctor tell me to stop swimming? This is really too much! (Diary, April 24)

Clearly, S. thinks it outrageous that an expert on the body should restrict the activity that most nourishes her body. Yet, unable to set boundaries between her self and her doctor's self, and believing him to be possessed of some higher truth, she takes his word as her order, leaving herself vulnerable to his mistakes.

At first the thought of swimming less was tolerable, because the doctor said not to stop but only to swim differently. The neck has mechanical limits, he explained; since bodies move so easily in the water people tend to overdo it, putting too much stress on the neck. The trick was to reduce that stress by swimming with a snorkel and mask, which obviated the need to turn the head, or by doing strokes other than freestyle, S.'s favorite. S. gamely accepts these suggestions with the comment, "I'll have to invent some new strokes, it seems" (Diary, April 27). A few days later she went out and bought the best snorkel and mask that money could buy.

Unfortunately, the swimming hypothesis gained some support. Reluctantly, S. admitted that the swimming might be exacerbating her pain:

> Last Wednesday, Thursday, Friday the headaches I had last weekend went
> right away after I . . . stopped swimming and doing the neck ranging exer-
> cises. I knew the swimming was contributing to neck pain; I had been
> swimming every single day, and, although I just love it—in fact it's the
> highlight of my every day—I could feel that it was creating pain in my
> neck. So I stopped and the headaches went away. (Diary, April 27)

But the headaches came back again a few days later. The doctor tried
adjusting the dosage of the sleep medications. When that experiment
failed he took drastic action: he changed the dosage of the drugs once
again and ordered the patient to cut out swimming altogether.

The Thin Line between Hope and Despair

S. was extremely discouraged by this total ban on her favorite activity:

> So, more bad news. It is very discouraging . . . The interdiction on swim-
> ming is the hardest to take, especially since I just went out and bought new
> snorkeling gear. It's really the only thing that predictably brings happiness.
> So, I have to be really brave . . .
> [It is so hard] to keep my spirits from sinking. There is a very fine line
> here between hope and despair; every day, every hour, my life seems to
> be about negotiating that line in a struggle to stay on the hope side of it.
> No wonder people lose heart and drop out [of D.'s treatment program];
> it takes extraordinary emotional and personal resources to stay optimistic
> in these conditions. (Diary, April 30)

S. tried to fight off depression by redefining what "counted" as
progress in overcoming her physical problems. Indeed, in a pitiful effort
to talk herself out of her dismay, she designated as progress her discovery that swimming was exacerbating her pain (Diary, April 30). Trying
to boost her sagging spirits, she also tried counting as "good" those days
in which she felt mentally alert all day long. How her life and her views
of it had changed: "Up and down, up and down. Today a small up . . .
I actually felt quite mentally alert *all day*. I really have to applaud when
things go well so that everything does not always seem so black" (Diary, May 2).

But the loss of her favorite form of exercise was a terrible blow. Along
with writing, swimming was the minimal definition of S.'s life. It was her
identity, what she was all about. In the past, no matter how bad her joint
pain had gotten, she had always consoled herself with the thought that
it was not a catastrophe because she could still swim. Now even that was
in jeopardy. S. felt her life slipping away from her. Struggling to contain
the anguish, she writes:

I had lots of questions [for D.] about exercise. *I really cannot hold onto anything,* even my oft-stated feeling that "at least I can still swim; it's one of the most important things in my life." Such statements are dangerous because, since my body has changed, activities that were good for me before may not be now. [What the doctor is saying is] that I shouldn't be swimming now and probably not much in the future. (Diary, May 2)

S.'s daily chart provides numerical traces of her descent into mental hell. In April, when she experienced improvements in her sleep and joint pain that offset the disheartening diagnosis and prognosis, her mood averaged 3.6, a little better than "so-so." During May, when her upper-back and neck pain emerged in full force and she followed her doctor's orders to stay out of the pool, her emotional state fell to 2.3, just above "moderately depressed." A more graphic statistic is the proportion of days spent seriously depressed (a reading of 0 or 1 on her scale of 0 to 5). When she coded a day as 0 or 1, it meant that she cried almost the whole day long. In April S. was morbidly depressed "only" 15 percent of the time. In May she felt that way nearly 40 percent of the time.

"Fibromyalgia Is Forever": Depression Becomes Despair

Dr. D.'s ban on swimming was rooted in his fibromyalgic interpretation of S.'s recent headaches and neck pain. It was not hard to identify that newly diagnosed disorder as the source of her distress. S. began to wonder what this meant for the future. How long would she have to stay out of the water? How long was fibromyalgia supposed to last? S. reread the notes on fibromyalgia that she had taken during appointments with her doctor. Strangely, he had said little about the duration of the condition. He had said that "fibromyalgia, left untreated, is almost always progressive." But what if it were treated? Then how long would it last? The notes were silent on that crucial question.

Dr. D. Gives a Public Lecture

One night in late May Dr. D. gave a public lecture in Seattle on his specialty disease. Hoping to learn something that would help alleviate her condition, S. made a special effort to go by scheduling a doctor's appointment, also in Seattle, the next day. S. arrived at the scheduled time and place, pencil and pad in hand.[1] Facing a packed room eager to learn about his favorite subject, her doctor was in his element. He spoke for almost an hour and then answered questions from members of the audience, most of whom seemed to be shopping for a doctor for themselves.

Dr. D. began by saying that joint diseases—the various arthritises—are not the most important problems in rheumatology. Why not? Because they are not the most important conditions he sees. Rather, the most serious problems he encounters are syndromes that are "periarticular" (around the joints) and "nonarticular" (not related to the joints). Of these, the most disabling is fibromyalgia. In published studies, he continued, about 20 percent of patients in rheumatology clinics have fibromyalgia. In his practice, however, 90 percent have the condition. Why so many? Because other doctors underdiagnose the disease. "Many doctors say it's all in your head," he declared, his voice rising excitedly. "But it's all in *their* head. It actually exists! They don't know physiology!" He then proceeded to explain referred pain, pain amplification, the need for "obsessive workups," and many other things S. had encountered before in examination-room lectures.

One subject S. had not heard D. talk about was the gender distribution of the condition. D. noted that about 80 percent of fibromyalgics are women. Why are women more prone to have this muscle syndrome than men? "If you're running after the kids all day long, fibromyalgia will interfere with function, so you're apt to note the pain. Men are often in occupations that allow them to overcome that function." Dr. D. had just revealed his views about appropriate gender roles. Indeed, every one of his examples of activities producing pain—from lifting a young child to touching a hot stove to paring potatoes—assumed a fibromyalgic who was not only a woman, but also a homemaker.

Dr. D. sought to reassure his audience—most of whom were older women with fibromyalgic-like conditions—that they could get better. Even though fibromyalgia "disables you and interferes with your life significantly," he said, if you follow my regimen of regular medication and restructured exercise and ergonomics, "you should get better, you should be more functional." Although his message may have been comforting to listeners who had long lived in pain, S. left the lecture deeply discouraged. The doctor had said patients would get *better,* but he had not said they would get *well.* The overall picture he had painted—of a disease more crippling than arthritis, one associated with significant work disability, debilitating mental as well as physical symptoms, and even anomalies in the biology of the brain—left her feeling that her problems were much worse than she had realized.

Biomedical Truths: "Fibromyalgia Lasts at Least Fifteen Years"

A few nights later, after a long day of torturous headaches and unrelenting fatigue, S. began to grow morbidly worried about her future. What would this new condition mean for her in the years ahead? She grew frantic. She wanted to call her doctor and hear him say that fibromyalgia was a temporary affliction that, with treatment, would eventually go away. But it was too late; his office was closed for the day. Desperate for some good news, S. set out for the science library at her university. She would consult the medical literature and find the answer she wanted.

She spent several hours poring over the journal *Arthritis and Rheumatism,* the official publication of the American College of Rheumatology. The journal contained a surprising number of articles on fibromyalgia. But what they said about the prospects for recovery was not reassuring. The most recent study, published in the April 1996 issue, indicated that fibromyalgia is of very long duration.[2] This was a prospective follow-up study in which patients initially diagnosed with fibromyalgia syndrome (FMS) were reinterviewed ten years later, regardless of whether they were currently being treated for it. In this study, the longest to date, twenty-nine patients were investigated in an effort to determine the "natural history" of the disease. In their own words, what the researchers found was that:

> FMS symptoms last, on average, at least 15 years after illness onset . . . All patients had persistence of some fibromyalgia symptoms, although almost half (48 percent) had not seen a doctor for them in the last year. Moderate to severe pain or stiffness was reported in 55 percent of patients; moderate to a lot of sleep difficulty was noted in 48 percent; and moderate to extreme fatigue was noted in 59 percent. These symptoms showed little change from earlier surveys. In 79 percent of patients, medications were still being taken to control FMS symptoms.[3]

Although many of the patients reported doing well, by the objective standards of biomedicine they were doing little better than at the time of their diagnosis ten years earlier.

This was not an isolated finding that S. could dismiss on some charge of poor science. To the contrary, this latest research confirmed and extended the findings of previous studies. For example, an investigation of seventy-two patients in England had found that, after four years, 97 percent still had symptoms and 85 percent met the criteria for the diagnosis.[4] Another study of fifty-six Swedish patients had shown that, after five years, symptoms of FMS persisted in all but one patient, and almost 50 percent reported a worsening of symptoms.[5]

The 1996 article also hinted at an association between fibromyalgia and serious mental problems. Of the original group of thirty-nine patients, two had committed suicide between the time of diagnosis and the research. Although the sample was too small for statistical inference, S. found the 5 percent suicide rate shocking nonetheless. Knowing that she should know the truth, but dreading what she might find, S. forced herself to read on. To her considerable horror, she discovered that the connection between fibromyalgia and "psychiatric disorder" was a well-known biomedical hypothesis.[6] A recent article in the same journal reported that a group of fibromyalgia patients had three times the number of lifetime psychiatric diagnoses as two control groups, one fibromyalgics who were not in treatment, the other healthy subjects. More than 50 percent of the fibromyalgia patients had been diagnosed with a major mood disorder, mostly depression, compared to 20 percent in the other groups.[7] Either something about the patients who sought care was different, or the care they received was depressing them. But the most unsettling news was yet to come. Tracking down some alarming-sounding references, S. discovered that fibromyalgia is associated with sexual abuse.[8] In the most recent study, 65 percent of women with fibromyalgia reported a history of sexual abuse. The figure for a healthy control group was 52 percent.[9] Although the difference was not statistically significant, the raw percentages jumped out at her from the page as hugely significant in a social sense. These statistics on depression and abuse were so disturbing to S. that she consciously put them out of mind as something she would deal with later, when her own mental health was more secure.

The stark conclusion about the duration of the disease—that its symptoms last, on average, for at least fifteen years—was a staggering piece of news. And this was just the longest study done to date; who knows, S. thought, it could be for life. Seeing herself as one of the patients in the studies, S. described the results of her foray into the biomedical literature this way: "I found that [fibromyalgia] was chronic and does not go away, despite daily medication, for 15 years . . . This just robbed me of my hope" (Diary, June 1).

Patient Advice: "No Thinking About How This Will Ruin Your Life!"

When she returned home from the library S. sent a distress e-mail to Dana, asking for her thoughts about how to cope with this new information.

If her message, reproduced below, sounds restrained, it is because S. did not want to expose the full horror of her fears to a friend whose fibromyalgia was much worse than her own. Here is what she wrote:

Hi [Dana],

. . . I've been thinking lots about you lately because I have good news and bad . . . [T]he bad news is, now that I'm no longer so focused on the constant exhaustion and joint pain, I am very aware of the fibromyalgia pain, especially in the neck. It is so depressing to experience improvement, only to have things fall apart again. I heard a lecture on FM on Monday night (by my doctor . . .) and was so depressed by what he did not say. He gave listeners, many of whom have FM, no hope that things would get much better . . . So, I determined to prove him wrong (i.e., to find literature showing improvement). I went to the [s]cience library and [found that]. . . , lo and behold, the condition is chronic and few patients get much better . . . Of course, statistical averages cannot predict individual circumstances; one can hold onto that, I guess.

This biomed lit really gets me: it says that depression and pain are totally interrelated, with one exacerbating the other and vice versa. Then it says the pain won't go away. So we have to stop being depressed even tho we are in pain, and tell ourselves this is fun and we can't wait for some more pain. I'm hoping you have more productive ways of looking at things than I do!!! . . .

Well, [Dana], I'm waiting for you to tell me this is just all dumb. Somehow I have to get over this stuff, mentally if not physically, so I can get back to my life. (I know, this is my life.) . . .

Love, S.

(E-mail, May 30)

Dana offered some sound suggestions for dealing with the sadness one inevitably feels after learning that one's life has been foreshortened by a chronic, debilitating illness:

First, [Dana says,] I have to stop thinking about the long run and concentrate on today, what strategies I am using now and how much better I am feeling today than yesterday. No thinking of how this will ruin my life! . . .

I asked how she deals with being unable to do things. The answer: her expectations have changed. She can go days without doing any work at all. She makes things, or otherwise keeps busy . . . I would say her coping strategies are so much better than mine even though her medical condition is so much worse. (Diary, June 1)

This was extremely sage advice—for someone with fibromyalgia. But the thought of scaling back her expectations about what she could accomplish in life just made S. all the more depressed. Try as she might, she could not stop thinking about how this new condition would ruin her life. During the next two weeks, as she prepared to leave for the East Coast, she struggled with some success to stay afloat on her sea of sorrow. Perhaps the anticipation of leaving a place that had brought so much unhappiness and pain helped to buoy her spirits. Whatever the reasons, in early June her overall emotional state remained unchanged from May's level of 2.3 on her scale, just above moderately depressed. And the morbid depression lifted a little, leaving a wet gray fog over "only" one-fourth of her days.

By mid-June, after eleven weeks of treatment, S.'s emotional health had fallen into a precarious state. Cleaving to the rules of biomedicine, her doctor had induced a major depression in his patient by diagnosing a second serious disease, instituting a treatment program that somehow begot the symptoms of the disease, and then sharply restricting the patient's activities to control the symptoms. The discourses of objectivity allowed D. first to precipitate a psychological disease and then to refuse to take responsibility for it on the grounds that it was subjective and therefore of no concern to him. These changes in her body and life were so demoralizing to S. because she had a long history of symptoms and restrictions from her arthritis. She knew only too well what it meant to have a chronic illness: it meant loss of the things that gave her life shape and meaning. It meant loss of "normalcy" and all that that entailed. And because the new condition was so much more debilitating than the old, the new losses, she believed, would be even more devastating than those she had already sustained. S. devoted massive energies to fighting off depression, but her efforts only deepened her psychic pain. Living by the codes of femininity, she silenced her doubtful self and took her physician's truth as her own. Subject to two powerful and mutually reinforcing silencing mechanisms, she allowed her doctor to invade her mind and replace her bright dreams for the future with his dark vision of disability and death as the inevitable future of the rheumatological patient. The voiding of the patient self was a logical outcome of the two codes being enacted. But it was a dangerous outcome, for it left the patient with no one to defend her when her doctor made mistakes. The mistakes were made in the spring, but their most serious consequences would emerge only later, in the summer and fall.

Part Four | A Losing Battle to Get Better

CHAPTER 7 **Struggling to Make the Treatment Work**

In mid-June S. left her home base in southern California to spend five months on the East Coast. Her plans called for passing the rest of June in her second home in New York's Hudson River Valley, followed by July and August in a lakeside cottage in the Maine woods. In September she would return to her New York home and remain there through the fall, returning to California around Christmastime.

Her main project for the summer and the fall sabbatical was to write a book on the birth-control program in China. She had worked hard for a good many years to create protected time to write this book. She had even taken a pay cut to get an early sabbatical. To be sure, during her months on the East Coast S. spent every hour she could working on that project. But her body was not well. Throughout the summer and fall her bodily ills kept intruding on her life, forcing themselves to the top of her mental and emotional agenda. When the body is not well, when sleep refuses to come, when the head throbs and the back and neck complain of pain, the mind loses its acuity. And so it was that her precious sabbatical came to be used up by her struggles to get well.

This chapter tells the story of S.'s battles to gain control over the physical symptoms of her new disease. In a mid-June appointment, Dr. D. had declared victory over the arthritis and fibromyalgic tender points. But we have seen how the notion that her illnesses had been vanquished rested on a peculiar discourse in which some symptoms simply did not "count" in the doctor's evaluation of how she was doing. Symptoms that troubled the patient but did not figure in the doctor's assessment included the sleep problems, which had been only partly resolved, and the new symptoms of "fibromyalgia," especially the headaches and back and neck pain. These complaints did not count, because the doctor had no "objective" measures of them and because, in the case of the headaches and back pain, they were not the problems he had set out to fix, but annoying new symptoms that had cropped up after the initial diagnosis had been made. Another reason that these symptoms did not count was that there was nothing else the doctor could do about them; by definition, then, they were the patient's problems, not the doctor's. Commuting the rhetoric of biomedical infallibility into a concrete blueprint for further treatment, scientific medicine had assigned the patient full responsibility for the symptoms that medicine itself could not measure or fix.

Because these physical problems had to be eased before S. could write, to say nothing of enjoy her life, S. found herself devoting most of the summer and fall to finding ways to reduce their severity. According to her doctor's microenvironmental theory of fibromyalgia, she could reduce the pain and become "more functional" by closely monitoring her activities and by cutting back or eliminating those that produced pain. The chapters in this fourth part of the book show how the logic of this treatment discourse worked itself out on the patient's body and life.

During the summer S. put this theory into practice, making it the cornerstone of her disease-management program. This chapter records the ups and downs of her struggle to make the theory work. The chapter moves chronologically through the summer months. It begins by describing the arrangements that S. worked out with her doctor to obtain care from afar. It then turns to the successes and failures of her summer of struggle. For the first month the disciplines of self-surveillance and self-restriction felt very empowering, as S. discovered activities that made her pain worse, eliminated them, and enjoyed temporary respite from the pain. But this high came crashing down in late July, when she suffered a seven-day headache that had no discernible cause. Early August brought a second high of self-discovery and apparent pain reduction. The summer ended on another low when S. used her charts to compute some long-term statistics on her success in putting her doctor's treatment discourse into practice. The numbers brought dismaying news: despite her mighty efforts, the symptoms were anything but under control.

Why the results of treatment fluctuated so wildly we discover only in a later chapter. Here we attend to the gendered, relational approach through which S. socially enacted her treatment from afar. We will see how her relationship-first approach kept her obsessively focused on making her doctor happy, even as her own health and sanity ebbed. In letter after worshipful letter, she worked to present herself as the ultimate in good patients, whose witty commentary on her self-treatment proved her doctor's therapy a stunning success. This other-directed ethic of care, however, entailed an erasure of self-other boundaries that robbed her of her critical faculties and left her feeling unhinged when the program she was so rigorously following failed to work.

Arrangements for Monitoring from Afar:
A Private Pact Based on Mutual Trust

Before leaving the West Coast, S. had worked out a detailed plan with Dr. D. for how he would monitor her health when she was too far away to make in-person visits. The importance of his continuing to oversee her health care was self-evident to both of them. The doctor had said he needed three to six months of aggressive treatment to bring her conditions under control. By the beginning of the summer only half of that time would have elapsed. Neither S. nor D. wanted to interrupt the treatment program before it had had time to prove its usefulness.

In a doctor's appointment in mid-April, S. raised the question of how she might remain in his care while living three thousand miles away. The doctor answered that she should find a primary care physician on the East Coast who was "in her pocket"—that is, who would "just write out the prescriptions that [D.] wants" (Diary, April 19). She should avoid seeing a rheumatologist, who might want to adopt a different treatment program, undoing all the work D. had done over many months (Diary, April 19). With its conspiratorial tone, her doctor's plan for the summer and fall left S. feeling that there was a secret pact between them. The pact was based on an implicit pledge of mutual trust: he would assume responsibility for her care, while she would keep their arrangements confidential and protect his unorthodox treatment program from the scrutiny of his professional peers. The creation of this undercover understanding made S. feel that her efforts to make herself a stand-out patient had paid off. She was so special that Dr. D. would trust her with safeguarding his trade secrets.

Before S. left the West Coast this plan was modified slightly to eliminate the primary care physician. Dr. D. himself would write out prescriptions for three months, with one refill, which S. would fill through a mail-order prescription service. While on the East Coast she would get her blood work done monthly at local laboratories, ideally ones with contracts with her insurer, and have the results faxed to Dr. D. They would talk by phone each month after the results of the blood work came in. S. would call the doctor if any problems should arise. If the problems were serious, she would either fly back to Seattle to see him or find another rheumatologist on the East Coast.

S. left for New York in high spirits. During an appointment the past spring her doctor had described how she could be empowered despite her fibromyalgia: "It is very possible," he had said, "to gain control over the disease and, in the process, to take charge of one's life again. Being able to identify the environmental . . . sources of increased pain is an important part of the process" (Diary, April 30). S. was more than ready to take charge of her medical conditions, to empower herself and gain control over her disease. And she had the perfect tool with which to tackle the task: her daily chart, which provided places to note a wide range of factors feeding into the pain. Moreover, her summer and fall locations would provide ideal environments in which to conduct her self-science. The New York country home and the Maine cottage afforded almost completely controlled climates in which all the social stresses of her life at the university would be eliminated, leaving only the strain of her own activities to produce pain. Armed with multiple copies of her chart and optimistic that she could track down the causes of her pain and slay the monster on her own, S. set off for the East Coast, happy at last to be her own medical boss.

Initial Successes

On June 17 S. flew to New York, with medical paraphernalia and writing materials in tow. Her husband would follow in a couple of weeks. The very next day she began surveilling her daily activities to see which of them contributed to her aches and pains.

Lessons for the Fibromyalgic: Issuing Orders to the Self

S.'s first task was to clean the large converted dairy barn that served as their home in the New York countryside. Unoccupied over the winter and spring, the barn had accumulated a respectable layer of dust, cobwebs, and mice droppings. On June 18 she spent five hours vacuuming, dusting, and generally restoring the barn to habitable condition. Her chart reads:

> June 18: General pain—Backache from housecleaning
>
> June 19: General pain—Backache from vacuuming

Two days later she began to take stock of the barnyard—five acres of original pasture and the lawn and flower beds she had put in over the years. Everything was crying out for attention. The tractor and hand mower needed to be readied for use. The lawn and pastures wanted to be mowed. Her flower gardens begged to be weeded, the flowers fertilized, the climbing vines trained to grow up their wires. On June 20 S.

spent one and a half hours weeding. Over the next few days she devoted half an hour to an hour and a half daily to mowing, weeding, raking, and otherwise tending her gardens. Under the category "General Pain" she made the following observations on her chart:

June 20: Backache all day from previous day of housecleaning and weeding

June 21: Moderate backache, some neck ache all day

June 22: Moderate ache in mid- to lower back all day

June 23: Wrist and back pain from weeding and hand mowing

June 24: Back protested the raking and weeding

Clearly, yard work was a source of muscle pain. She would have to limit her gardening to short stints.

S. could scarcely wait for the local county pool to open for the summer season. On the day the pool opened S. drove over, eager to dive in. But it was a public pool, and pool rules, she discovered, prohibited using a snorkel and mask. Because of her neck pain, S. could no longer swim without them. (In California she had not faced such restrictions, because she swam in a private pool.) Being kept out of her beloved pool was hugely discouraging, for it meant that she could no longer swim when she was living in her New York home.

Determined not to be deterred from getting her exercise, S. decided to walk instead. It was the summer solstice, and the sun was setting late. To enjoy the sunsets S. began taking long country walks, setting out after her favorite news program ended at 8:00 P.M. These strolls took her under a range of rock-clad mountains, past a small bucolic lake, and down a wooded lane that wound its way alongside a noisy mountain stream. The air was crisp and clean and invigorating. Yet the exhilaration she felt was not to last long. Puzzlingly, the same week that S. began taking walks, her sleep deteriorated and her headaches returned. At the end of the week she studied her chart and made a striking discovery: the poor sleep and headaches occurred in every case just *after* her late-evening walks. Here is the pattern she spotted:

June 24: Exercise—Walk, 8:00–9:00 pm

June 25: Sleep—10:00 to 5:30, not enough

How Feel—Tired, drugged all day

June 26: Exercise—Walk, 8:00 to 9:00 pm

June 27: Sleep—Poor sleep, 11:00 to 3:30 to 5:30

How Feel—Slight headache due to poor sleep, tired from early afternoon

June 28: Exercise—Walk, 8:00 to 9:00 pm

June 29: Sleep—10:45 to 3:30 to 5:30, poor sleep in early morning hours

General pain: Mild to moderate headache all day, from poor sleep

The connection was so clear! Her late-evening strolls had disturbed her sleep, causing fatigue and headaches the next day. The following week she shifted her walks to early evening, and the sleep problems and headaches vanished. S. felt so empowered!

Yet it was not only exercise that produced problems. Any slight deviation from her standard routine seemed to disrupt that precious sleep and bring on headaches and/or back and neck pain the next day. On July 2 her chart says: "*Poor sleep,* 10:30 to 3:30 to 6:20; Awoke with slight headache, [which developed into] splitting headache [lasting] all day." What could possibly have induced the headache? The only change in her routine was the addition of a root beer float late in the afternoon. S. reasoned that the root beer float had created the problem by making her wake up in the middle of the night to go to the bathroom, after which she could not get back to sleep. Evidently, she would have to closely monitor and control diet and drink.

On the night of July 5 S. slept poorly and awoke with a bad headache. Her chart records the following information: "Sleep—10:15 to 5:15, doze[d] to 7:15, awoke with bad headache; How Feel—*horrid;* How Function—[Unable to write,] reduced to yard work and housework; General Pain—Massive, splitting headache *all day long,* neck and back of head painful." What could have caused these problems? The only change she had made was to adjust the timing of her sleep medications ever so slightly, taking one pill ten minutes later than usual and the other thirty minutes earlier. Lacking any other explanation, she concluded that this minor change in the timing of her medications had produced the headache. Clearly, she would have to impose a rigid discipline on her pill-taking schedule.

After a few weeks of observation and study, S. began to write down what she had learned from her research in the form of "lessons." She wrote these at the bottom of her charts, using a shocking pink felt-tip pen to make them stand out as urgent messages. Her charts for late June and early July include the following commands to herself:

Lesson: Must wear wrist splints when [use the] hand mow[er]!

Lesson: Must not bend back—anything that requires it (for example, vacuuming, weeding) produces same-day and next-day back pain.

Lesson: Mid-evening walks seem to produce poor sleep! Walk earlier in the day!

Lesson: No late afternoon drinks!

Lesson: NEVER, under *ANY* circumstances, change sleep meds!

These orders may strike the reader as comical in their excessive strictness, and indeed, there was an element of self-mockery in S.'s project. Yet at the most basic level, this program of self-restriction was an act of true desperation. S. issued these orders to herself in a dead-serious effort to do whatever was necessary—including imposing a straitjacket of temporal and physical disciplines on her life—to rid herself of the noxious symptoms.

Although S. worked hard to keep her spirits from sagging, these new limitations on her life were hard to swallow. The hardest to take was the restraint on gardening. Making things grow, maneuvering her sturdy old farm tractor around the pastures, smelling the sweet aroma of freshly cut grass—these things were a source of supreme pleasure to her, second only to swimming. S. had gardened vigorously for years, with no untoward effects on her body. But now, it seemed, the gardening had to be sharply circumscribed to keep the fibromyalgia under control.

An Upbeat Letter to Dr. D.

Despite these discouraging developments, S. was happy to be on her own, making discoveries and finding ways to gain control over her aches and pains. The doctor's promise that she could feel empowered seemed to be coming true.

On July 8, a few days after her husband returned from the West Coast, S. rented a car, filled it with her computer, books, and writing materials, and drove nine hours to the cottage in north-central Maine that she would be renting for the next two months. The cottage was on the lake where she had spent her childhood summers. Just a stone's throw away was her parents' cottage. S. chose to pass her summer in this location because of the happy memories it evoked. After a springtime of distress, she needed to be in a place that would be emotionally nurturing. Her parents, who were deeply concerned about her failing health, promised to provide that sustenance. They also offered to feed her "good home-cooked food," something S. badly needed to fill out her thinning frame. S. would also be able to swim again—and in her favorite lake. Because she was planning to devote the summer to working on her book, S. went to Maine by herself. Her husband would join her there for a few days in September, after which they would drive back to New York together.

Accomplishing the move to Maine with little ill effect (only one day of "moderate mid-back pain") boosted S.'s confidence that she was conquering her symptoms. A week later she wrote a letter to her doctor to report how well everything was going. The timing of the letter had a hidden logic: mid-July was when S. would have had her next doctor's appointment had she been on the West Coast. She used the letter to tell her doctor the things she would have communicated in person. I quote the letter in full, because it reveals both the precariousness of her quest for symptom control and the trickiness of communicating these contradictions within the relationship-first approach to her health care that she had established during the spring.

13 July 1996

Dear [Dr. D.],

Since I wasn't able to see you this month, I thought I would drop you a line to let you know how I have been.

The answer, in a word, is great. All joints seem to be in fine working order. I'm sure *you* could produce some joint pain, but, left on my own, I feel none. Even my left wrist, which was mercilessly injected and re-injected by my doctor earlier in the summer, refuses to complain.

The sleep and mid-back pain remain sometimes-problems. But, by being ultra-analytical, I've figured out which activities from the previous day are responsible for the problems. Should you wish to feel lousy some day, here are some strategies guaranteed to produce the effect:

1. Take a brisk walk in the countryside . . .

2. Have a root beer float . . .

3. Change the timing of your sleep medications . . .

4. Weed a flower garden . . .

5. Drive for nine hours straight.

I've come to liken good health (i.e., sound sleep and the absence of pain) to a carefully constructed house of cards; so fragile is it that if you try to replace the Six of Clubs with a Seven of Clubs, the whole thing comes crashing down. The good news is that, by leaving the Six of Clubs in place, you can feel well practically every day.

On the personal front, I'm renting a quaint little cottage on a lake in north-central Maine . . . I'm getting some writing done—which was the whole point of this caper—but the close proximity of my favorite lake does provide certain distractions.

It was so nice to hear your voice on the phone the other day; sometimes I think it is not the new medical regime but the new doctor that is making me feel so much better.

Hoping everything is looking bright in [Seattle] . . .
Until next time,

Warm regards,

S.

This letter lays bare the tensions surrounding S.'s strivings for symptom control. She describes her overall health as "great," but goes on to note that the sleep and back pain continue to be "sometimes-problems." She uses the metaphor of a house of cards to convey how vulnerable she feels in her new life, in which the tiniest deviation from her daily schedule can turn the next day into a nightmare of agonizing headache and pain. These feelings of fragility and closure of a life were to grow as the summer wore on and as more and more parts of her life had to be suspended.

Continuing to follow her relationship-first approach to care, however, S. is careful to maintain an upbeat tone and witty style throughout the letter. She mentions the negative but highlights the positive. Her house-of-cards image, for example, alludes to the fear that "the whole thing [may] come crashing down," but ends with the "good news" that, if she leaves the six of clubs in place, she can "feel well practically every day." Hoping to endear herself to her doctor, S. makes her communication clever and entertaining. She teases D. about producing the pain in her joints, jokes about his having to redo an injection that did not take the first time, and frames her own lessons about what to avoid as programs of action her doctor could follow if he "wish[ed] to feel lousy some day." That her project was to secure her doctor's medical attention by retaining his personal affection is clear from the penultimate paragraph. In cloyingly sweet language, she writes: "[S]ometimes I think it is not the new medical regime but the new doctor that is making me feel so much better." So deep and sincere was her belief that she could garner good health care by making her doctor happy that she did not even flinch when she wrote that line. As the summer wore on, she would continue to follow an ethic of care that placed her doctor's happiness above everything, including her own emotional and physical well-being.

The First Big Failure

No sooner had S. mailed this letter to her doctor than the house of cards did come crashing down. The first week in her new lakeside location had gone tolerably well, with only occasional mild back pain and headaches. Then, on July 18, the headaches descended and refused to go away. On the first, second, and third days, according to S.'s charts, the headaches remained "mild." On the fourth day they grew worse and were accompanied by dizziness. Her chart for that day notes: "Persistent headache feels chemically induced; [Managed to work] despite headache, [though] very hard to think and write effectively; Headache stayed, turning to notable dizziness in late afternoon" (July 21). On the fifth, sixth, and seventh days the low-grade headache developed into a middle-grade one. Her chart reads: "Total breakdown; Low- to mid-grade headache all day (July 22);" "Persistent mid-grade headache" (July 23); "Moderate, throbbing headache all day" (July 24).

S. had had headaches in the past few months, but they had been manageable because they rarely lasted beyond one day. These were different. They went on, day after day, with no break and with S. not knowing when—or if—they would ever go away. Try as she might, S. could not figure out what had caused them. Neither her friends nor her family could make heads or tails of them. Desperate for relief, she finally called her doctor in Seattle. Here is her report of that conversation:

> Well, my honeymoon with my body is over. For the first five weeks of my time on the East Coast, I felt wonderful and, when I did not, I was able to analyze the situation and figure out what I was doing wrong. Now I cannot figure out what is going wrong. I have had a *low- to mid-grade headache for seven days running,* and nothing I do seems to make a dent. I finally had no choice but to call [D.].
>
> The lesson: pushing it produces peril, pain, and punishment. It is not worth it. (I pushed it because I just cannot stand to feel so dis-abled and incapable of doing *anything*. And I thought it was time to start thinking about self-strengthening. I was wrong.)
>
> What to do? Well, [the doctor] gave me six changes to make:
>
> 1. Get a larger base pillow for the neck-roll casing.
> 2. Turn the pillow over so the neck roll is up.
> 3. Take 1 and 1/2 Flexeril tablets so I don't wake up early.
> 4. Take maximum dosage of Tylenol with codeine [12 tablets a day].
> 5. Stop swimming for a few days.
> 6. Wear a neck brace.
>
> Well, I'm trying those I can here. The first night I did not sleep more and awoke with exactly the same kind of headache. What did I ever do to deserve this??? That is the question that distresses me no end. (Diary, July 24)

Effective treatment depended on correct analysis of the underlying problem. S. thought the headaches felt chemically induced—that is, related to her medications. But when she shared that idea with her doctor, he dismissed it, insisting that the headaches were connected to her fibromyalgic neck problems. S. admitted that possibility but could find nothing in what her doctor said to explain the neck problems. The only explanation that made any sense was that her swimming had exacerbated the neck pain, which in turn had produced the headaches. S. was frustrated beyond belief. She had begun to swim daily, because she could no longer stand feeling disabled by her disease. The result was greater disability than before. "What happened?" she asks herself in anguish, "I wish to god I knew."

The doctor suggested six changes that she should make, all based on the assumption that the headaches were fibromyalgic in nature. Over the next few days S. tried all of them, driving forty miles to the south to get a neck collar, going ten miles north to get a new pillow base, and calling her husband in New York to ask him to send her vial of Tylenol with codeine. Some of the strategies proved counterproductive. For example, when she increased the dosage of the sleep medication, she felt drugged all day. After two days she returned to the original dose. She tried turning her pillow over so the neck roll was on top, but doing so produced new pain. Before she could implement even half the doctor's strategies, however, the headaches disappeared just as miraculously as they had appeared. Inexplicably, they returned a few days later and, just as mysteriously, vanished again. Although these headaches continued to come and go throughout the summer, they usually lasted for only one or two days. S. learned to live with them and to focus her energies on other, more tractable symptoms.

More Successes, More Restrictions

S. was only too happy to put the baffling seven-day headache behind her and get on with her project of self-monitoring and self-regulation. During late July and early August she remained hypervigilant about her activities and made a host of discoveries about things that increased her discomfort. As her findings multiplied, her list of lessons grew.

More Lessons for the Fibromyalgic: Self-Orders Become Self-Abuse

Exercise continued to be a major item on her list. Here are some of the new lessons S. learned on that front:

Lesson: Rowing leads to back pain.

Lesson: Canoeing produces a lot of neck pain. No canoeing!

Lesson: Best to cut out backstroke altogether—[it is] really hard on the neck.

Lesson: One form of aerobic exercise a day is *enough*.

The orders she issued to herself regarding sleep were especially numerous. Here are a few:

Lesson: Don't use neck roll [pillow]. Leads to shoulder/upper back pain.

Lesson: Stay on sleep schedule no matter what.

Lesson: Go to bed by 10:30—meds don't adjust to your variable bedtime schedule.

Lesson: Be in bed 1/2 hour after taking Ambien!

Lesson: Waking up one hour early can mean (mild) headache! So sensitive!

Lesson: Don't disturb your daily schedule in any way.

Even S.'s eating habits seemed to be implicated in her sleep problems and, in turn, the headaches. These too came to be subject to self-commands:

Lesson: Don't eat anything more than a small dinner—*EVER!*

Lesson: Don't snack just before bed, dummy!

What is striking about these lesson-commands is how harsh S. had become toward herself. The doctor's microenvironmental theory had identified her daily activities as the source of the fibromyalgic headaches and neck pain. Ever the good patient, S. had accepted the blame and begun scouring her life to discover what she was "doing wrong" (Diary, July 24) to cause the problems. We saw in chapter 3 how, during the spring, the doctor had used threats, accusations, and trivializations of her suffering to get her to follow his orders. Now, in applying his treatment program to her life, S. reproduced his punitive tone in her orders to herself. With the boundaries between her doctor's self and her own self blurred, she began to issue punishing commands to herself—"No canoeing!" "Don't disturb anything!"—even calling herself abusive names like "dummy" to bring her self into line. In taking her doctor's approach to fibromyalgia to its logical conclusion, S. turned on her self like a stern patriarch-physician. With her care focused on her doctor, there was no one to protect her from this double dose of abuse.

S.'s close relatives did everything in their power to help her. To amuse and distract her, her husband ghost wrote precious letters from her beloved cat, filled with tales of butterflies chased and mice gobbled down on the run. Her sisters offered suggestions and support over the phone. Her parents fed her wholesome dinners and provided companionship whenever she wanted it. But S. remained obsessed with her symptoms, her body, and her doctor, adhering to the doctor's program of self-discipline as though her very life depended on it. Her family members could only look helplessly on as their loved one's life continued its downward spiral.

Another Adoring Letter to Dr. D.

When the orders to the self worked and the pain dissipated, S. felt a renewed sense of empowerment. In mid-August, about the time of her second missed appointment, she wrote another letter to her doctor to tell him how well she was doing. I quote this letter at length because it shows the extremes to which she took the ethic of care.

15 August 1996

Dear [Dr. D.],

A Canada high sits over northern Maine today, bringing a brisk breeze from the north, spectacular sunshine, and shimmering waves that play on the lake. And so I thought of you. You wanted to hear good news. Today seems like a good time to write with some.

The elevated sed rate you reported on the phone a couple days ago (29) does not map onto my perceptions of my bodily reality. My joints have been enjoying a nearly painfree summer, and when fibromyalgia-related pain or poor sleep occurs I can always trace it back to something I've done . . .

I like to have pain *some* days because it provides an opportunity to learn more lessons about what to avoid. Last week my wrists began to complain a little—soaping in the shower, for example, became a bit of a trial. I figured the only thing that could be causing them to act up was the swimming: pulling against the water puts quite a bit of strain on the wrists. So I started wearing wrist splints while swimming. Voilà! The wrist pain has almost disappeared. All this figuring-out-of-stuff of course makes me feel greatly empowered. All you had to do was say two words—"environmental" and "mechanical"—and a whole new way of analyzing and gaining significant control over my life opened up. I am so grateful to you for those verbal magic carpets!

I've been having fun devising new swimming strokes that diversify my exercise routine and spread the stress over a larger number of joints . . . Because I swim with a snorkel and mask, it's possible to use the water to relax my neck/head in a way I would not be able to if I had to worry about breathing when waves roil the water surface (a frequent occurrence here). A Maine lake is not a Caribbean coral reef, but it's still fun to watch the fish . . . Why am I telling you all this? Mostly in hopes that my experiences might give faith to other patients who want badly to swim even though swimming seems bad for their joints . . .

I've been sleeping very well (7 to 8 hours a night), except for nights when my routine gets disrupted (which are invariably bad ones) . . .

I do want to say that I think this heavy-medication approach to the psoriatic arthritis was a brilliant move. I'm remembering with a smile how I was willing to "suspend judgment" last March, but basically could not let myself believe I could get better. Of course, I am living in a rose-colored bubble here, suspended up and away from most of the stresses of normal life. The real test will come in January when I have to return to [my university in southern California] . . .

Well, I hope that news was good enough to lift your spirits at least a little bit. I truly hate to spend all this time writing about myself, but I did want to stay in touch and there was no other obvious way to do so.

Signing off, for now . . .

Your grateful patient,

S.

This sugary letter was a product of older patterns of communication and of a new development as well. In late July, when S. was stricken by the seven-day headache, her doctor had neglected to return her first phone call, forcing her to call again four days later. Humiliated and fearful that her doctor had already forgotten about her, S. began to invest all the more heavily in her relationship with him, using her letters and phone conversations to bind him more closely to her. This letter shows the extremes to which S. took that strategy. Whereas during the spring and early summer, S.'s goal of making her doctor happy had been kept in the background, here it is foregrounded, becoming the explicit, indeed, the sole aim of the communication. S.'s desire to make her doctor happy literally frames the letter, providing both opening and closing statements. "You wanted to hear good news," she declares at the outset. "Today . . . [I] write with some." And at the end she writes, "I hope that news was good enough to lift your spirits." In addition to sharing her feelings of health and empowerment, S. expresses strong gratitude to her doctor, praising his heavy-medication approach to the arthritis as "brilliant" and thanking him for his "verbal magic carpets," which gave her a "whole new way of analyzing and gaining significant control over [her] life." The doctor must have been very happy to read this letter. In her efforts to find beguiling formulations, however, S. goes overboard, writing that she "like[s] to have pain *some* days because it provides an opportunity to learn more lessons about what to avoid." This line, which sounds less funny than pathological, provides an early hint of the mental dis-order that would descend in the fall as she continued to destroy her life to make her body better, only to watch it get worse.

The Statistics Show Not Success, but Failure

So far S.'s summer project of controlling her new symptoms had produced mixed results. Only a few days after she posted that happy letter to her doctor she began to wonder if things were quite as good as she had represented them—to her doctor and, perhaps more important, to herself.

After more than two months of medical self-management, S. was beginning to feel that there was a point beyond which her interventions were doing no good. For example, no matter how closely she monitored her activities and how many of them she excised from her life, the headaches kept on coming. Nor could she ever guarantee a good night's sleep. Moreover, S. had been managing her medical conditions daily. She had been so focused on the micropicture of which activities today caused what problems tomorrow that she had little idea of the overall trajectory of her conditions. How much better had she actually gotten since she had begun to see Dr. D.? Because her memory had played tricks on her, she had only a vague idea. Her mind had blurred the pain of the past to focus on the improvement of the present. Though this forgetting helped her make it from day to day, it had also distorted her sense of how her conditions had changed over the long run. Finally, the emergence of the new symptoms of fibromyalgia, a subject S. found so distressing that she tried very hard to push it out of her mind, kept coming back to trouble her. Was she gradually gaining control over the symptoms, or were they coming to control her?

In late August S. determined to face up to these difficult questions and find the answers. It seemed an apt time to take stock, because it was just six months since she had started seeing Dr. D. That was the amount of time he had asked for to bring her symptoms under control. One fine morning she pulled out all the charts she had kept between April and August, got out her calculator, and began to compute some statistics. Whenever possible, she used her recollections of her bodily conditions in February, before she began seeing Dr. D., as a baseline. She omitted March, because it had been devoted to the dreadful drug experiments and, aside from her drug chart, she had no record or even much memory of what had happened then. What was certain was that, however

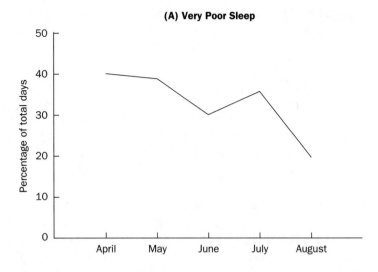

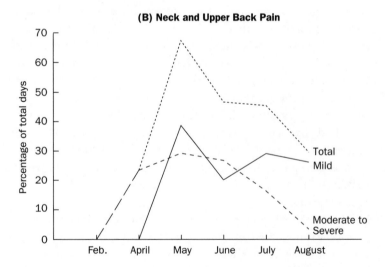

Figure 2. Patient Success in Controlling the Symptoms of "Fibromyalgia"

wretched she felt in February, she felt massively more so in March. The
results of her calculations can be found in figure 2.

The statistics showed that there had been substantial, if far from complete, success in alleviating the sleep problem (see panel A). The proportion of nights of very poor sleep—those producing debilitating fa-

(C) Headache

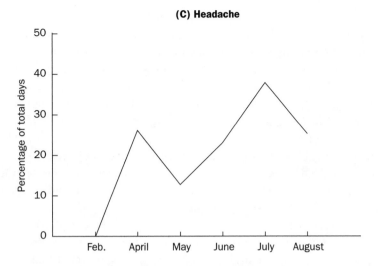

(D) Functional Incapacitation

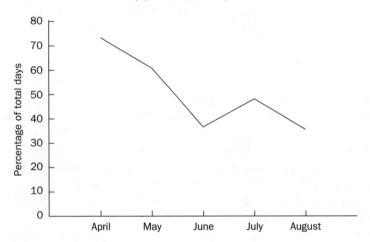

Figure 2. *(continued)*

tigue the next day—slid from about 40 percent in April and May to 30 to 35 percent in June and July, before declining sharply to 20 percent in August. Though the trend was promising, the numbers showed that on one day in five S. still got far too little sleep. And the proportion of nights of truly restful sleep remained too low even to count.

When S. tracked the new symptoms that had emerged after treatment began, the numbers showed that she had legitimate grounds for concern. The neck and back pain, plotted in panel B, showed a pattern of marked worsening in the spring, followed by improvement as the summer wore on. Overall, the proportion of days on which S. suffered neck and/or back pain surged from none in the months before treatment to a high of 68 percent in May. The overall prevalence of pain in this region then began to fall, slipping to three days in ten by August. S.'s statistics allowed her to distinguish between mild and more severe degrees of neck and back pain. Here the news was better: during these same months, pain of moderate-to-severe intensity grew worse and then better, becoming negligible by August. At the same time, the prevalence of milder forms of pain grew, rising from nil in April to a high of almost 40 percent in May, then falling slightly to 20 to 30 percent in the ensuing months. Despite S.'s mighty efforts to reduce the back and neck pain, the extent of mild pain in that region had shown virtually no change over the summer months.

The most debilitating new symptom was the headaches. While severe headaches made it impossible for S. to do anything, even mild headaches took the edge off her mind, making it difficult to concentrate on her writing. The figures, graphed in panel C, showed a worrying increase in headaches over time. From a headache-free condition in the months before she had fallen under the "gaze" of Dr. D., the fraction of days marred by headache inched up to one in four in April. That number dipped in May and rose again to reach a high of two in five in July, before sliding back to one in four in August. The figure for July was particularly bad: in that month S. had a headache an average of three days a week.

To see changes in functional capacity, something her doctor had promised she could improve, S. added the number of days with headaches to the number of days with serious fatigue. The combined number gave the proportion of days in which she was essentially unable to do her professional work. The calculations, pictured in panel D, showed that during April S. was functionally incapacitated an appalling 75 percent of the time. In May that figure fell to about 60 percent. The extent of functional incapacity dropped to about 35 percent in June, climbed back to 50 percent in July, and then slid again to 35 percent in August. The decline between July and August was small comfort, for what the figures said was that, even in the best of times, S. was losing as many as one-third of her days to her fibromyalgia.

Overall, the statistics were hugely discouraging. They said that, even after she had cut everything fun out of her life and imposed rigid disciplines on what was left, she continued to suffer debilitating symptoms a significant amount of the time. Pursuing a doctor-centered ethic of care, she had followed her doctor's theory to a letter, yet, for some unfathomable reason, that theory had failed to make her better.

We track S.'s reactions to these discoveries in chapter 9. First, though, we take a detour to tell the story of the other well-body project that S. pursued during the summer. Although S. did not yet doubt the veracity of her doctor's theories, she knew the limitations of the biomedical approach to health care and wanted to do everything in her power to rid herself of the symptoms. She was also keenly aware of the risks of her doctor's drug-intensive strategy and hoped to supplement the drugs with less harmful methods of making the body well. It was with such fears and hopes that she turned to alternative medicine to learn how to mobilize her mind to heal her body.

CHAPTER 8 **"Accept It!"**

Alternative Medicines Offer Medicine for the Mind

During the spring S. had struggled unsuccessfully to shake off the depression that enveloped her life like a dark fog. With the arrival of summer and, with it, breathing space from her university obligations, she determined to tackle the emotional and even spiritual dimensions of her new life condition head-on. Instinctually, she turned to books for insight and inspiration. Over the months, she had collected a good number of books on subjects as diverse as meditation, visualization, aromatherapy, and stress management. Some had fallen into her hands serendipitously, as she perused local bookstores for inspirational texts. Others had been sent or recommended by concerned friends and family members. What tied these books together, what made them into treasures in her personal quest for spiritual gold, was their common concern with understanding the mind-body connection and using these understandings as resources for self-healing.[1]

About a month into the summer, when she was finally ready to face up to these emotionally difficult issues, S. began reading and thinking about the books she had gathered. She soon discovered that, despite the differences in topic and tone, all the books she had collected propagated a set of ideas that has become a powerful current in American culture. These ideas are that the mind and emotions have profound effects on the body; that the individual is in charge of the state of his or her mind and emotions; and that the individual, therefore, is also in good part responsible for her health—and, by implication, her illness. What is wrong with contemporary culture, the critique goes, is the constant striving and struggling against what is. Americans need to learn that the first and most essential step on the road to healing is to *accept what is,* including disease, discomfort, symptoms, and pain. People who "fight it" only hurt themselves and make it harder to get well.

S. found this advice paradoxically empowering and disempowering.

It was empowering, because it offered hope that she could regain control over her body and her life. Yet it was disempowering, because it placed the responsibility both for causing and for curing or "healing" her medical conditions on her. In locating the cause of the problem in the individual patient, the books on alternative and New Age medicine neglected the possibility that larger structural forces—the inequalities of race, class, and gender, for example, or even biomedicine itself—might be partly at fault in many cases. And by counseling acceptance of what is—the symptom, the disease, the diagnosis—they embodied the powerful assumption that scientific medicine does not or cannot err in its labeling and treatment of disease. At the same time, these approaches ruled out the possibility that continued struggle and search for the source of the problems outside the individual might be a better route to healing in some cases.

This chapter describes the messages S. took away from these books and the helpful and less-than-helpful things she did in a desperate attempt to make the mind-cure work where the body-cure had not. Fighting to push the monster of depression away, she struggled to stay focused on the positive, empowering message that if she just followed the right strategies, she could use her mind to conquer the pain in her body and remake her life along new and happier lines. It was a hopeful message, and she threw her energies into it for about a month. By the end of the summer, however, S.'s enthusiasm for mind work had fizzled out. Try as she might, the philosophy of acceptance and the techniques of creative visualization did not take her symptoms away or even help her forget about them. In the end she had to find her own way. That way was to keep fighting what everyone—from her doctor to the books to friends and family who echoed popular medical advice—said was the "truth." That way was to continue searching for the source of her pain in locations outside herself. As she pursued her own alternative-to-the-alternative route, S. found that the pervasive cultural discourse of acceptance and individual responsibility, intended to help people, became yet another obstacle she had to overcome. These cultural messages were a hurdle on the road to healing, because they left her feeling accused and ashamed. She was to blame both for her pain and for her failure to get rid of it through mental techniques. Because she felt accused, her experiences with the cultural discourses on mind-body connections also left her feeling isolated from family, friends, and society at large. In the end she felt all alone in her struggle for survival.

"Stop Fighting It!" Alternative Medicine and New-Age Philosophy Render Advice

As she began her search for new ideas and practical solutions to her problems, S. found inspiration and solace in her books. In contrast to the radically reductionistic discourses of biomedicine, the books on alternative and New Age medicine were full of evidence of the power of the mind and emotions to heal the body. And they contained a wealth of ideas, some more practical than others, on ways to use the mind and soul to promote healing and wellness. The books were encouraging in other ways as well. Relying on mental strategies and herbal remedies, they offered a welcome alternative to the potentially dangerous drugs her doctor had prescribed. In contrast to Dr. D.'s ultracontrolling approach, the new philosophies placed the patient in charge, promising a level of patient empowerment that could never be achieved with biomedicine. Finally, the books offered an uplifting, hopeful view of a future in which things could improve. The contrast with her doctor's dark, pessimistic outlook on the future could not be more striking. In turning to the self-help brand of alternative medicine and New Age philosophy, S. hoped not to supplant conventional medicine, but to supplement it with treatment strategies that were less noxious and, perhaps, ultimately more effective. She found three of those books especially helpful. Just below I give her readings of these texts at the time. The reader should remember that these were the readings of a very sick person desperate to get well. S. read for helpful ideas, skipping over those that seemed unhelpful or problematic.

Spontaneous Healing

One of S.'s favorite books was Andrew Weil's *Spontaneous Healing: How to Discover and Enhance Your Body's Natural Ability to Maintain and Heal Itself.*[2] In this popular best-seller, Weil, a medical doctor by training, argued that the body has a natural healing system that, when activated, can lead to spontaneous healing of even the most serious diseases. "Medicine that takes advantage of these innate mechanisms of healing," he wrote, "is more effective than medicine that simply suppresses symptoms."[3] His book provided detailed practical advice on how to optimize the natural healing system and improve the management of illness.

Conventional medicine attends only to the body, but the body and mind are intimately interrelated. By attending to matters of mind and spirit, belief and emotion, Weil advised, one can often unlock the process of spontaneous healing.[4] If only the depression that people with serious illness feel could be "accessed and moved," he wrote, "it [could] be a catalyst for spontaneous healing."[5] The master key to natural healing, Weil argued, is a mental shift to an attitude of acceptance, submission, surrender. "Most people . . . are in a state of perpetual confrontation, trying by the imposition of will to shape events and control situations."[6] But the author's many interviews with people who have experienced healing revealed that fighting one's disease was counterproductive. More productive is accepting one's life as it is, disease and all: "Acceptance of illness is often part of a larger acceptance of self that represents a significant mental shift, a shift that can initiate transformation of personality and with it the healing of disease."[7]

In his concluding chapter Weil identified seven strategies that underlie patient success. "Successful patients," he advised, not only cultivate self-acceptance; they also refuse to take no for an answer, actively search for help, seek out people who have been healed, and form constructive partnerships with health professionals. In the mental and emotional domain, they regard illness not as a misfortune but as a gift, because it provides an opportunity for personal growth. Finally, they are willing to make radical changes in their lives in order to "open the blocks" to spontaneous healing.[8]

In these terms S. was already well on her way to becoming a "successful patient." She had worked hard to make her relationship with Dr. D. a close if hardly equal partnership. She had actively searched for information on her diseases and their treatment. She had construed her "DD&PP" as a gift and was ready to make big changes in her life to heal her ills. The only task that remained was to cultivate self-acceptance. Keeping that in mind, she set Weil aside and moved on to the next book in the pile.

Mindfulness Meditation

S. knew from her own body and life that stress made her conditions worse. For ideas on stress reduction as a route to illness abatement, she turned to *Full Catastrophe Living: Using the Wisdom of Your Body and Mind to Face Stress, Pain, and Illness.*[9] This book was a practical, step-by-step guide to relaxation and coping with stress through "mindful meditation." Its author, Jon Kabat-Zinn, was a medical doctor and director of the Stress Reduction Clinic at the University of Massachusetts Medical Center.

Taking his lead from Zorba of the novel *Zorba the Greek*, Kabat-Zinn likened life to a "full catastrophe"—full of joy as well as sorrow and disaster, tragedy and irony. Given the inevitability of chaos and calamity, the only way to respond to life was to embrace it, to celebrate it, and to laugh at it and at one's own foibles and follies.[10] The trick was to live life as if every moment, even moments of pain and despair, counted and could be "worked with."[11] "This 'work,'" he wrote, "involves . . . the regular disciplined practice of moment-to-moment awareness or *mindfulness,* the complete 'owning' of each moment of your experience." Through mindfulness, you take the "scattered and reactive energies of your mind and [focus] them into a coherent source of energy for living, for problem solving, and for healing."[12]

Mindfulness, Kabat-Zinn maintained, is best cultivated through meditation. To tap into the healing power of mindful meditation, one needs to develop new attitudes toward learning. In the stress reduction clinic, Kabat-Zinn and his colleagues teach that seven attitudes promote the practice of mindfulness. These are nonjudging, patience, a beginner's mind, trust, nonstriving, acceptance, and letting go.[13] Acceptance does not mean that you have to like what is or be resigned to the fact that things always have to be as they are now. Rather, "[a]cceptance . . . simply means that you have come around to a willingness to see things as they are."[14]

In meditation, patients with painful symptoms are urged to experience those symptoms fully to learn from them:

> By sitting with some discomfort and accepting it as part of our experience in the moment . . . we discover that it is actually possible to relax into physical discomfort. This is one example of how discomfort or even pain can be your teacher and help you to heal.[15] The way of mindfulness is to accept ourselves right now, as we are, symptoms or no symptoms, pain or no pain, fear or no fear. Instead of rejecting our experience as undesirable, we ask, "What is this symptom saying, what is it telling me about my body and my mind right now?"[16]

Healing, a major aim of mindful meditation, is not the same as curing. Healing is a transformation of view, a profound mental shift "brought about by the encounter with one's own wholeness."[17] This shift toward acceptance promotes feelings of inner peace, control, and optimism. And "sometimes . . . it is also accompanied by a major reduction in physical symptoms."[18]

Kabat-Zinn's book was full of encouraging ideas. S. especially liked the thought of putting laughter and self-levity to therapeutic use. She took up meditating and promised herself that she would continue to pursue this form of relaxation. But before committing to any particular program of meditation she wanted to finish her reading.

Life as a Work of Art

It was the third book, Shakti Gawain's *Creative Visualization*, that truly captured S.'s imagination.[19] Although the book was not about health per se, Gawain, a well-known New Age guru, described techniques for improving one's life that could readily be applied in the domain of the body. Gawain's short book outlined a philosophy of life according to which the world is made up of energy, which can be harnessed, through techniques of the imagination, to make changes in one's physical, emotional, mental, or spiritual being. She explained it this way: "In creative visualization you use your imagination to create a clear image, idea, or feeling of something you wish to manifest. Then you continue to focus on the idea . . . giving it positive energy, until it becomes objective reality."[20]

When we are negative and fearful, Gawain writes, we often attract into our lives those things we most fear, whereas when we are positive and hopeful, the good things we want come to us. In other words, our often unconscious negative thoughts have produced the negative things in our lives; by bringing these fears to light and replacing them with positive ones, we can remove the blocks and help ourselves get the good things we want.[21] In a short chapter on healing, Gawain applied these same ideas to health and disease. People get sick, she wrote, because:

> [T]hey believe on an inner level that illness is an appropriate or inevitable response to some situation . . . because it in some way seems to solve a problem for them, or gets them something that they need, or because it is a desperate solution to some unresolved and unbearable inner conflict.[22]

Echoing a theme sounded by Kabat-Zinn, she declared that the first step in healing is to ask what message the sickness is sending about parts of the consciousness that need to be recognized, acknowledged, and healed. Remember, she cautioned, "not all ailments are meant to be 'healed' in the sense of getting well . . . Some may serve an important purpose in our lives, or in our soul's journey, and may stay with us for a long time, or for life."[23]

For Gawain life is full of surprises, things that happen in ways that no one plans. To make room for the unexpected to happen, one must accept what is and understand that life knows no losses, only gains.[24] With this insight, one can use every moment as an opportunity to create what one wants in life, all the while remaining open for new things to happen that may be better than those imagined:

> In . . . hanging onto what we have, we fail to keep the energy moving and we don't make space for new energy [and surprising things] to come to us.[25] *Always remember that you are creating something new and fresh.* You are not trying to redo or change what already exists. To do so would be to resist what is, which creates conflict and struggle. Take the attitude that you are accepting and handling whatever already exists . . . and at the same time taking every moment as a new opportunity to begin creating exactly what you desire and will make you happiest.[26]

Gawain offered many imaginative and fun techniques for putting her ideas into practice. The most important was meditation, a practice that is enhanced through imaginary processes such as creating a sanctuary, meeting one's guide, and using "pink bubble techniques" (described below) to symbolize the letting go of thoughts. She also recommended the use of "clearing," the bringing to consciousness of old, self-defeating fears and thoughts, and "affirmations," strong positive statements that something desired already exists. Other techniques included goal setting, methods to deepen self-acceptance and self-appreciation, and a variety of listing and meditational techniques to get the energies moving in more positive directions.

S. liked this book right away. She read it several times, underlining and highlighting in multiple colors passages that made sense of her life. Gawain's outlook was optimistic, positive. She had said that there are no losses, only gains; that the world is trying to give us everything we want; that life is basically good and abundant; that having what one wants, without struggle, is part of one's natural birthright; and that through a change of consciousness we can effect change in our bodies. To S. these were comforting and encouraging thoughts, words of hope after a spring of despair.

"Accepting It": The Good Things List

Shakti's book (Shakti encouraged readers to call her by her first name) apparently provided the stimulus S. needed, for two days after reading it she began the painful task of facing up to the emotional consequences of her new diseases. In the spring, after deciding that her doctor's DD&PP was a gift because it forced her to make big changes in her life, S. had created a loose-leaf notebook to accommodate all the ideas, images, and information she planned to gather on how she might compose a new life. She called it her "Make-a-New-Life Book" (MANL Book). Now, with Shakti's ideas as catalyst, she began adding to that notebook. In her first entry of the summer, she described her resistance to confronting the emotional issues and how that very resistance had allowed the depression to maintain its grip on her:

> Boy, I *really* have to do some headwork, some selfwork . . . I guess that's why I came to Maine—to figure some things out, to self-strengthen in a safe, comfortable place. Well, the space is that, but I've been avoiding the self-work like the plague. Trouble is, since I refuse to come to grips with this stuff, the depression—from a million things, but especially from the illness stuff—just hangs on. I put on a cheery face and fight it off for as long as I can. But then, in weak moments, or when a new set of symptoms sets in, I just fall to pieces, give in to the eternal sadness of life, cry myself to sleep. I know this is really unhealthy. I've got to shake this depression, which has been hanging over me like a dark shadow . . . for years. . . . I know I *have* to get control of this, to turn myself back into that happy person I used to be. . . . After all, I really don't want to spend the rest of my life like this. (MANL Book, July 28)

But how was S. to gain control over her depression? All the books she had read counseled accepting her illnesses as something that had happened, something that had become an undeniable part of her new self. So she tried to accept it:

> I got the first glimmer that I had to "accept it"—the ill, imperfect body— the spring of 1996, when I was forced to come to terms with [D.'s] "dismal diagnosis and poor prognosis." I came around, within only a few weeks— though horribly bad . . . weeks they were—to seeing this DD & PP as a *gift.* Yes, indeed. *BUT,* I had nothing positive to put in the place of the old image of the-body-beautiful, the-body-lithesome . . . So the sadness, the feeling of deep loss, lingers on, maintaining its firm grip on me, totally taking over my life too, too often.
>
> Now I'm seeing that I can create something new to put in its place. So, the feeling will be not only of loss, but also of gain. Hey—[D.] and I can be co-creators, collaborators in the making of a new, better body for my late 40s, 50s, 60s, 70s, 80s, and 90s! That is a nice thought. I'm not alone in this! I have a wonderful, caring, smart person to work with me on it . . .
>
> [Yet] I have to . . . *really grieve* the things I have lost—the healthy body . . . and probably other things, too, [that] I haven't even thought of. I have to truly, emotionally accept that I have lost them, before I can open the space to . . . allow in something else. (MANL Book, July 28)

Throughout the spring S.'s depression about her illness was rooted in the feeling of loss, the feeling that her life, her dreams, and her hopes were being snatched away from her, never to return. S. found Shakti's idea that one never loses anything, but only gains, extremely comforting. As if to make the feeling of gain more real, S. listed for herself all the "good things" that had emerged from the dis-ease:

Lots of Evidence Already of Surprising, New,
and Good Things to Emerge from "Dis-ease"

So, let's list some of the good things that have come out of my dis-ease(s).

1. I just kept getting "worse and worse" . . . which induced me to work hard to find a new doctor, one who cared and would help arrest the [process]. In a totally unexpected turn of events, I mentioned to [the laboratory technician] that I had always wanted a friend with psoriatic arthritis, she connected me to Anna, and Anna urged me to see [D.], and so I found a wonderful new doctor/co-creator of my new body. In a word: I found [Dr. D.].

2. [D.'s] "DD&PP"—just wonderful, in the end. It scared me into taking responsibility for my health and agreeing to a rather drastic, high-chemical-input approach to making the well-body. My [arthritis] is now so [controlled that] the inflammation level is within normal range. This is a dramatic turnaround . . . In a word: a new body—in many senses indeed!

3. . . . The DD&PP also "scared" me into realizing that I need to make some drastic changes in other parts of my life. This is much to the good—a conclusion I've been trying to suppress for years. . . .

Not all the changes, however, could be construed as "good." The restrictions on her swimming are a case in point:

4. So, my latest "distressing discovery"—that is how I experienced it—is that swimming (daily, rapid build-up) is NOT OK. What good will come of this? Here I need to keep an open mind, an open heart . . . (MANL Book, July 28)

S. saw in her own body striking evidence for Shakti's point that life was full of unexpected turns and surprising outcomes. Speaking of the disease, she writes, with wry humor: "Here is a prime example of something I did not plan!" She goes on to list yet more "wondrous, wonderful things" that have come out of becoming ill, concluding, with perhaps a touch of overexuberance, that it was better to have been ill and enjoy improvement than to have never been ill at all:

Life Is Full of (Often Wonderful) Surprises

Hey—I used to think the development of all these symptoms and medically-labeled "conditions" was just BADBADBAD. But now I think:

Wow! Think of all the surprising, wondrous, wonderful things that have come out of these physical changes. I got to have two operations, fascinating insight into the operations of the medical establishment, new understandings of the workings of the body and its connections to the mind, . . . a chance . . . to . . . reorganize [my life] along quite different lines at midlife, and new, deep empathy for people with medical conditions . . . Oh yes, and one more surprising outcome—after . . . feeling wretched for so many years, I can now enjoy the profound pleasure of feeling well! Surely, it will turn out that it is better to have felt pain and then wellness, than to never have had a change in bodily well-being at all. (MANL Book, July 31)

"Removing the Blocks": The Negative Thoughts List

Recognizing the good things that had come from her illness was an important part of the process of creating a new life. But before she could "move on" and create that life, S. had to "remove the blocks" to "get the energy flowing." Both Gawain and Kabat-Zinn had insisted that it was necessary to ask, What is the illness telling you? What message is it trying to convey? So S. asked herself those questions:

> Let's ask another question: what "message" is this six-year period of almost progressive dis-ease sending me? And/or, what . . . purpose is it serving in my life? Surely, "it" is telling me it is time to make a change! To set my life off in a different direction. Different from what? From pushing way beyond the limits of the bodily/humanly reasonable. The two-handed carpal tunnel surgery [followed by] immediate resumption of professional travel—such a wonderful example of an old self I need to remake. (MANL Book, July 28)

S. had determined that the old self had to go. But what was preventing her from getting rid of that old self? For quite some time she had been stuck, glued into a state of depression by a host of mostly unexamined fears about what her diseases might mean for her life. She decided to bring those fears to light in hopes that doing so would reveal them to be not only unhelpful but also untrue. That is what Shakti had promised. S. ransacked her mind in search of her deepest fears about disease. The list she compiled shows that most of them centered on "disability" and loss of function:

What are My (Mostly Negative, Self-Defeating)
Feelings Around Body/Dis-ease/Health?

1. I am so "dis-abled!" I can no longer do any of the things I've done so easily and well all my life!

2. My life is just one big list of "No's"!

3. The number of things I can do is shrinking daily! Pretty soon all I'll be able to do is sit . . . and look straight ahead [at a book or computer screen].

4. All the things I enjoy, I can't do anymore!

5. Life is just a daily struggle. Every little thing has become a huge chore.

6. I can't swim any more! Swimming is the second most important thing in my life, coming just after being able to do my writing . . .

7. A major part of my identity has always [revolved around having] a [nice] figure [and] agile body. Now I have been robbed of my identity. (MANL Book, July 28)

"Moving Forward":
The Personal Goals and Protective Bubbles Lists

Now that she had brought these fears out into the open and, she hoped, relaxed their hold on her, the next step was to decide on a set of personal goals. Having a clear set of aims was crucial, for they provided a focus and direction in which to channel one's energies. Shakti had emphasized the connection between imagination and reality, between forming goals and realizing them: "As soon as I have a very clear, strong intention to create a particular thing, it manifests almost immediately."[27]

S. had never asked herself about her health goals. She had seen herself as a victim of a bad body and a nasty disease; since she had no control over the process, of what use was it to speak of goals? But now she realized that she was not a victim of her body or her ills. To the contrary, she was an active agent of her own life who could use her mind to change the course of her disease. With these new understandings, she got into the goal-setting mood with ease. Here are her ruminations about that change of attitude:

Body/Dis-ease/Health: Personal Goals

This is a new question! What to say? Mostly I try not to ask or find out about the future—that is, the prospects for improvement, according to medical science—because I am afraid the answer will be bad, discouraging, depressing . . . [But actually] science is its own world, and it's only one. The mind has other ways of healing that are invisible to scientists and their methods. So, I'll let science . . . do its thing, and I'll do something else. Let's . . . accept the idea that the mind and imagination have powerful effects on the body. From this it follows that, by creating a new mindview,

I can create a new body . . . Therein lie[s the rationale for] my bodily
goals . . . What might some be? (MANL Book, July 29)

A few days later S. set some short-term goals for her two conditions. She
"gives them energy" by telling herself how eminently achievable they are
and how capable she is of achieving them:

Body/Dis-ease/Health: Personal Goals

1. This summer the arthritis has miraculously disappeared! . . . So, my
   short-term goal ([for a] few months) is to keep the joints happy and
   well and to lower my sed rate further—to make [Dr. D.] happy! This
   is very do-able . . .

2. On the fibromyalgia, my short-term (this week, a few weeks) goal is
   to reduce the proportion of days I have a headache (most common) or
   back and neck pain. I do this by constantly being aware of and noting
   things that promote headaches, then avoiding them on future days. This
   is not a matter of "suffering ever-more limitations on living"—it is a
   matter of feeling better, going through each and every day feeling fit and
   fine. I *can do* that! . . . (MANL Book, July 31)

To help ensure realization of her goals, S. used some of the creative
imagery techniques that Shakti had suggested. Here she describes an
"imaginary bubble" she can use to heal her ailments:

Protective and Healing Bubbles

I need some bubbles to start throwing energy into and moving me forward,
so that when I leave my wonderful cocoon [in Maine], I won't be subject
to all the down-pushes of the real world. Here [is one].

"Peach Healing Bubble:" I often awake with an unpleasant, unwelcome
headache. Here's how to urge it away. In the morning, just after I awake,
I'll create a beautiful peach-colored . . . bubble. First it will surround my
head. Then I'll move it upward until it floats on top of my head. It will sit
there for awhile, collecting together all the aches of the head, concentrating
them *outside* of my head. Then, when I'm ready, it will float away with a
breeze. (MANL Book, September 2)

A Failure Twice Over: Blame, Shame, and Isolation

This burst of enthusiasm and creative energy for alternative techniques
came in late July. For a few days S. busily filled her notebook with lists
and plans and devoted herself to meditations, visualizations, affirmations,
and self-appreciations. But her zeal for the imaginative techniques of New
Age teaching soon petered out. Somehow they did not feel quite right.

And mostly they did not work. For example, S. tried to use the healing bubble on a number of headaches. She felt a little silly, but figured she had nothing to lose and everything to gain if the peach bubble alleviated the pain even a tiny bit. Unfortunately, it brought not a modicum of relief. Discouraged, she stopped using the bubble technique.

Other techniques proved counterproductive. S.'s attempt to construct a "good things list" only reminded her that some things, such as the loss of her swimming, were simply *not* good and that the gap between how she really felt about this "distressing discovery" and how she was trying to feel was too great to be papered over with imagining techniques. Similarly, listing all her "negative, self-defeating feelings" about illness did not make S. see that her fears were "unhelpful and untrue." To the contrary, her fears that she was becoming "dis-abled" and that her life was becoming "one big list of 'No's'" were rooted in a bodily reality that was only too real and true. Bringing these fears together in one place simply reminded her of how bad things had gotten.

Despite the efforts S. poured into the task, she could not trick her mind into accepting her diseases and her symptoms. The "master key to natural healing" was said to be shifting to an attitude of acceptance, submission, and surrender. But S. could not make that mental shift. Her mighty efforts notwithstanding, she could not rid herself of the feeling that she was "suffering ever more limitations on living" and replace it with the view that she was "feeling better, going through each and every day feeling fit and fine." The idea that she was supposed to "relax into physical discomfort" seemed especially cruel. How could she "relax into" weeklong headaches that came from nowhere, responded to no treatment, and then went away for no discernible reason? How could she accept these debilitating symptoms that she had never had before? Try as she might, she could not quiet her questioning mind.

As she tried again and again to make her mind heal her body and failed again and again to make it work, S. felt like a personal failure. Indeed, by the standards of the fields she was consulting, she was at fault twice over. Not only had she not succeeded in mobilizing her mind in service of her body, but she was also making things worse by continuing to struggle against "what is." And her bigger wrongdoing was causing her illness in the first place. Gawain had placed the blame squarely on her shoulders: "People get sick because they believe . . . that illness is an appropriate or inevitable response to some situation."[28] Weil had emphatically distanced himself from the view that patients cause their illness or are responsible if they do not get better.[29] But he had said nothing about why alternative healing methods work for some but not for others. What sorts of factors might prevent some patients from enjoying the benefits of non-conventional therapies? On this topic he was silent. Moreover, his book was filled with cases of "successful patients," creating the impression that all readers could be successful if only they tried hard enough. The implication was that those who do not succeed had not done enough.

S. deeply believed that her mind and emotions were deeply implicated in her bodily ills. Internalizing the cultural blame that books like these placed on her, implicitly if not explicitly, she felt blamed for her illness and blamed for her failure to heal it. The feeling of being accused grew more acute every time a well-meaning person in her social world repeated some of the dogmas of alternative or New Age therapy for her benefit. These people were trying hard to help, but the effect was the opposite of what they intended. It happened rarely, but it took only one person telling her she wasn't "letting herself get better" to make her feel that everyone was secretly thinking the same thing. Her feelings of guilt were accompanied by feelings of shame—shame about her illness, which made her "damaged goods" in a culture obsessed with the perfect body, and shame about her lifestyle or personality, which evidently was faulty or she would not be ill. S.'s decision to reject the mind-cure directives and follow a different course also left her socially isolated. Feeling subtly accused by intimates and experts alike, she was all alone in her struggle to restore her bodily and emotional health. Although self-help alternative medicine and New Age therapy contained productive insights about mind-body connections and promising strategies for empowering patients with more body-friendly methods, this encounter with them turned out to be another obstacle on S.'s long road to relief. In the long run they were to help her, but in the short run they compounded her suffering by adding the emotional pain of guilt, shame, and isolation to the physical pain of her symptoms.

At the end of the summer S. set the alternative therapies aside and returned to her single-minded focus on the self-disciplining techniques of biomedicine. We will see in the next chapter that those failed her too, leaving her in a perilous emotional and physical state.

CHAPTER 9

A Life Shrunk, a Mind Gone Nearly Mad

During the summer months S. had followed her doctor's treatment program closely, monitoring her activities to find the source of her fibromyalgic symptoms and limiting those that seemed to contribute to the pain. But that strategy had yielded limited success: at summer's end the new symptoms remained dismayingly serious. Finding alternative therapies of little use and desperate to rid herself of the debilitating headaches and insomnia, in the fall S. redoubled her efforts to make her doctor's discourses work. This chapter shows the lengths to which she took that project and what happened when it failed.

In mid-September S.'s husband drove to Maine to fetch her. After a brief vacation on Vinalhaven, a charming island off the coast of Maine, they returned together to their New York country home, where S. had planned to spend the fall working on her book. But things did not work out as planned. As S.'s bodily and emotional health declined, she drew away from people into an inner universe of terror and dread. Her husband, the only person who saw her regularly, grew increasingly worried about his wife's mental stability. Yet he could not find the way into her inner world. To his intense dismay he was helpless to stop the erosion of her life.

Carrying the discourse of self-surveillance and self-restriction to an extreme, in the fall S. began to slice off more and more parts of her life, until not only her activities but her whole personality was put on the chopping block. But instead of getting better she grew markedly worse. Beginning in September she suffered recurring headaches, tenacious fogginess, and cognitive distortions that ravaged her ability to work. By October, when she had lost everything *but* the symptoms, she began a steep descent into insanity. Unable to halt the decline, she shut everyone out of her life, drastically reduced her intake of food, and drowned herself in tears, edging ever closer to the brink of madness, before a small miracle occurred that saved her life.

The madness that came on her in the fall was the logical result, the end product, of the discourses and practices that had been applied to the patient's body since she came under the gaze of Dr. D.'s brand of bio-medicine. The treatment discourse that did not work pounded the nail into the coffin of S.'s sanity, but the coffin was built of other discourses that had been put in place earlier in the process. Among the most im-portant was the *symptom discourse* that attributed all the new symptoms to fibromyalgia and then omitted them from the evaluation of the doc-tor's success. Another critical plank in the coffin was the *diagnostic dis-course* that bestowed on her "tender points" where usually there was no tenderness and defined her as "fibromyalgic" when she lacked the con-dition's cardinal symptom. Last but most fundamental was the *discourse of objectification* that dismissed S.'s emotions as irrelevant to her bod-ily state and named the doctor the sole expert on the patient's health. In the spring the gap between the lived reality of her body and the medical discourses imposed on it produced a profound sense of epistemological and ontological invalidation. In the fall the gap widened, leading to men-tal disintegration.

The chapter also records the doctor's continued use of rhetorics that furthered the biomedical cause but impeded doctor-patient communica-tion by silencing the patient. Faced with escalating complaints in the early fall, D. opted not to listen to them, but to deflect them with the same sorts of linguistic devices he had used to create a perfect patient in the spring (see chapter 3 for details). Foremost among these were accusations, threats, and trivializations of the patient's concerns and rhetorical aug-mentation of the doctor's own prowess in conquering the patient's dis-ease. Finally, this chapter charts S.'s slow, halting realization that her doc-tor might not be the solution to her problems but the cause of them. Slowly and sputteringly, the growing gap between her doctor's rhetorics of "stu-pendous success" and her own reality of emotional and physical distress began to undermine the trust on which everything had depended. In this void between the two truths—doctor's and patient's—lay the seeds of S.'s eventual revolt against biomedical authority. But that is a story for a later chapter. Here the main plot is the obliteration of a patient's life.

A "Profound Revelation":
My Personality Is Causing the Fibromyalgia

As we saw in chapter 7, at the end of August S. calculated the long-term statistics on her symptoms. The results came as a shock: she had thought she was getting the fibromyalgia under control, but the numbers said otherwise. Dejected, she drafted a letter to her doctor. She wrote that instead of improving, she had "traded one set of unpleasant symptoms for another." And the new symptoms were worse than the old. "With the old set of problems I remained extremely active . . . Now my activities are sharply restricted" (Draft letter, September 1).

The letter reveals S.'s growing concern with finding answers to her frequently asked question of why the new symptoms had appeared. She wanted an elaboration of the doctor's standard but uninformative reply that new symptoms tend to emerge after the sleep problems and fatigue are brought under control. She demanded to know the mechanism by which this occurs. And she raised the possibility that the medications might be at fault. The letter's tone conveys S.'s growing desperation about whether anything could be done to ease her symptoms:

> I hate to ask this because I'm afraid there may be no more answers. For the muscle pain, as I understand it, all one can do is to continue to monitor one's activities and then limit those that create pain. More limits. But the headaches are really not nice. Are there any medications, aside from Tylenol . . . , which do[es] not work for me? Mine seem absolutely invulnerable to treatment. (Draft letter, September 1)

But S. never sent this letter, for after a few days of despondency she had a "profound revelation" about her life and body. Following her doctor's treatment discourse, S. had eliminated more and more activities from her life. Although the strategy had not yet alleviated her symptoms, S. did not trace the problem to the strategy itself; rather, she traced it to the program's still incomplete implementation. What she did next was to carry the discourse one step further toward its logical conclusion. It was not just her daily activities that were causing the problems, she reasoned, but the configuration of her entire personality. All her life she had been a go-getter, a high-energy, hyperactive person who could never relax. It was this ingrained habit of always "pushing it," of stretching the limits of endurance, that underlay all these symptoms. By changing her whole approach to living, she figured, she could conquer the symptoms and make them disappear at last.

This was such an exciting personal discovery that she wanted to share it with her doctor. In mid-September S. drafted another letter to him describing how this breakthrough occurred. Although she never sent the letter—because things got much worse, rendering the enthusiasm inappropriate, to say the least—it is useful to quote from it, because it provides direct insight into S.'s mind-set at the time.

12 September 1996

Dear Dr. D.,

I write to share some data and an insight. [She begins with a recitation of the discoveries of late August.] . . .

After getting over the shock, I sat down to figure out what was going on. On reflection, it became clear that the continued symptoms were reflecting something about my whole personality, my whole way-of-living-in-the-world. What was that way of living? It's a bit inelegant, but you might call it pushing-it-all-the-time. If I thought I could work 8 hours, I would work 9; if I thought I could walk 3 miles, I would walk 4. I realized that I was doing precisely that this summer: always swimming that extra distance. So, I decided to try something different: doing less than I thought I could. (Draft letter)

To test her new hypothesis S. began to drastically restrict her activities. She cut out all exercise for five days in a row, then began to exercise again but at half the duration or intensity to which she was accustomed. Instead of swimming her usual half mile, she swam only a quarter mile, ten minutes in all. The results were dramatic: for two full weeks she had no headaches (at least none she was willing to "count" in her chart) and no back or neck pain. Her sleep was not much improved, and the fatigue came back, but the headaches and neck pain seem to have been vanquished. The item "General Pain" on her chart reads as follows: September 3: "None at all, feel really just fine"; September 4: "None; whole body feels good being at rest"; September 6: "Strategy feels so *right*. Whole body feels so healthy!"; September 11: "None, felt just great. Did not get tired all day."

S. thought that, after months of agonizing struggle, she had finally solved the problem. Her (unsent) letter to her doctor hints at the euphoria she felt at finally getting her new symptoms under control: "This sounds, in retrospect, like a quite mundane piece of self-discovery. For me, though, it was like a revelation. And honestly, from the first of September, I have felt wonderful physically. I mean, I've felt like what I imagine it feels like to feel healthy" (Draft letter, September 12).

The Larger Picture Becomes Clear: My Life Has Shrunk to Nothing

The ebullience did not last long, however. After getting over the thrill of tasting success, S. began to realize what a huge sacrifice she had had to make to rid herself of the noxious symptoms of fibromyalgia. Essentially, she had given up everything that had brought pleasure and fun into her life. And each of these activities—gardening, boating, swimming—was imbued with special meanings and memories. Every time she gave one up, part of her died.

This realization—that she had to change her whole personality and give up all the pleasure in her life to rid herself of a condition that had emerged just a few months earlier—provoked a major reevaluation of what had happened to her under D.'s care. This reconsideration actually had its roots in late August, when S. discovered that improvement in some conditions had been accompanied by long-term deterioration in others. Her failure to send the September 1 letter is one of the first signs of her loss of faith in the doctor she had worshiped for months. But the doubts and anger S. felt at the end of August had not lasted long. They had been whisked away by the personal revelation of early September. It was only in mid-September, when the larger picture of how much her life had shrunk began to emerge, that she began to sustain doubts about the course of treatment. This would turn out to be a major turning point, when S. started to question what had gone on all those months and to wonder whether the whole thing might not have been a monstrous mistake.

As S. began to rethink her doctor's management of her case, her old anxieties about the strong drugs he had put her on returned. She made no secret of her concerns. In a phone conversation on September 9, she fretted about becoming addicted to the sleep medications and proposed that she try weaning herself off them. She was worried, she said, because she had discovered that she could no longer get to sleep on her own. The doctor pooh-poohed her concerns:

> No [he said]; what would happen if the fibromyalgia symptoms return?—
> [They] would be too hard to manage from afar. [We] cannot worry about
> this—there are tradeoffs, as always. [It is] better to accept any long-term
> side effects (about which [D.] had nothing to say) than to mess up the
> pattern of sleep, which is great. (Diary, September 12)

One night in early September, when S. was reading in bed, she sensed that her vision had deteriorated. She tried closing one eye, then the other, and discovered that the near vision in her right eye was terrible. Her right eye had always been weaker than her left, but the blurriness of the printed words was more pronounced now than it had ever been. She grew alarmed, thinking that the Plaquenil, which she was taking for arthritis, might be affecting her eyesight. The next morning S. called Seattle and left a message of alarm. The doctor called back that evening. Again, he reassured her that everything was fine. He said that blurred vision is rarely seen in connection with Plaquenil. He told the story of his own experience of losing visual acuity and eventually coming to wear eyeglasses as a matter of habit. He evidently enjoyed the thought that his older patient was having to come to grips with the effects of aging too and seemed to think it was funny that she was worrying about Plaquenil toxicity when she was merely suffering from old age. "A case of aging, pure and simple," he declared confidently. What solution did he propose? "Get a good strong light!" (Diary, September 13).

S. was not reassured. Her near-distance vision had deteriorated too fast to be caused by "aging pure and simple." And she remained concerned about drug addiction. All the books she had read warned about addiction to Ambien, the medicine that helped her get to sleep. Yet her doctor would hear nothing of it. He resolutely refused to use the word *addiction*, saying it was meaningless in cases of multiply ill patients such as her.

A Six-Day Headache from Hell

While S. was struggling to deal with the enormity of her losses, she was struck by another prolonged period of headache, dulling, and fatigue. For no discernible reason, on September 21 she felt tired and drugged all day. The fatigue and heaviness in her head persisted for three days, during which she was unable to do any writing. Even reading proved impossible. This was a new development. Amazingly, during the summer, no matter how bad the headaches had been, she almost always had managed to work at least part of the day. Now she could hardly think. Lacking any other explanation, S. seized on the idea that the problem lay with the sleep medications. In the spring, when the doses of those drugs were too high, she had felt dulled and drugged, too tired to make it through the afternoons without naps. The same thing seemed to be happening now. For one night, the second of six, she slept almost nine hours, two more than usual, then had to take a nap the next day.

Determined to solve this problem on her own, on the fourth day S. sliced off a tiny sliver of the pale yellow Flexeril tablet, removing roughly 15 to 20 percent of the pill. This was the amount she figured she needed to remove to get to a dosage that would give her the right amount of sleep. Unfortunately the pill slicing had no effect on S.'s waking time. But it had a distinct impact on the quality of her sleep—for the worse.

On the fourth day, she wrote in her chart, she felt "tired all day," and on the fifth she felt "tired, dull head all day." On the sixth day, she "awoke with a big headache: like a balloon in the head."

S. was beside herself with anguish. Unable to do any work for six days in a row, unable to figure out why this was happening, and feeling her head exploding with pain, she descended into despair and began to think the unthinkable: that there was nothing left to live for. Her mental state was so perilous that she could not even bring herself to write about it in her diary. Here is how she recapped that period four days after it ended:

> Last week [I] went through six days of hell: on the first three I felt totally lousy—tired, heavy head, virtually unable to work. . . . [F]or [the next] three days . . . I got insufficient sleep and again felt lousy . . . I fell into a state of absolute despair, thinking that life was not worth living if I could do neither physical work nor mental work. I mean, it was really bad . . . (Diary, September 30)

The Doctor Says Everything Is "Stupendous"

Unable to bear it any longer, on the sixth day of the hellish headache S. called her doctor. Because he was very busy they did not connect for several days. During that time S.'s sleep problems and the "balloons" in her brain went away on their own. But S. remained deeply concerned about what had happened. While waiting anxiously for D.'s call she developed a long list of questions for him. She wanted to know why such a headache should occur and why she was not getting better, even though she was devoting all her waking hours to following his treatment program.

The phone call finally came on the fourth night. After hearing what had happened, the doctor indicated that the headache was probably viral: she had caught a cold, which had knocked her out for a few days. Because she was on so many medications, he explained, the symptoms of colds tend to be suppressed, so she was probably unaware of what was happening. S. thought about this for a minute and, remembering that she had been sneezing a little, accepted his explanation as probably correct:

> He finally reached me last night, and gave me the best news I've had in so very long: it was most likely a virus, a viral infection—the symptoms I described are not distinguishable from those of a slight flu or cold! Come to think of it, I have been sneezing for about a week and a half. Maybe I even got it that day we went to Vinalhaven. I think he is right. Another way to tell [that] it might be a cold or virus is when it happens out of the blue. One has to look at the context. If you suddenly get worse and then

just as suddenly get better, it is most unlikely to be a medication problem. That is what happened. I was great, I was awful, and then I was great again. When it is just "one day out of a whole lot," the thing to do is just sit it out. (Diary, September 30)

Trying to talk his patient out of her evident distress, the doctor told her that the "cold episode" was very good news indeed: it meant that she was normal again. If she could have colds and then recuperate so fast, that meant that his overall strategy of gaining control over her diseases and then building a physical reserve was working. The rhetorics of physician heroism had come around again. Dr. D. was so confident that his design for her disease management had been a success. His enthusiasm was boundless: "That is astounding information!" he said; this is "stupendous news!" S. badly wanted to believe him, even though his view of her situation diverged so wildly from what she knew to be the truth of her body:

> But the good news, [D. says,] is I recovered, like a normal person. For many patients, this would be just another setback that contributed to a larger downward spiral. But I got over it. This is exactly what was supposed to happen as a result of building up a reserve: I responded the right way. This is "astounding information," "stupendous news." He was so happy!
> This is good news for me as well: it means that every little thing that happens to me is *not* related to these conditions. I can have colds, too, and suffer them like everyone else. It means that the fibromyalgia and psoriatic arthritis are just fine—the medications are working. (Diary, September 30)

While waiting four days for D.'s call, S. had prepared a list of serious concerns she wanted to raise with him. Her anger, suppressed for so long, reemerges in her list of questions: "*WHY so fucking many headaches and days of NO SLEEP???* Why the increase in fibromyalgia? Where is the lit[erature] on that? Why is the sleep problem [still so serious that I am] losing *significant* amounts of work time? Why is it always two steps forward and two steps back, with no overall improvement?" (Post-it note, late September).

But D.'s absolute certitude that her worries were baseless and that everything was fine threw S. off guard and off track. All her concerns had just been obviated by his rosy reading of the facts. Once again, she had tried to send a distress signal, and once again her doctor had refused to pick it up. With his rhetorics of physician heroism and patient benefit, he had effectively silenced her, replacing her concerns about the causes of her symptoms with his self-congratulatory hype about the brilliance of his approach to their treatment. The issues S. wanted to raise had been bulldozed out of the conversation.

She did, however, find a space in the conversation to alert her doctor to the sharp decline in her emotional well-being. Although her emotions had been declared irrelevant to her condition, in this discussion S. forced them back onto the agenda. She felt that the downward tilt in her physical health had left her mental and emotional balance in a precarious state, and that her doctor, who was in charge of her health, should know this. She tried to explain how the diagnosis of fibromyalgia had been a two-edged sword for her: while it helped her name and find a solution to her sleep problems, it made her feel twice as sick as she had felt before. This comment produced silence on the other end of the line. Pressing the point, S. wondered aloud about the possibility of returning to the status quo ante. Overall, she asserted, she had been better off *before* the doctor's treatment program had gotten underway. She proposed that they now simply "forget about" the fibromyalgia, drop the sleep medications from the drug regimen, and treat only the arthritis. The doctor must have been very disappointed to hear this, for it signaled his patient's lack of confidence in everything he had done. He replied, lamely, that "after a certain point there is no going back." His comment ended that discussion.

Having made little progress with this suggestion, S. shifted to a different topic. She next tried to convey her feeling that the important benefits she had enjoyed from her doctor's treatment were won at significant cost. What she was doing here and in the conversation just described was mapping out her contradictory feelings about the treatment in hopes of opening them up for discussion so that together she and her doctor could decide how to deal with them. But her communicational strategy did not work. The doctor responded in characteristic fashion. Dusting off the rhetorics of biomedical infallibility, he told her that her feelings were part of her problem; they were obstacles that had to be removed before bodily healing could occur. How was she to overcome the emotional difficulties? By reading Elizabeth Kübler-Ross's book, *On Death and Dying*. This book, he explained, "deals with issues that are always raised with chronic illness," namely, that illness is a precursor to death, which is right around the corner. Once again D. was telling S. to think not of life, but of death. Apparently he was oblivious to the possibility that his death talk might worsen the patient's emotional state, as it had done in the spring, or even become a self-fulfilling prophecy. Here is S.'s brief record of that part of the conversation:

I did tell him about the problems I am having dealing with this stuff, accepting it. It just uses up a huge amount of psychic energy, I said. "You can't let it control you," was his reply. Right [S. says to herself]. So, there is more emotional work to be done. He recommended Elizabeth Kübler-Ross's book on death and dying: it has nothing to do with arthritis or fibromyalgia, but deals with issues that are always raised with chronic illness. The most important thing is to move beyond asking "Why me?" to ask "What can I do?" I have taken that step, but it still gets me way down. (Diary, September 30)

The morning after that conversation S. figured out why her worsened physical condition was wearing her mental health so thin:

Now I know why this stuff is getting me so down. It is seriously compromising my ability to pursue my life projects. I don't have a life, I have life projects, and they are TO WRITE. I live to write. And when I have headaches for six days on end, I cannot write at all. (Diary, September 30)

Now not only had all the joy and pleasure been removed from her life, but her ability to work was also being undermined. Her research and writing were the minimal definition of her life: Without them, what was left?

The Mind Begins to Malfunction

Fogginess had been S.'s regular companion since the spring. At the beginning she felt like she had been hit by a truck. Those feelings soon subsided, however, and were replaced by more occasional and subtle sensations of mental fogginess. These sensations appeared off and on throughout the spring. But they were manageable. Since they did not impair her mental functioning she decided that she could live with them. The doctor was not concerned about them, so S. was not either.

In the summer the mental fogginess turned into a sense of distancing, as though S. were separated from the world, perceiving people and objects through a light gray haze. S. figured this was part of her new life condition to which she had to grow accustomed. Deep in her heart she suspected that the fogginess might be related to the sleep medications. But she needed the sleep so much that she did not consider dropping the drugs, a step her doctor would not have agreed to in any case. The sense of distancing was so common an occurrence that S. did not bother to record it in her chart, except on the occasional day when the fog was so thick it kept her from working. On July 1 she wrote in her chart: "Awoke with mild headache, which turned to notable dizziness in late afternoon." The August 13 entry reads: "Felt tired and dulled all day—definitely down; low energy."

In the fall, however, the fogginess became more noticeable and obtrusive. Often, when S.'s husband would ask her a question, she would reply that she couldn't answer with any certainty because she felt distanced, cut off from the world he was asking about. The grogginess and dulling had become so normal a part of her life that she made a special note in her chart when she did *not* feel that way. September 4 was such a day: "Wonderful sleep, not even groggy, dulled feeling from sleep meds." She also noted occasions on which the fogginess was especially apparent. September 20: "Some spaciness at night." October 6: "Subtly dulled, mentally." The fogginess grew more noticeable as time went by. October 7: "Spacey by 1:00." October 18: "Chemically, drugged feeling all day—no clarity." November 2: "Very spacey, especially from mid-afternoon." November 3: "In a fog until 3:00, then lifted; mental acuity low."

The fogginess, disturbing though it was, was trivial compared to the other neurological symptom that developed during the fall: mental distortion. These disturbances of cognitive function crept up on S. so slowly and insidiously that she almost didn't notice when they came and went. Mostly these distortions entailed difficulties with concentration, comprehension, and memory, especially of words. As a scholar and writer, S. was hypersensitive to any changes in her intellectual capacities. Yet because the changes were subtle, she could not decide whether they were really occurring or whether she was going crazy. Was the dysfunction real or a figment of her imagination? Was it evidence of disease, or just "aging, pure and simple," as her doctor might put it? She could not say for sure.

One day, October 12, she had no doubt that the cognitive disturbance was real. That day she awoke with a splitting headache. The headache had moderated somewhat by noon, but all day she felt "in [a] total fog, out of touch with reality." Unable to think or write, she sat outdoors in the fresh air and sunshine and tried to read. But she found she could not comprehend the words on the page. She had to read the sentences three times to make sense of them. And then, when the meaning of the sentences became clear, the point of the paragraphs they made up would elude her. S. was hysterical with worry. This is for real, she thought: now my mind is going too. Her husband tried to calm her by reasoning out what might be happening. But S. could not be calmed. She was in such bad mental shape that she could not bring herself to make a record of how bad things were. Yet she left clues about her mental state on her daily "well-being" charts. On October 19, a very bad day, she wrote: "Felt *wretched* all day. Totally bummed out—so frustrated and *angry* [underlined three times]. My life is just *wasting away*."

Fear of Food

Throughout the fall S. continued to experience on-again-off-again problems with sleeping. These problems were undoubtedly made worse by the depression that had descended over S.'s life. Nights empty of sleep were followed by days full of fatigue. As time went by S.'s work time began noticeably to shrink. In the summer she had often been able to work eight or nine hours a day, from early morning until 5:00 or 6:00 o'clock in the evening. By mid-October her workdays had shrunk to five or six hours. By 1:00 or 2:00 in the afternoon her head would crash, the fatigue would set in, and she would have to put aside her work. S. saw her writing project going up in smoke. With such short days, how could she ever finish her book?

With her work—her core identity—jeopardized, S. became obsessive about trying to track down the causes of poor sleep. That was often hard to do. On October 19, for example, she went to bed at 10:15, awoke at 2:30, and never went back to sleep. "WHY?" she wrote in her chart in distressed pink. A week later she began to reason that her dinners might be causing the insomnia. Eating had been a problem for many months. Like many people, when S. grew depressed she tended to lose her appetite and stop eating. In late June, when she was living alone in the barn, she had lost interest in eating. In no time at all she lost seven or eight pounds. Thin to begin with, she began to look gaunt. Her loved ones were deeply concerned. In the summer her parents had tried to revive her interest in eating by serving her home-cooked dinners that were always balanced and tasty. In the fall her husband tried to nourish her body and soul with gourmet, multicourse dinners. His servings were larger than those S. had grown accustomed to during the summer. Maybe, S. began to think, the more generous helpings of food were sitting in her stomach like lead, impairing her sleep. One night in late October, after a heavier than usual dinner, she slept very poorly. The cause-and-effect relation seemed transparent. So S. begged her husband to make smaller dinners. And she herself began restricting her intake, eating only tiny portions of every course. Anxious about how she would sleep, she became deeply fearful of eating. She would do anything—including skipping dinner altogether—to rid herself of the insomnia. And yet this drastic step did little to fill those troubled nights with sleep.

"Progression into Serious Mental Deterioration"

By October S.'s physical and cognitive problems had taken on grim emotional dimensions. Her emotional problem was not just depression; it was verging on mental disorder. Desperate, S. struggled to get a grip on things. She took long walks in the countryside to calm down and talk herself out of doing something crazy. Only too often she would return sobbing uncontrollably. Through the tears and little comments on her mental state, S. kept trying to convey messages to her husband about her disintegrating mental condition. Her husband was dismayed beyond words. But he was unable to find a way into her mental world to bring her out. Her sisters and friends knew from the hysteria in her voice that things were going from bad to worse. But they were thousands of miles away; what could they do to help? Once in a while S. would scratch notes to herself on little pieces of paper. She wrote things like:

> OK, S., things are going to turn around, NOW: That is, YOU are GOING TO TURN THEM AROUND . . . Just look: . . . you have made unbelievable progress . . . You have turned everything around. (MANL Book, October 2)

Would that these words had been true.

As she watched her world shrink and her life veer further off track, S. began to lash out at people, including strangers who accidentally got in her way. She was so angry at the world that her life was being destroyed, she did not care that her social graces were falling away. Her husband grew very worried as his once sociable wife became increasingly socially dysfunctional. Even people she knew hardly recognized her, so introverted and brooding had she become.

In early November S. mustered the courage to return to her charts and calculate another round of statistics. She discovered that although her neck and back pain had eased somewhat, the other problems had either remained unchanged or grown worse. During September and October her head ached one day in four, the same amount of time as in August. During those fall months she slept very poorly almost two days in five. That was twice as bad as in August. And she was functionally incapacitated two days in five. That was also worse than in August, when she was unable to work one day in three.

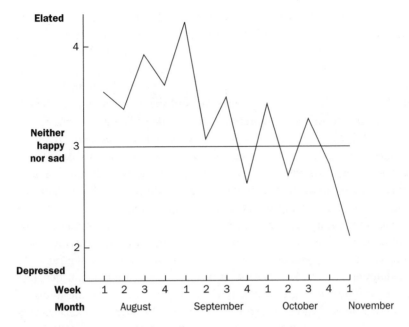

Figure 3. An Emotional Free Fall

Her major reason for checking the charts, however, was to see whether her suspicion that she was growing ever more depressed was true. She calculated her mood scores and found frightening confirmation of her fears: from August to early November her spirits had been in an absolute free fall (see figure 3). In August her mood on an average day ranged from 3.5 to 4.0—reasonably happy. By the second week of September it had sunk to just above 3.0, neither happy nor sad. By the first week of November her spirits had fallen another full point, to 2.1, indicating pervasive depression. As her overall emotional well-being slid downward, the number of days S. suffered serious depression rose. August was blissfully free of such times. In September, she spent 10 percent of her time crying off and on the whole day. In October that figure rose to 23 percent, and in early November S. was morbidly depressed 60 percent of the time. These numbers forced her to see that she was teetering on the edge of madness. Without them she might have never taken steps to arrest the decline.

S. did not call her doctor. For one thing, he was not in Seattle; he was out of town for two weeks and had had only a few minutes to talk to her before leaving. But even if he had been in his office, S. would not have called him. For by now she no longer trusted him. She knew he would deny her reality, substituting his for hers. Every time she had brought up mental or emotional problems, he had replied with the discourse of objectification, which made the body the sole object of biomedical concern. The negative emotions were her problem, he had said; she had to deal with them on her own. And she was just causing herself more problems by being depressed. As recently as September 30, S. had tried to tell her doctor how hard it was for her to cope with the emotional consequences of having fibromyalgia. He had told her to get over it. If anything, his advice on dealing with the emotions made things worse. In that conversation he had reminded her that "we are all dying all the time anyway," implying that what was happening to her made no difference in the grand scheme of things. S. had read the book on dying he had recommended, but thinking about dying rather than living—D.'s counsel all along—made her all the more despondent. As she reflected on that September conversation, it began to dawn on her that her doctor and his advice might be part of the problem rather than the solution. Not for a second did she suspect that her doctor might be exacerbating the physical as well as the emotional problems. That discovery was to come later. In late October the problem was being heard. S. no longer trusted her doctor to be on her side: he would whitewash her story and tell her that everything was "stupendous," when she knew only too well that it was not.

A Way Out?

For months S. had been slowly sinking in a thick black muck of despondency and despair. In the first few days of November she sank to the bottom of the pit. As if to record how her life had ended, she took a piece of scrap paper and scribbled this cryptic description of her emotional state:

> Progress[ing] into serious mental illness—*am going insane*. Situation
> is OUT OF CONTROL—totally losing grasp of reality. Now slightly
> calmer—can see more clearly. I feel so lousy physically—so emotionally
> *weak and vulnerable.* ***Mentally—lost in FOG!!! [Things are so bad]
> I cannot even get a clear picture of what I should do about it. (Scribbled
> note, early November)

Then on the fourth day of the month, a miracle occurred. For some mysterious reason that no one will ever unearth, that morning the fog lifted from her head. S. could feel it rising and marveled at how clear-headed she felt. Instead of working on her book, she let her mind roam and began thinking back on how her life condition had changed. As she thought back over the past eight months of growing mental fogginess, distancing, and dysfunction, it suddenly hit her what had been happening: all those months her mind had been so clouded and dulled that she hadn't even been able to figure out what was wrong, let alone take steps to make things right again. All along S. had thought she had been perceiving reality clearly enough. Now she knew she had been wrong. Not only her body, but her *mind* had not been working: *that* was the fundamental problem. This was a truly frightening thought. Yet it was also a thrilling idea, for it meant there might be a way out of the muck. But what was that way? S. did not know. But she knew she needed professional help. She also realized that she might have only this one day of clarity. So that day she took decisive action to try to regain control of her life.

The first thing she did was to call her former rheumatologist in New York City and make an appointment to get a second opinion. Blessedly, Dr. K. was able to fit her in at the end of the day on November 6. S.'s husband had been urging her to get a second opinion for weeks. But S. had resisted his suggestion because she felt that doing so would be disloyal to Dr. D. After all, she had agreed to undergo six months of aggressive treatment, giving him an essentially free hand to treat her in the way he deemed best. Also, Dr. D. had advised her not to see a rheumatologist while on the East Coast, fearing that another specialist might meddle in his treatment program. A good and faithful patient, S. felt protective of her doctor's program, which she knew very well was unorthodox, and didn't want another physician looking into the private world that she and D. had created together. Even in September and October, when she became aware of the trade-offs she had made during her treatment, she never dreamed that the treatment package she was guarding so closely might actually be causing her problems. By early November she had become too desperate to worry about her promises to Dr. D. She needed help, and now.

S. spent the afternoon of that day of clearheadedness on her tractor, mowing the pastures and trying to figure out what else she needed to do. That evening she called a friend in California to get the name of a therapist who might be able to help her work out her emotional troubles. Then she called the therapist and made an appointment to see her in mid-November, when S. would be on the West Coast for a few days. The next day the fog descended again but, without knowing it, S. had prepared the way for the haze to lift for good.

Thus it was that a chance event, coming at a time of growing skepticism about the biomedical view of her life and the documentable disintegration of her mind, enabled S. to unlock the prison of "fibromyalgia" and discover that it was her doctor's brand of biomedicine itself that had led her to the brink of insanity.

Part Five | Rebellion and Self-Renewal

A Second Opinion

The Unmaking of a "Fibromyalgic"

On November 6 S. traveled to New York City to obtain a second opinion on her case. This chapter tells the story of that visit and its life-restoring effects on the hapless patient. Dr. K., the reader will recall, had been S.'s rheumatologist for five years before she moved to California. Dr. K. provided a radically new perspective on S.'s treatment. Without criticizing D., Dr. K. said that, in her opinion, the diagnosis of fibromyalgia made no sense, the prognosis was overdrawn, and some of D.'s practices were unorthodox and risky if not outright dangerous to the patient. And Dr. K. identified the source of the headaches and fogginess as Indocin, the antiinflammatory to which Dr. D. had insisted on tolerizing his patient. Dr. D. had presented his story as the only true story of S.'s ills. But Dr. K. told another story that made more sense.

This chapter relates how the visit with K. turned S.'s life around. At last rid of the diagnosis that had caused her such psychic and physical torment, she left the office on a cloud of ecstasy, jettisoning her "fibromyalgic" identity on her way out the door. The next day she went off the offending drug, and the neurological symptoms vanished into thin air. And she realized for the very first time that her faith in her ultrascientific doctor had been badly misplaced. Jolted out of her lifelong belief in the mystique of medicine, she saw that her doctor's science of the body was anything but infallible, disinterested, and invariably beneficial for its objects. Dr. D. was neither hero nor medical miracle worker. He was but a technician of the body who had rhetorically exaggerated his abilities and made serious mistakes at her expense. D.'s medicine had lost its luster.

Dr. K. also outlined a new theory of the female-body-in-pain that transformed S.'s understandings of her physical problems. K.'s account employed a new, postbiomedical discourse on the body that recognized the contributions of gender, the emotions, and larger societal forces in the development of bodily ills. Dr. K. posited a syndrome of symptomization of psychosocial stress and traced its roots to women's childhood socialization into pleasantness. Because it pointed to the larger social roots of the syndrome, the theory provided a way out of the trap of self-blame in which S. had been caught for so long. Although Dr. K. herself relied exclusively on drug therapies, her theory of the roots of women's pain suggested new strategies for pain alleviation that centered on addressing the underlying psychosocial sources of symptoms rather than simply suppressing them with strong drugs.

If D.'s story had shortcomings, so too did Dr. K.'s. It may have overstated the role of childhood socialization in adult behavior. It failed to specify the mechanism connecting personality and symptom. Its psychological therapies might have been incapable of eliminating symptoms rooted in such deeply embedded structures of the personality. The theory might have applied only to certain ethnic or class categories of women. Yet at the time S. did not see these possible weaknesses of K.'s theory. In her neediness, she clutched onto the gender story like she might grab onto a lifeboat in a raging flood. The gender story was attractive in part because it fit S.'s life and intellectual predispositions like a glove. It also gave her fresh hope at a time when she desperately needed it. If she seems to heroize K. and demonize D., it is for these personal, intellectual, and emotional reasons. Dr. K. gave S. what she needed at the time: new understandings of her symptoms and new hopes for a future without them.

Another Story of the Suffering Body

S. had spent a long time preparing what she would tell Dr. K. in the November 6 appointment. Her planned presentation, sketched out in detailed notes, is highly revealing of her mind-set at the time. Dr. D. had represented his story of S.'s ills—the multiple diagnosis, the dismal prognosis, the drug-intensive treatment—as the only credible story that could be told. S. had taken it as the final truth of her body. Believing her doctor to be a scientific genius and a medical miracle worker who could do no wrong, she had come to believe deep in her heart that she had his specialty disease and that her condition was serious and growing worse. Given these convictions, S. intended to start by telling Dr. K. the bad news about her fibromyalgia and what it had meant for her life. The questions she prepared for Dr. K. concerned only the third part of the story, the treatment program, and whether it contained hidden risks of which D. had not apprised her.

S. began the appointment by explaining briefly what Dr. D. had done. She then went on to relate, with emotion, how her once rich and rewarding life was slipping away from her at a frightening pace. Alarmed to see her former patient in such a dire state, Dr. K. interrupted before S. could finish her presentation. Starting with the diagnosis, she went over every step of D.'s evaluation and treatment of S.'s case, giving her own professional opinion of what he had said and done. What she said undermined everything S. had believed to be beyond question for eight full months.

A Diagnosis by an Overeager Specialist

Dr. D. had attached five disease labels to S.; Dr. K. shrank the list back to one. She quickly dismissed the osteoarthritis as "normal aging" and the scoliosis as so mild as to be clinically irrelevant. Psoriatic arthritis was, of course, S.'s major rheumatological condition—that diagnosis remained. But fibromyalgia was a different matter. Dr. K. said she was "really reluctant" to give this diagnosis. S. just did not fit the pattern. Most important, she did not have the main symptom of the disease, widespread pain. Moreover, her exercise habits and personality were different from those of most fibromyalgic patients, who, in Dr. K.'s experience, tend to dislike exercise and to have "whiny and dependent" personalities (both no doubt related to their constant pain, which is rarely taken seriously).

The idea that she did not have fibromyalgia came as a complete shock to S. How could she not have fibromyalgia, she demanded to know, when she had the tender points and the sleep disorder associated with the disease? It was on those bases that Dr. D. had diagnosed the disease. He was a specialist on fibromyalgia, so how could he make a mistake? Dr. K.'s answer to this question blew her patient away. These symptoms, she explained, are not uniquely diagnostic of fibromyalgia. Rather, they are free-floating symptoms that can be associated with any number of conditions, including psoriatic arthritis. Dr. K. felt strongly that it was better for S. to think of herself as having one condition, arthritis, with a number of related symptoms. This approach was easier on the patient, who, if faced with numerous diagnoses, would tend to feel "overburdened," "like she was falling apart."

But if S. did not have fibromyalgia, why would D. diagnose the disease? Dr. K. reminded her that specialists in given conditions often overdiagnose their specialty diseases. S. felt her stomach turn. Had her Seattle doctor unconsciously put his interests in promoting his specialty disease above her interests in improving her health? This was simply unthinkable. Had her presumption that "he cared," an assumption that had led S. to put her health and life in his hands, been wrong?

An Overblown Prognosis

Dr. D. had stressed the seriousness of S.'s diseases. This, together with the prognosis of imminent deterioration of her skeletal system, was the rationale for putting her on a cocktail of potent drugs. Now S. wanted another opinion on this. "How serious is my psoriatic arthritis?" S. asked Dr. K. The answer? "Serious, but only in a few joints." Then what about Dr. D.'s prognosis that S. would progress into serious deterioration in five years if she did not take drastic action immediately? "No one can predict the course a disease will take." In other words, D. had presented as indisputable scientific fact something that science does not and cannot know.

A Risky and Unorthodox Treatment Program

S. had many questions about Dr. D.'s treatment strategy. She wanted to know whether the high dosages of the three drugs he had prescribed for her arthritis had associated risks or dangers that D. had not told her about. Dr. K. assured her that the arthritis treatment was standard rheumatological practice. All the doses Dr. D. had prescribed were acceptable, as long as no side effects emerged.

S. did not ask specifically about her antiinflammatory, because she never suspected that it might be the cause of her many problems. But she did ask what might be producing the neurological symptoms that had been causing her such grief. Dr. K. immediately identified the likely culprit as Indocin and suggested that S. go off the drug for a few days to see if the headaches and mental dulling went away. Here is what she said, as reconstructed by S. the next day:

> It could very well be the Indocin that is causing the headaches and fogginess . . . It is very poorly tolerated by patients generally. Yes, it's the strongest antiinflammatory, but it is not my drug of choice for anyone . . . What is the best drug for a patient is the one that works for that patient. You should try switching back to Oruvail for . . . at least three days, [and] maybe up to a week to see if the fogginess and headaches go away . . . Take 200 mg. a day. (Diary, November 7)

At last S. had a possible answer to the question that had plagued her for eight months. It seemed that Dr. D. had put her on a drug that almost always causes problems. But that was not the only questionable practice he had engaged in.

From the beginning S. had been concerned about becoming addicted to her sleep medications. Dr. D. had refused to use the word *addiction,* dismissing it as a trivial concern. S. asked Dr. K. for her views on the matter. K. replied in no uncertain terms that drug addiction was a serious issue. For someone in her forties to be totally dependent on sleep medications was "really bad." This was a phrase Dr. K. did not use lightly. S. had never fully realized just how unorthodox some of D.'s methods and ideas were.

A Gender Theory of Chronic Pain

Following the discourses of biomedicine to the letter, Dr. D. had said little about the causes of S.'s conditions. Splitting her body from her mind and emotions and reducing her ills to pathologies of the tissues and cells, he had stressed that her diseases were genetically rooted and biologically based. As such, they would respond only to treatments that altered the biochemistry of the body. This view of her problems left S. no alternative to a lifetime of dependence on drugs—and, not incidentally, on the doctor who dispensed them.

Dr. K. placed the discourses of scientific medicine within a broader framework that demoted science and the body from their status as Truth and Nature, making them instead parts of society that are responsive to social, political, and cultural forces. Broadening the scope of discourse on the body, she was willing to talk about causes and to recognize the role of emotions in the genesis of bodily ills. While not denying the importance of genetics and biology, especially in arthritis, she highlighted the contribution of psychosocial forces to the development of arthritis, fibromyalgia, and other musculoskeletal disorders. This view expanded the range of strategies that the ill person might employ to ease her pain.

This critically important discussion started almost by accident. S. had mentioned the shocking statistic she had discovered in the medical literature: two-thirds of fibromyalgic patients, almost all of whom are women, have a history of sexual abuse. Reference to this statistic led Dr. K. to launch into her own theory of the psychosocial origins of fibromyalgia and other poorly understood rheumatological conditions. K.'s theory placed gender at center stage. In her view the problem was not abuse per se but something more insidious because it was more commonplace. The fundamental problem lay in the social roles that women are expected to play in today's society. As girls, they are socialized to think they must please everyone. Then a time comes when pleasing someone important in their lives leaves them no choice but to abnegate themselves, to stifle their thoughts and silence their desires. The psychological stress of having to erase one's self comes out in the form of physical symptoms. In other words, many women have no way to deal with the anger they feel from having to deny their needs, so they take it out on their bodies. This syndrome, Dr. K. suggested, might be particularly active in the genesis of fibromyalgia, which has no clear organic basis yet is well known to be related to stress. But such dynamics contribute to other symptoms as well, including sleep disturbances and even arthritic flares. K. proposed that such patterns might even be operative in S.'s case. S.'s arthritis had grown much worse during her last two years in New York, a time when she had reported growing difficulties with her supervisor at work. Little did Dr. K. know how well her gender theory of stress and symptoms fit S.'s life after she moved to California!

If the social construction and psychological repercussions of gender were significant contributors to these conditions, a new type of treatment program was called for. In addition to drugs for symptom relief, Dr. K. recommended that the chronically ill consider counseling or stress management programs to help them both understand how they deal with stress and develop new methods of managing it. Although such methods cannot be expected to eliminate diseases such as arthritis, which have biological and genetic bases, they should help to alleviate the symptoms, which are worsened by psychosocial stress.

S.'s Life Is Transformed Overnight

S. literally danced out of Dr. K.'s office. Finally she had heard a doctor say something that validated her views of acceptable risks and affirmed her lived experience of the connections between social stress and bodily health. At last a physician had given her hope for a future other than dependence on drugs and doctors. The effects were immediate and dramatic. She cast off the label "fibromyalgic," her headaches and mental distortions disappeared, and she began to reconsider everything that had happened to her under Dr. D.'s care.

The Headaches and Fogginess Disappear in Days

S. was thrilled with the notion that the antiinflammatory might be causing the headaches and fogginess. Full of hope, the next day she filled a prescription for Oruvail. That first day, as Dr. K. had suggested, she took Indocin in the morning and Oruvail at night. On the second day she had a mild headache. That day she went off Indocin altogether, taking Oruvail instead. On the third day, the second under the Oruvail regimen, she detected a marked change in her head: her old mental clarity had returned. Her chart says: "Mental acuity—great all day and all night. *Huge* change. *No more fog!*" The clarity persisted into the fourth, fifth, and sixth days. The chart says it all: "[Head] so clear—day into night" (day four); "Fogginess gone; head so clear. Dramatic change in [mental acuity]" (day five); "[Head] crystal clear—felt great all day" (day six). The fogginess had gone, never to return.

It was not just the spaciness and cognitive distortions that went away. The headaches departed too. From the day she dropped the Indocin, S. never had another big headache like the ones she had endured during the summer and fall. When she was taking Indocin her head always felt hypersensitive, as though any slight change in activity or environment might make it start throbbing. Now her head felt different—it was more solid, less vulnerable. Her own perceptions of her body told her that the headaches would not return.

S. Discards Her "Fibromyalgic" Identity

The most far-ranging effect of the visit to Dr. K. was to rid S. of her "fibromyalgic" label. It was not just that the label had never felt quite right. It had had devastating emotional consequences of which the reader needs no reminder at this point. And through a peculiar causal pathway, the diagnosis of fibromyalgia was also responsible for the bodily symptoms that had caused S. such discomfort. From the beginning, her doctor had viewed her case through the larger interpretive lens of "fibromyalgia." All her new symptoms—from the neck and upper back pain to the headaches to the sleeplessness—came to be viewed as related to the fibromyalgia. Now Dr. K.'s reinterpretation of the headaches as caused by Indocin—an interpretation that was empirically supported by S.'s experiment—made S. see that Dr. D. had missed the well-known connection between the arthritis drug and the headaches, because he was so intent on reading the headaches as fibromyalgic. It was not that the doctor had seen the headaches as the cost of controlling the fibromyalgia; again and again he had tried to alleviate the headaches, with no success.[1] What had transpired was more complicated. Because of his conviction, his unshakable certainty that his patient "had fibromyalgia" and that the headaches were part of the syndrome, he had overlooked the role of his arthritis drug in producing these debilitating symptoms. Dr. D. had erred, and S. had suffered unspeakable misery as a result.

S. had been doubtful about the diagnosis of fibromyalgia because she lacked the "pain all over" that was the cardinal symptom of the disease. But she could not reject it, because her doctor had discovered all eighteen of the fibromyalgic tender points. Despite her vague suspicions about these tender points—something the doctor had made a big deal of but had failed to correspond to any sensation she felt—he was the expert on fibromyalgia, and she had no basis for thinking he was a fraud. S. had also puzzled over some contradictions in her doctor's explanation of the course of her disease. He had said that fibromyalgia was a chronic condition that never goes away, yet over the spring he had, according to his own reckoning, reduced the number of tender points in her body from eighteen to six. It was as though, at the first appointment, he had reported all the tender points to make her think she had the disease and then gradually reduced the number to convince her that he had made her better. But even if one did not accept the story about the tender points, there was still the "sleep disorder," which is almost universal in fibromyalgics and which S. had come to believe that she had. Despite her sense that there was something odd about the diagnosis, for these reasons S. had come to accept it.

Now Dr. K. had solved the mystery of the diagnosis that both did and did not fit: the tender points and sleep problem were not unique to fibromyalgia. To the contrary, they could be associated with any number of conditions, including psoriatic arthritis. To be sure, some of Dr. D.'s theories about the dynamics of the disease had gotten some support from S.'s life. The hypothesis that worked best was the one tying her back and neck pain to exercise. But the connection between pain and muscle use could well have been due to physical deconditioning, deconditioning the doctor himself had produced by ordering his patient to stop swimming and to cut back on many other activities. Now, at last, the pieces of the puzzle were beginning to fall into place.

New Understandings of the Social Roots of Bodily Symptoms

Freed from Dr. D.'s demoralizing diagnosis, S.'s depression lifted and her spirits soared. The psychological uplift also had happy effects on her physical well-being: she began eating again and took up her beloved swimming with a new fervor.

Conceptual changes were also underway. Because Dr. K.'s account of the role of gender socialization and stress in the development of musculoskeletal problems mapped so perfectly onto S.'s life, S. was able to see how larger social forces had worked to create in her—and probably in many other women—a syndrome of somatization or symptomization of gender-based psychosocial stress. Now the Cornell neurologist's diagnosis of her problem as "pleasantness," which she had so angrily rejected a decade before, made eminent sense. Indeed, S. had struck more than one doctor that way. She was astonished to find, upon reading her patient file in California, that her first West Coast rheumatologist had described his initial impression of her in these words: "Pleasant white woman." The Cornell neurologist was wrong to hurl that adjective at her as an insult and send her away, denying not only the role of biological factors but also the presence of bodily pain. But he had been onto something that S. had not understood at the time. Dr. K. made the same point in a more sophisticated and helpful way. She added the gender component to the explanation, tying individual personality to its social roots, and she suggested how women entangled in these damaging patterns might find their way to a better life.

For S. the gender theory provided a way out of the trap of self-blame that had kept her from coming to grips with these issues earlier. That trap had been set by thoughtless doctors like the Cornell neurologist, who had accused her of causing her own illness. His charge left her with feelings of guilt and shame that made it difficult to react in any way but denial. Well-meaning practitioners of alternative medicine and New Age philosophy unwittingly participated in this cultural blaming by exaggerating the power of the mind to heal the body and by neglecting larger structural forces that impinge on mind and body alike. We saw in an earlier chapter how S. ended up feeling like a failure after trying to apply the ideas of a few alternative practitioners to her own life. Dr. K.'s theory led S. out of this trap of self-blame that S.'s personal experiences with the larger culture of illness had led her into. The syndrome was not a result of her personal failing. Rather, it was a result of the failings of a society that trains girls to be sugar and spice, then gives them no way to deal with the anger they must suppress to stay ever sweet. S. had been given new ideas about how to treat her ills and new hope for a future that might be different from the past.

Dr. D.'s Science Loses Its Sheen

Dr. K. had taken care not to criticize S.'s Seattle doctor. But her radically different view of S.'s physical state and how it should be treated forced S. to see her ultrascientific doctor in a new, more critical light. In this harsh new light the science that Dr. D. had purveyed and of which S. had been so enamored quickly lost its sheen. That science had presented itself as a disinterested set of knowledges and practices that was based on irreducible truths, incapable of error, and worthy of the utmost patient trust. Now all that fell away.

An Interested Science of the Body

Dr. K. had reminded S. that specialists in a given disease tend to over-diagnose that condition. S. knew that was true but had not realized how true it was in Dr. D.'s case. Curious, she checked her notes from the public lecture he had given in the spring (for details see chapter 6). In that lecture he had stated that, in most rheumatological practices, roughly 20 percent of patients were diagnosed with fibromyalgia. In his practice 90 percent of the patients were given that label. At the time S. had smugly accepted D.'s interpretation of the figures to mean that other doctors were too ignorant to know when their patients had fibromyalgia. The numbers now took on a different meaning. The most innocent explanation for the high proportion of patients in D.'s practice with fibromyalgia was that D.'s reputation as a specialist attracted large numbers of people with muscle pain to his practice. Perhaps many of the patients who traveled some distance to see him did so because of his specialization. D.'s reputation was certainly part of it. But there was more. Of course, S. now realized, D. had seen fibromyalgia in her because that is the diagnostic lens through which he views all rheumatological complaints. Vague symptoms that other rheumatologists might ignore he collected together and labeled as "fibromyalgia." But there was even another, darker side to Dr. D.'s unconscious "fibromyalgia-ization" of his patients. D. had also "given" her fibromyalgia, S. now recognized, because that was the disease he specialized in treating. The diagnosis provided the rationale for her, and patients like her, to go to Dr. D. As long as she "had" fibromyalgia, it followed that he was the best doctor to treat her ills. If she had only psoriatic arthritis, even with some associated conditions, it made little difference which rheumatologist she saw, since all rheumatologists are experienced in the treatment of arthritis. It was now clear that D.

was anything but a disinterested scientist. To the contrary, his economic interest in attracting patients to his practice had subtly colored his clinical judgments.

"Scientific Facts" Rhetorically Enhanced

Dr. D. had presented key aspects of his story about S.'s case as hard scientific facts, indisputable truths that he, with his superior knowledge of her body, was merely reporting to her to the best of his ability. Key narrative facts included the reality and significance of the tender points, the seriousness of her conditions, and the chronic, progressive nature of her diseases. Faced now with different readings of her bodily reality, S. was forced to see that D.'s facts, while always based on some empirical evidence, had been rhetorically enhanced so as to exaggerate their facticity. The phrase "frank not brutal," murmured in self-deprecating tones each time the doctor said something that seemed to S. cruel, conveyed the message that he was merely the bearer of bad tidings, the innocent, even "humble" reporter of the regrettable truths of her flawed body. With phrases such as this, S. now realized, D. had not *told* so much as *stretched* the truth, magnifying the facts to make them seem more real than they were. His rhetorics now exposed, the whole interpretive grid he had placed on her case began to collapse.

Not Always in the Patient's Best Interest

All along S. had believed she could trust her doctor always to do what was in her best interest—that just went without saying. She had come to trust Dr. D. absolutely, even putting off getting a second opinion until her life was at risk, because she did not want to betray that trust. She knew her doctor was pursuing a high-risk strategy, but it was only after the discussion with Dr. K. that she realized how far outside the medical mainstream some of his practices were. She now saw that D. had followed some procedures that were deemed unacceptable by many if not most rheumatologists because they are dangerous to the patient. Prime examples were the lack of concern about drug addiction, the heavy reliance on strong drugs that are notorious for producing debilitating side effects, and the habit of "tolerizing"—that is, forcing—patients back onto drugs that their bodies resist the first time. While risk is always an issue in medical treatment, what was problematic was the absence of discussion of acceptable risk. The doctor made all the decisions, withholding from the patient information about the true dangers. By no stretch of the imagination could this be considered "in the patient's best interest."

A Fallible Science That Denies Its Fallibility

On many occasions Dr. D. had rhetorically emphasized his infallibility. But obviously he could and did slip up. Although S. could understand how his entrapment in the discourses of fibromyalgia and his enchantment with the rhetorics of heroism could lead him to miss the side effects of the arthritis drug, in the end his failure to trace the headaches and spaciness to Indocin was a medical error, pure and simple. Dr. D. was not a miracle maker but a maker of mistakes for which she the patient had paid the price.

Dr. K. had revived her former patient's optimism and eliminated the troubling neurological symptoms, but S. still had a host of other physical and psychological problems with which to cope. Her first task, though, was to confront Dr. D. with what he had done.

CHAPTER 11

The Final Meeting

A Tale of Decline and a Denial

The myths of medicine's infallibility and beneficence shattered, S. was finally able to see what had been happening all those months. Her newly acute vision was enabled by an underlying transformation in her gender identity. We have seen how, early in treatment, S.'s critical feminist voice was silenced by a highly controlling physician. Desperate for help with her illnesses, she unconsciously adopted a "feminine" identity with which she sought to obtain medical care, not through the direct means of voice and action but through indirect "girl games" of sweet self-subordination and silent consternation. That feminine self lacked the political, intellectual, and emotional resources needed to resist the encroachments of biomedical power on the patient's body and life. Resistance had to emerge from another more "feminist" identity. Mercifully, S.'s verbally assertive and politically aware gender identity reappeared now because crisis was imminent—the feminine self was dying—and the emotional, intellectual, and political resources with which to recompose such a self were now at hand. Armed with such weapons, the "feminist" S. not only openly resisted biomedical authority by "speaking truth to power" in a final meeting with her doctor; she pressed on, beyond resistance, to undertake the publicly political act of writing this book.

This chapter tells the story of that final, high-drama meeting that S. staged with Dr. D. It relates S.'s sad yet angry tale of how her life had come undone and D.'s dogged refusal to hear her pain and his resolute denial of responsibility for anything that had gone wrong. Freshly empowered, S. was trying to talk a new language of the body in medicine and in society. But the doctor knew only the language of biomedicine—a language that sees itself as speaking the Only Truth—and could not or would not hear her words. It was not only the conceptual apparatus of biomedicine that kept D. from hearing S.'s critique of his handiwork, however. Although he probably was not fully conscious of them, he had real professional, material, and legal interests in not hearing what S. had to say. Dr. D. had every reason for not recognizing his mistakes.

Preparing for the Big Meeting: The Resistant Self Is Reborn

S. would be in California for ten days in mid-November. On one of those days she planned to fly up to Seattle for an appointment with Dr. D. The twelve days between the visits with Dr. K. and Dr. D. were filled with revelations and transformations. S. found the critical voice that had been silenced. She developed the mettle to talk back to the doctor who had unwittingly done her such harm. And she plotted out what she would say at that much-anticipated appointment.

Tools of Self-Empowerment

S. was able to restore her earlier, more politically aware identity quite quickly because it had never fully disappeared; it had only been submerged, waiting for an opportune moment to regain expression. Equally important, over the months that S. had passed under the "gaze" of Dr. D., she had been quietly accumulating a wealth of intellectual and emotional resources with which to fashion that newly outspoken, resistant self. Crucial tools of empowerment included Dr. K.'s gender theory of chronic pain as well as wider scholarly critiques of science and medicine that supported and augmented it. S.'s power toolbox also contained the anger that had been nurtured by her friendships with other patients and the information and insights she had recorded in her diary and daily charts. The theories and data provided the intellectual means with which to create another story about her body, as well as the confidence to challenge her doctor on his own turf. The long-suppressed anger gave her the energy and animus to do what she had to do.

Getting Angry, Plotting Strategy

After eight months of suppressing her concerns or expressing them obliquely, S. finally allowed herself to vent the anger that had been seething below the surface of her ever-pleasant exterior. Still lacking access to the object of that anger, she filled her notebook with the rage that came pouring out of her soul. Although that fury had been dress rehearsed in her spring conversations with friends, the intensity of the feelings that now bubbled to the surface surprised even her. "HOW DARE YOU?" she scrawled in huge black letters. "How dare you take advantage of people when they are most weak and vulnerable, destroy their self-esteem . . . [make them] surrender control over their lives to you, and then use them as guinea pigs and feed them poison? And then make them pay thousands of dollars of their own money for it!" Behind the tirade was a deep sadness at the loss of her faith: "I trusted you—and you massively betrayed that trust. I put my life in your hands, and look at what happened: my life has immeasurably worsened." What she most wanted to say came last: "This is monstrous! You owe me eight months of my life back!" (Notes, November 14).

Yet S. did not plan to strut into her doctor's office, tell him off, and storm out. That would be counterproductive, she thought, and it just was not her style. What she really wanted to accomplish was to get through to her doctor, to make him hear her pain and suffering and see that he had made mistakes. Angry denunciations would not accomplish those ends. Attacked, the doctor would reject everything she said out of hand. Through careful persuasion and rational argument, she felt certain she could get him to acknowledge her pain and apologize for all the suffering he had caused. How sorely she had underestimated the power of biomedicine over the imaginations of its practitioners!

Deep in her heart S. also harbored a tiny hope that she could open her doctor's eyes. By using her skills as an educator, she thought, she could bring him around to seeing how the myths of science and the practices of gender had thwarted their combined efforts to heal her ills. By sharing the insights of the humanities and social sciences, she could convince her doctor to modify his practices so that she could continue to be his patient. But if she was to keep seeing him, the trust that had been so badly damaged had to be restored. A new relationship had to be negotiated in which the doctor allowed the patient to define her own reality. What she needed was "full disclosure: I want to be given the whole truth and I want to be given a fully informed choice" (Notes, November 14). In her innocence, which is touching and even quite sweet, S. thought she could topple the biomedical paradigm with a few well-chosen words.

Would her doctor be willing to work out such a relationship? S. remained cautiously hopeful. The upshot of the meeting would depend on how he reacted to what she said. S. outlined three possibilities. From best to worse, these were contrition and apology; denial and insistence that he was right; and anger and hostility. S. sketched out how she would respond to each of these reactions. If he was contrite and apologized, she would agree to continue seeing him, but only if he radically reinterpreted her diagnosis. Moreover, she would insist on a new modus operandi in which he was more sensitive to her definitions of her problems. If he denied everything and continued to insist that he was right, S. would say,

"Okay, I will look for another doctor, but I want you to continue monitoring my blood work and writing prescriptions until I find one." There would be no physical exam. Finally, if the doctor became angry or hostile, she would announce, with satisfaction, that his behavior just proved her point—that he was so adamant about dominating the interaction and reducing his patient to a body without a mind that he could not even hear her pain and pleas. The medical relationship would then end (Notes, November 14).

The Big Meeting Takes Place: S. Finds Her Voice at Last

On the appointed day S. flew to Seattle and took a taxi to Dr. D.'s office, arriving promptly at 1:00 P.M. She was eager and anxious, happy and afraid at the same time. The appointment started at 1:15. After the usual "how are you's" and the inevitable stories about the doctor's children, D. asked S. to list the medications she was on. S. did not want to give away the end of the story before she had a chance to tell the beginning. So she said that that was part of a larger story she wanted to tell. He asked another question and got the same reply. Realizing that he wasn't going to get anything from her without the story, he reluctantly agreed to let her tell it.

S. began by announcing that she had come to do her doctor a favor. "Most patients in my situation," she declared, "would just walk away and never look back." The doctor looked alarmed. His patient had never talked like this before. But, she said, because she respected him as a professional, she wanted to tell him in person what had happened to her under his care. She wanted to let him know the harm that had been done in the name of doing good. The doctor tried hard to look calm.

"Remember Your Hippocratic Oath"

Speaking from notes, and trying hard to hide her anxiety and trepidation, S. began her speech by reminding the doctor of his Hippocratic oath: *above all, do your patients no harm.* She went on to refresh his memory of his own qualified version of that oath: he had promised to do "no harm in the long run." She continued: "I don't know your definition of 'the long run,' but in my view eight months certainly counts as the long run." The doctor, probably shocked, said nothing.

"Four Consequences of Your Care"

Here is what she said next, as reconstructed from her notes:

"I want to trace the trajectory of my health since March 8, the day I first came to see you. I'm going to describe four sets of consequences that flowed from your treatment, unfolding in roughly chronological order. Two of these are physical, one is cognitive, and the last is emotional. Some of these consequences emerged in the summer and fall, that is, after I left the West Coast. But I am certain that things would have been substantially the same if I had been on the West Coast and seeing you in person.

"Let me begin by reminding you of the basic facts of my case. When I first came to see you, you diagnosed five conditions. Most important for the story I am going to tell, you diagnosed fibromyalgia, even though I lacked the main symptom of the condition, pain all over."

Unable to control himself, the doctor interrupted his patient, saying that yes, she *did* have pain all over at that first meeting. Once again he was silencing her, claiming to know her body better than she herself did. S. ignored the interruption and went on.

"In your prognosis you said I would 'progress into serious deterioration' within five years if I did not take drastic action now. That statement was pure speculation, since no one can predict the future course of a disease."

This assertion evidently angered the doctor, for he interrupted again to contradict the patient: "Your arthritis *is* erosive; I was right to say that!" S. ignored him and went on to finish her point: "Then, based on this scenario of rapid deterioration, you administered strong drugs to treat the diseases and prevent the decline.

"What effects have this diagnosis, prognosis, and treatment had on me? The first set of consequences can be described as physical effects that were contradictory. Here the effects were helpful but they came at high cost. One such benefit was your naming my 'sleep disorder' and giving me medicine to alleviate it. I appreciated that immensely. But the drugs are nowhere near 100 percent reliable; many nights I still do not get enough sleep. And this sometimes-improvement in my sleep has come at great cost, for now I am totally dependent on these drugs to sleep. I can no longer sleep naturally! I cannot fall asleep at night and I cannot take a nap in the afternoon. And, in contradiction to common medical advice and to common sense, you refused to even consider the possibility of drug addiction." The doctor did not contest this representation of his views. S. went on.

"Another benefit has been from the treatment of psoriatic arthritis. The arthritis has been brought under control. This too I greatly appreciate. But the cost of suppressing the joint inflammation is dependence on extremely elevated levels of potent drugs." Perhaps seeing these risks as unremarkable, the daily stuff of medicine, the doctor let S. go on.

"The second set of results of your treatment is also physical. But in this case the consequences were not good *and* bad, but just bad, that is, harmful to my physical well-being. I am talking, of course, about that whole new complex of painful symptoms that you always attributed to 'fibromyalgia': the headaches and the upper back and neck pain. As you know, the headaches were terribly debilitating, especially when they went on for six or seven days without cessation. In addition to discomfort, these new symptoms imposed other costs that you should know about. I lost one-third to one-half of my working time to these headaches. But lost work time was just the beginning. Around the first of September I finally figured out that, in order to get rid of these symptoms, I had little choice but to eliminate everything in my life that gave me pleasure. In particular, I had to stop swimming and gardening, activities that also kept me fit generally. That meant there was nothing left to my life but my work. And there was another cost as well. In order to avoid suffering these awful symptoms, I had no choice but to become ultra-vigilant, ultra-careful. As the list of 'don't do's' became longer and longer, my life grew increasingly constricted; I became fearful of doing anything lest it produce yet another painful symptom.

"As if that weren't enough, beginning last spring another set of essentially cognitive side effects began to set in. These cognitive changes emerged the very day I began taking Indocin." Showing the doctor the charts she had brought along, she announced earnestly, as though her doctor was eager to see the evidence: "Look, here on the charts I have been keeping, it says, 'April 4, New drug, Indocin; [Felt] spacey, hit by truck;' 'April 6, Still light-headed;' 'April 7, Spaciness;' 'April 8, Spacey all day.' I complained to you about this spaciness. You interpreted it as part of the fibromyalgia rather than as a by-product of the drug. This fall things got much, much worse. The spaciness turned to mental dulling. It crept up on me slowly, making me feel like I was losing my mind. And then the mental dulling turned into cognitive dysfunction. While the cognitive problems came and went, I felt distanced from the world, in a fog all the time. Even as everyone kept telling me to accept it, that it wasn't as bad as I thought, I was gradually becoming hysterical—my work and source of livelihood, the only thing I had left, was now being undermined.

I thought I was on the verge of totally losing it mentally." The doctor remained voiceless. Perhaps he was thinking that these were common side effects of the drug. Whatever the case, he kept his thoughts to himself, so S. went on.

"And that is not even the end of it. There were also profound emotional effects, namely, sustained, chronic, clinical-level depression. As I saw my life shrink and slip out of my control, I grew terribly depressed. I mentioned to you many times that I was depressed by your multiple diagnoses. Getting five diagnoses rather than one made me feel five times sicker than I had been before. You had redefined my identity as a person with five disorders that you and only you could treat. It seemed that everyone in my social world and every book I read told me that I had to accept it, that by resisting the truth I was making things worse. "Relax into it," they kept telling me. "Accept it," you kept saying, again and again, adding that we are all dying anyway, so why did it matter? This advice, you will note, presupposes that the doctor's diagnosis is right. But I never thought the diagnosis of fibromyalgia quite fit me. I was never fully comfortable with the idea that I had it." D. looked mildly disgusted. S. ignored him and proceeded with her presentation.

"As I told you on the phone, struggling with these new images of myself and fighting the depression used up huge amounts of time and emotional energy. I cried constantly. I lost 10 pounds because I did not feel like eating."

Unable to restrain himself, the doctor interrupted to correct the patient, saying that S. had lost only five pounds. S. countered that, in fact, her weight had fallen by ten pounds, from 118 to 108. Visibly annoyed, the doctor retorted that, according to his records, S. had previously weighed 115 and now weighed 108, bringing the loss closer to five pounds. With disdain she did not bother to hide, S. pointed out that the scale in the doctor's office was inaccurate and weighing her fully clothed produced numbers of little value in any case. The doctor retorted that the numbers from his scale were the only measures he had, implying that his numbers on her body, however dubiously derived, were more accurate than S.'s own record of her weight. This matter could not be settled, so S. went on.

"I told you about the weight loss in July when I talked to you on the phone." D. interrupted again to say that, aha, the weight loss happened *after* S. left the West Coast, so it was not his responsibility. His next thought was that, of course, the drugs metabolize more rapidly when the patient loses weight, a fact that might explain the worsened side effects.

S. had raised the issue of weight loss to highlight the depths of her depression. Characteristically, the doctor had remained deaf to her message about her emotions, translating her point back into the language of the body, which he understood and controlled. Not to be so easily defeated, S. returned to her story, trying to get out the larger point she wanted to make. "I was in a state of absolute despair. After the mental dulling set in, things were really out of control. I thought for sure I was going to lose it altogether and 'progress into serious mental illness.'" Trying to calm herself, S. reached for a glass of water. Her hands were visibly shaking.

"One Day the Fog Lifted"

"Then two good things happened," S. continued. "One day, for some inexplicable reason, I got a good night's sleep and the fog lifted. I realized that I had been knocked into such senselessness by the drugs that I hadn't even been able to figure out what was happening to me, let alone take steps to do something about it.

"A couple days later I saw my previous rheumatologist in New York City. She has known me for five years and cares very much about my welfare. She was positively alarmed to see me. She thought I seemed desperate—and I was. I described how distressed I had become from the constant fogginess and headaches. She immediately traced these symptoms to the Indocin, noting that the drug is notorious for causing precisely these problems. On her suggestion I switched antiinflammatories, and the fogginess and headaches instantly disappeared."

Dr. D. interrupted to say that he "probably would have recommended a switch" off Indocin if he had known about the mental effects. S. was appalled at how lame his response was: she would expect a physician facing a patient experiencing such damaging side effects to immediately take the patient off the drug causing them. Putting her feelings about the Indocin in the strongest possible language, she declared emphatically, "I've been taking poison!" She repeated the statement to make sure it had the intended effect. Dr. D. replied, unhappily, "I don't know how you can say that."

S. went on: "My New York rheumatologist also was skeptical of the diagnosis of fibromyalgia. I don't have the major symptom of the disease and my personality and exercise configurations are nothing like those of people with fibromyalgia." Again looking slightly disgusted, D. interrupted once more to say that there was no such thing as a typical fibromyalgic personality. Of course you would not think so, S. thought to herself, when 90 percent of your patients are labeled fibromyalgic.

"You Made Two Big Mistakes"

S. was not to be deterred by the doctor's repeated attempts to dismiss her account. She went on to tell him point-blank that he had made serious errors: "You made two big mistakes in my case. First, it was wrong to force me back on the Indocin, using a sustained-release form of the drug, when my body had said no! the first time around. You should have listened to my body the first time!" Perhaps stunned at his patient's nerve, Dr. D. remained silent.

"The second mistake was the diagnosis of fibromyalgia. It was no mere academic matter, since you consistently interpreted all the side effects, including those from the Indocin, as symptoms of fibromyalgia." There was no reply to this charge either, perhaps because the doctor had already denied that he had made any mistakes.

"A Fundamentally Disempowering Experience"

S. also told her doctor about her new views of his promise of patient empowerment. Back in the spring D. had tried to persuade her that she could gain control over her fibromyalgia by monitoring her activities and eliminating those that caused pain: this would make her feel empowered. Now S. saw the process as a form of microempowerment that could be achieved only within a larger context of disempowerment, in which the patient lost control over her life. She tried to explain these new understandings to her doctor:

"In some of my letters last summer I described how empowered I felt from gaining control over the activities that caused pain. But now I've come to realize that these small empowerments, which I genuinely felt, existed within a larger process of disempowerment in which you, the doctor, took control over my life. You did this by quintupling the number of diagnoses and destroying my self-esteem; telling me I was falling apart and would progress into serious deterioration unless I took drastic action; saying only you knew how to manage the situation (other rheumatologists deserved ridicule); and insisting that effective treatment required high levels of strong medication whose interactions only you could track and understand. In this way I was made profoundly dependent on you, the doctor. And the dependence was not only pharmacological. You essentially reached in and remade my identity, redefining me as a chronically sick person, thus taking charge of not only my physical, but also my emotional life!"

Dr. D. hooted with disbelief. He dismissed the argument about disempowerment entirely. He flatly denied that he had taken charge of her life: "I am not in control! It's been a partnership!" Evidently the distinction between micro- and macrolevels of power was too subtle for him to grasp. He was right that it had been a partnership. S. had played an important role in much of what had transpired. But the word *partnership* implies a helpful relationship between relatively equal parties. The partnership between D. and S. was dysfunctional and hierarchical at best.

After this long disquisition S. stopped, not sure where she wanted to go next. So she threw out a challenge: "I'd like to know what you have to say for yourself."

Dr. D. Defends Himself in Characteristic Fashion

Untypically, Dr. D. was at a loss for words. He appeared genuinely baffled by what S. was saying. He had thought this patient adored him. Now she was saying that he had ruined her life.

"You Are in Great Shape! Look at the Numbers!"

Dr. D.'s first reaction was to ask what on earth S. was talking about. Waving the most recent lab reports in the air, he cried out animatedly, "Look! The numbers are great!" He went on to read them out, exclaiming in all earnestness at how good the white blood cell count was, how low the sedimentation rate had fallen. And it was not only the blood work that was good. His numbers from the spring showed that the arthritis and fibromyalgia had been greatly alleviated. "You are in great shape!" he exclaimed. "We did everything we were supposed to! When you came in, you were in terrible shape. We did a lot to make you better!" To prove his point, he cited his own statistics on S.'s tender points: "When you first came in you had all eighteen of the tender points. By June that number had dropped to six. Today you probably have none."

S. found these comments hilarious. She was reproaching him for reducing her to a body and ignoring the emotional and cognitive aspects of the disease. Even as she complained about his discourses of objectification and quantification, he continued to deploy them, missing her point entirely. She was also protesting his silencing of her views of her own well-being. Yet he persisted in ignoring her account and insisting that his was the only knowledge that counted. S. tried several times to joke about this miscommunication, but D. could see nothing to laugh about.

"I Thought You Were So Happy with Me!"

Looking truly perplexed, Dr. D. said he was confused, since he thought S. was enthusiastic about his treatment. He pointed out that her summer letters were very positive. Pulling the August letter out of her patient file, he read some of her own words out loud, focusing on the passages about feeling empowered. "I take very seriously what you wrote in those letters," he said. With hurt in his voice, he added: "You said you felt empowered, now you say I'm abusive."

The doctor was right about the letters, but there were other communications that were less enthusiastic. True to form, Dr. D. had focused on the good news, selectively filtering out the bad. S. replied that the letters had to be weighed against the phone calls, which detailed major problems she had encountered—a weeklong headache, deterioration of her eye sight, and so on. (During the summer and fall there had been eight phone calls, four of them placed by S. to report problems, compared to three generally enthusiastic letters.) The doctor had no reply except to reiterate his earlier statement that he could only respond to feedback he got from the patient. In response to this comment, S. tried to explain how her own interpretations had come to be shaped by the doctor's worldview, in particular, his fibromyalgic interpretation of her conditions. But D. did not understand her argument about the power of medical science to reshape patients' perceptions of their bodies' reality. He simply rejected the notion as contrary to reason.

To ensure that the doctor did not misunderstand her, S. explained that she was not questioning his motives, which she thought admirable. But, she said, outcomes can differ from intentions. "No," the doctor insisted with feeling, "everything I do is intended. Nothing happens that is unintentional!" S. replied, with irritation, "Of course things can happen unintentionally. That is just the way the world works." That ended that part of the conversation.

"I Cannot Look after You on the Phone"

S. realized she had made a mistake in not clarifying at the outset what she did and did not hold her doctor responsible for. She did not hold him directly accountable for the cognitive dysfunctioning that occurred in the fall; indeed, she had not even called to tell him about it, because the problem was too serious to deal with over the phone. But she did deem him *in*directly responsible for virtually everything that happened, even after she had left California and Washington. During the spring the doctor had set the treatment out on a particular path, which largely predetermined what would happen in the months to come. Almost everything that occurred during the summer and fall represented the long-term consequences of the diagnosis and treatment plan that had been established early on. Therefore, as S. saw it, the doctor *did* bear substantial culpability for symptoms and side effects that emerged later. But her failure to articulate her reasoning left a space into which he immediately moved. From there he declared his innocence: "You've indicted me. That isn't fair! I cannot monitor your conditions by phone!"

Dr. D. went on to insist that he wasn't responsible for what happened when patients were too far away to make regular visits; that things could be caught in face-to-face meetings that cannot be conveyed over the telephone. S. replied, heatedly, that the course of treatment and side effects would not have been substantially different had she been on the West Coast. She was certain about that, because she had timed her letters to coincide with what would have been regular, mid-month appointments and because she had told the doctor on the telephone and in her letters everything she would have told him in person. It wasn't that she hadn't told him; it was that he hadn't heard her. A shouting match soon ensued. In a rare raised voice, the doctor retorted angrily that S. "could not say that things would have been substantially the same." S. responded, in an even louder voice—ah, the anger at last—that, if *he* could say she would "progress into serious deterioration," then *she* could say things would have been substantially the same. Both statements involved a measure of speculation.

To bolster his argument about not being able or willing to monitor his patient's conditions from afar, the doctor insisted over and over that: "I kept telling you to find other doctors when you were away." Rehearsing once again the rhetorics of biomedical infallibility, D. was suggesting that this mistake, like all mistakes, was the patient's, not the doctor's. But in this case the doctor's statement simply was not true. S.'s medical diary records the conversation in which he instructed her to find a general practitioner who was "in her [that is, D.'s] pocket." The diary also registers their amendment to this discussion in which D. agreed to write out prescriptions for six months and to monitor S.'s blood work monthly if she had the results faxed from the labs. The doctor's statement that he had urged S. to find another doctor was either a fabrication or a misrecollection. They had agreed that Dr. D. would continue to monitor S.'s health, unless and until a serious problem arose. And that is what they did; when a serious problem developed S. found another doctor. If D. had been truly adamant that his patient consult another physician, he would not have continued to review her blood work and return her phone calls.

"There Was No Philosophy or Perspective!"

Part of S.'s argument about how the doctor had assumed power over her body and life rested on her conviction that he had a particular approach to rheumatological problems, a worldview, as it were, that the patient had to accept to work with him. In response to the doctor's question, "What happened?" she said, "I played the game until I realized it was hurting me."

D.'s reaction was instantaneous: "There is no game!"

"Okay," S. said, "let's cancel the word 'game' since it trivializes something important. Let's use 'distinctive approach' or 'perspective' instead." But the doctor refused to acknowledge those terms as well, insisting that each patient is treated on the basis of her particular conditions. S. tried the word *philosophy*, which D. also rejected. Now she began to grow angry, insisting that *philosophy* was the doctor's own word, and going on to remind him of the conversation in which he had used it. In that conversation—in which he had sought to dissuade her from dropping the sleep medications—the doctor had insisted that "we have to get together on philosophy." Once again, the doctor was denying that his philosophy was a philosophy, instead claiming its status as The Truth.

"I Was Right about Everything!"

Throughout the conversation the doctor continued to assert that he had been right in everything he had said and done. Perhaps to salvage his image of himself as a hero, someone who makes patients healthy and happy, Dr. D. had to protect himself from uncomfortable truths. But ignoring

S.'s uncomfortable truths meant refusing to acknowledge the pain and suffering that she was disclosing.

Regarding the side effects of the Indocin, the doctor agreed that the cognitive dysfunction might well have been due to the drug. But he refused to concede that S.'s headaches were connected to his favored anti-inflammatory. This, despite S.'s declarations that her headaches had disappeared and that her head felt different after she stopped taking the drug. Similarly with the diagnosis of fibromyalgia. S. had rejected that label, insisting that she had never felt the "pain all over" of the disease. The doctor's response was to dispute the patient's account of her bodily condition, saying that, to the contrary, at the first appointment she *did* have pain all over. In other words, his biochemical and clinical readings of her physical state were more plausible than her own perceptions of her bodily reality. The discourse of objectification was alive and well. As if to make the diagnosis more real, he reminded her that her "sleep disorder," a prominent part of her fibromyalgia, was biologically based; it was physical, therefore real, therefore part of a bona fide, diagnosable disease. "I was right all along," he insisted; "you *do* have all the conditions I said you had." Similarly with the prognosis, which S. had rejected. "The psoriatic arthritis *is* erosive," he declared, continuing to indulge in the rhetorics of reification, treating as proven fact a claim that was nothing more than an educated guess. "I was right to say you would progress into serious deterioration." He had heard nothing she had said.

"How Could Anyone Ever Say I Made a Mistake?"

The discussion continued in this vein, with S. speaking one language and D. speaking another, for almost two hours. Evidently, the doctor would not be conciliatory and contrite, the first and, to S., best possible reaction. He was not even going to recognize that she had endured extreme suffering and pain, let alone admit that his treatment had had anything to do with it. Despite her best efforts to get him to understand her, S. began to realize that she was not getting through, that she had not disturbed his discourse in the least. Even as she tried to explain how harmful his discourses, rhetorics, and practices had been, D. had refused to hear her, continuing to treat her in the same domineering, objectifying, quantifying—in short, scientizing—ways in which he had dealt with her throughout the eight months S. had been in his care.

Sensing that they were getting nowhere, S. observed with a note of regret in her voice that the conversation appeared no longer productive and perhaps should be brought to a close. With visible reluctance, Dr. D. agreed. "There's nothing else I can say," he said plaintively. "The last thing in the world I ever expected to hear from a patient is that I ruined her life!" The doctor seemed to think he was infallible.

Realizing that Dr. D. would not change his controlling, medicalizing ways, S. decided that she no longer wanted to have him as her physician. Following the scenarios she had worked out earlier, she asked him to continue writing her prescriptions and checking her blood work until she found another doctor. The reply was out almost before the question was finished: "No," he said, adding sarcastically, "If you think I've been so harmful to you, it would be dangerous for me to continue treating you."

S. shot back immediately: "Boy, you really have the rhetoric down," she said heatedly, "*I* asked you to do this and you say it's not good *for me?*"

"Okay, okay," he said in disgust. "I'm not going to do it *for me,* is that better?" And that was the end of the consultation. The doctor did not charge S. for the appointment, which was fortunate, since she had no intention of paying him a penny more.

A Danger to Society? Postmeeting Concerns

S. left the office deeply disappointed that a doctor she had liked so much and considered so caring did not have the decency to own up to the pain he had caused or even to show some empathy for the suffering she had endured. At first she interpreted his refusals to hear her and his denials of responsibility as products of the narrowness of the scientific mind-set. She had wanted to open his eyes, to help him gain a broader understanding of the impact of his approach on his patients. The teacher in her was saddened, but she could understand how someone so completely inside the worldview of medical science, a discourse that denies its status as a discourse, might not be able to hear the critiques of the social sciences and humanities, which insist that biomedicine is but one discourse and a power-laden and interest-ridden one at that. Clearly, S. had underestimated the hold of biomedicine over its practitioners.

Later, as she mulled things over, she realized that the highly litigious environment in which medicine is practiced today may also have contributed to her doctor's stubborn refusal to budge (Diary, November 28). This possibility was suggested by Dr. D.'s complaint during that final meeting that S. had unfairly "indicted him." Dr. D.'s fear of liability could explain the pure fabrications and flat-out denials of things that were documentably true. Statements such as "there is no philosophy" or "I said I could not care for you over the phone," which were contravened by the evidence in S.'s own diary, might have represented the doctor's attempts to protect himself in the case of a lawsuit.[1] (More generously, they could also have been the result of selective memory, which filtered out things that did not support the doctor's image of himself.)

Recognizing the legal constraints within which D. worked helped S. understand what seemed to her like a palpable lack of humanity on her doctor's part. But it also made her see how formidable the obstacles to changing his practices were. The barriers to reform were deeply embedded not only in the culture but also in the legal system, the political economy of health care, and the professional culture of biomedicine. Based on her own experience, S. had come to see her doctor's scientistic, controlling approach to medicine as dangerous. If the impediments to change were so great, how could she ensure that what happened to her would not happen again? How could she know D. was not giving the diagnosis of fibromyalgia to all his patients and then producing in them the symptoms he thought they should have? Believing that the only way to prevent a repetition of the mistakes was to hold D. accountable for what had happened, S. consulted several rheumatologists about the possibility of filing a complaint against him with the Washington Board of Medicine. Their reaction was to downplay the seriousness of the error and to discourage her from pursuing any action against the doctor. One urged her to "forget about it," because it was "only eight months of her life." Another actively defended D. Counseling her to keep quiet, she suggested that Dr. D. had probably changed his procedures as a result of his experience with S.[2] Clearly, some members of the rheumatological community were not eager to find fault with a colleague.[3]

While S. had originally hoped to be able to hold Dr. D. accountable, now she felt that she had no choice but to relinquish that idea and instead direct her efforts to writing a book that would raise public and professional awareness of the problems with the general style of medical practice typified by Dr. D. The larger issue she faced was how anyone outside the medical community can bring such problems with medicine to the attention of those with the power to change things. She tried tapping mechanisms of discipline in the doctor's professional community, but these established channels for airing complaints and getting redress urged her to keep her grievance to herself. She turned to writing a book because neither Dr. D. nor other rheumatologists she consulted would hear her out or suggest a way forward. S.'s experience addresses the important issues, central to this book, of accountability and reform. Indeed, this book is not only about one person's story, but also about how we as a society can go about changing a health care system that has serious defects. Incidentally, S. never seriously considered a lawsuit. She did not want the lawyers to silence her the way the doctor had. She wanted to tell her story in her own words.

S. was disappointed with the outcome of the meeting, but she was elated as well. For she believed that, even though he had refused to show it, her doctor had heard her pain and suffering. Although he evidently had not understood her larger analysis of the power of scientific medicine not only to heal but also to harm a person's body and soul, he had been forced to see that something had gone terribly wrong in S.'s case. There was no other possible motive for her to make a special trip to his office and tell her sad story than to share the truth of her experience with the person most centrally involved in her care.

S. was also gratified that the doctor's behavior had confirmed her views about what had gone wrong. Even as she criticized him for turning her into a body without a head or heart, he continued to deny the importance of the depression and cognitive dysfunction in her experience of her illness. Even as she chided him for controlling the definition of the problem, he continued to dismiss her perceptions, insisting again and again on the correctness of his own view of the patient body. Even as she complained about being disempowered, he remained unwilling or unable to see the larger power structures in which he had occupied the dominant position. Their final meeting presented a perfect cameo of what had been happening all along. The only thing that had changed was S. herself. With her more vocal, politically astute self now dominant, she could see how the power of biomedicine had left her little choice but to abandon that critical, political self, and she was newly aware of the damage that loss had caused.

With this final meeting S. closed a tortured chapter of her life. She had rid herself of the harmful doctor, but she was left with the aftereffects of his "care" on her body and soul. The most damaging physical consequences were the new symptoms of "fibromyalgia" that had emerged early in treatment. Blissfully, two of these, the headaches and mental dulling and dysfunction, had vanished when she changed antiinflammatories. But the third new symptom, the upper-back and neck pain, remained as noxious as ever. Her sleep difficulties, one of S.'s initial complaints, had never been fully resolved, and now, thanks to Dr. D., she had the additional problem of addiction to sleep medications. Troublesome as the physical problems were, they were trivial compared to the psychological aftershocks of eight months in Dr. D.'s care. The doctor's powerful discourses had reached deep into her psyche, rearranging her sense of her self, her body, her life, and her future. How would she undo all the damage that had been done? How would she get out from under the medical gaze?

CHAPTER 12 **Out from under the Medical Gaze**

Dr. D. had undertaken eight months of "aggressive treatment" to fix his patient's ills. It took the patient six more months to heal the physical wounds he had inadvertently inflicted on her. The psychological damage would take much more time to undo. There were no doctors who specialized in curing iatrogenic disease, biomedicine's technical term for physician-induced illness; nor were there practitioners who treated the psyche and soul of the ill-treated patient. So S. had to improvise her own path to healing, calling on friends, family, and many kinds of specialists to help.

This chapter describes some of the paths she followed and what she learned along the way. Routes to self-healing included conventional strategies as well as less conventional means—religious rituals, psychotherapy, and more. It was a project not only of healing the body but also of building a new subjective self. Now free of Dr. D.'s control, S. realized how deeply the diagnostic gaze of medicine had penetrated, disconnected, and redefined her inner being. The attendant treatments had then expunged so many core parts of her identity that there was barely a shred of her former self left. S. now faced the urgent task of creating a new self, one strong enough to resist the incursions of biomedicine in the future. In her quest for self-renewal S. discovered how wrong many of her taken-for-granted assumptions about scientific medicine had been. She had already lost her faith in the mystiques of truth, objectivity, and beneficence surrounding D.'s practice. Now she was forced to see that medical science at large was not at all what she had imagined. Her experience made her realize that guidelines created by the scientific community may be ignored by community members at no peril; that medical science as an institution takes no responsibility for the errors of individual practitioners; and that scientific medicine routinely damages the patient's self yet leaves reconstruction of the fractured person to other social institutions. These insights suggested broader problems in the practice, accountability, and ethics of American medicine. I return to these in the conclusion. The winter and spring brought week after week of such disturbing discoveries, until one day S. woke up knowing that the long journey from night to day was over.

Unraveling the Diagnostic Difficulties

Knowing now that the root cause of all her problems was Dr. D.'s diagnosis, S. hastened back to the science library to find out the official diagnostic criteria for her erstwhile disease. It was curiosity that sent her back to the library; she wanted to see how her doctor's practices compared with the internationally accepted guidelines established by the American College of Rheumatology (ACR). The thought that Dr. D. might not have followed those criteria never crossed her mind. He was a specialist in the disease; how could he not know, or not adhere to, the guidelines of his professional association? But that is precisely what she discovered had happened.

The official diagnostic criteria for fibromyalgia are listed in table 3. What they indicate is that, for a diagnosis of fibromyalgia to be correct, two conditions must exist: the patient must have complaints of pain lasting for at least three months in all four quadrants of her body and the physician must detect by palpation methods eleven of eighteen clearly specified tender points. Dr. D. had not followed these criteria in deciding that S. had fibromyalgia. He had slighted the "subjective" pain criterion and based his diagnosis on his tender-point count as well as on the presence of a common symptom of the disease, the "sleep disorder" and associated fatigue. That these were the criteria he used is clear not only from S.'s notes on the appointment, described in chapter 1, but also from the report he wrote for her patient file after the initial consultation: "She has associated fibromyalgia with accompanying nonrestorative sleep pattern and 18 out of 18 tender fibrositic points" (Dr. D. Report, March 8, 1996).

Reading further in the biomedical literature, S. discovered that the diagnosis of fibromyalgia, which Dr. D. had presented to her as a straightforward matter, was a hugely contentious subject among his colleagues. A number of them complained about problems of tautology in the interpretation of the tender points. (I return to this issue in the book's conclusion.) Still others worried about methodological problems. A major difficulty was that of clinician bias: the results of the tender-point assessment can be influenced by the amount of pressure exerted by the ex-

Table 3

The American College of Rheumatology
1990 Criteria for the Classification of Fibromyalgia*

---

1. History of widespread pain

   Definition. Pain is considered widespread when all of the following are present: pain in the left side of the body, pain in the right side of the body, pain above the waist, and pain below the waist. In addition, axial skeletal pain (cervical spine or anterior chest or thoracic spine or lower back) must be present. In this definition, shoulder and buttock pain is considered as pain for each involved side. "Low back" pain is considered lower segment pain.

2. Pain in eleven of eighteen tender point sites on digital palpation

   Definition. Pain, on digital palpation, must be present in at least eleven of the following eighteen tender point sites:

   Occiput: bilateral, at the suboccipital muscle insertions

   Low cervical: bilateral, at the anterior aspects of the intertransverse spaces at C_5–C_7

   Trapezius: bilateral, at the midpoint of the upper border

   Supraspinatus: bilateral, at origins, above the scapula spine near the medial border

   Second rib: bilateral, at the second costochondral junctions, just lateral to the junctions on upper surfaces

   Lateral epicondyle: bilateral, two cm. distal to the epicondyles

   Gluteal: bilateral, in upper outer quadrants of buttocks in anterior fold of muscle

   Greater trochanter: bilateral, posterior to the trochanteric prominence

   Knee: bilateral, at the medial fat pad proximal to the joint line

   Digital palpation should be performed with an approximate force of four kg.

   For a tender point to be considered "positive" the subject must state that the palpation was painful. "Tender" is not to be considered "painful."

---

*For classification purposes, patients will be said to have fibromyalgia if both criteria are satisfied. Widespread pain must have been present for at least three months. The presence of a second clinical disorder does not exclude the diagnosis of fibromyalgia.

SOURCE: Wolfe et al. 1990: 171

aminer as well as by his interpretation of the patient's verbal and behavioral response.[1] Devising a "gold standard" for telling how much discomfort a patient feels on being pinched is an inherently difficult matter. In the 1990 ACR study, researchers used the following guidelines to assess the presence and extent of pain:

o = no pain

1 (mild) = complaint of pain without grimace, flinch, or withdrawal

2 (moderate) = pain plus grimace or flinch

3 (severe) = pain plus marked flinch or withdrawal

4 (unbearable) = patient "untouchable," withdraws without palpation

The study then went on to define *grimace, flinch*, and *withdrawal*.[2] As clinical experience increased, other articles were published suggesting ways to streamline the process.

Although the ACR criteria did not include consideration of associated symptoms, since fibromyalgia is a syndrome rather than a disease proper, its diagnosis properly involves judgment about what disease label makes the most sense of the patient's signs and symptoms. It was clearly appropriate for Dr. D. to consider the presence of related symptoms, such as the sleep disturbance, in diagnosing S.'s disease. However, she discovered, there were many more characteristic symptoms of fibromyalgia that she did not have at the time of the initial consultation. She did not suffer from morning stiffness, paresthesias (abnormal skin sensations), anxiety, headaches, or irritable bowel syndrome, all common in people with the disease.[3] Furthermore, the symptoms that she did have were not unique to fibromyalgia. In the ACR study, for example, sleep disturbances were found in 75 percent of fibromyalgics but also in 27 percent of the controls, who were patients with other rheumatic diseases, primarily arthritis. Eighty-one percent of fibromyalgics suffered from fatigue, but so too did 39 percent of the controls. "Widespread pain," from which, mercifully, S. did not suffer, was found in 98 percent of those diagnosed with fibromyalgia but also in 69 percent of those with other musculoskeletal problems.[4] Even the tender points were found among the controls: fibromyalgics were found to have 19.7 of 24 tender points, the controls 8.0.[5]

Moreover, a variety of "modulating factors," which typically reduce pain in the fibromyalgic, had no effect in S.'s case. Virtually none of the characteristic pain modulators—warmth, massage, rest—eased her pain. Although the effectiveness of these pain alleviators is not required for diagnosis, their absence might have helped to rule out the presence of the disease. Yet Dr. D. had not inquired about them.

S. did not conclude that Dr. D. had deliberately misdiagnosed her. She had no doubt that he was doing what he thought best to help a patient in evident distress. But, she now realized, there were many points at which biases such as those his colleagues worried about could have entered into the evaluation. The doctor may have used greater pressure than stipulated in the tender-point evaluation, or he might have exaggerated S.'s reaction to the stimulation. It is also likely that S., sensing that her eager new doctor hoped for a response to his pinching, compliantly gave him one. In neglecting the patient pain criterion, Dr. D. clearly violated the official guidelines. But it was unlikely that he consciously overlooked this factor. Probably he simply felt that his own "objective"—that is scientific and quantifiable—assessment of her tender points provided more important and reliable information than his patient's "subjective," unquantifiable report of pain (or lack thereof). Putting the tender-point count together with the symptom evidence, he made the brave leap to diagnosis.

To check her understanding of how the diagnosis had been reached, S. contacted the organization that had sponsored D.'s public lecture on fibromyalgia the previous spring and learned that it had been taped. On the tape D. stressed that, technically speaking, the ACR criteria are not diagnostic guidelines but standards for classifying patients as fibromyalgic or nonfibromyalgic for purposes of study. (Dr. D. is correct here, but he ignores the 1990 article's suggestion that the criteria have diagnostic utility.) Although "everyone treats the criteria as diagnostic guidelines," he continued, he himself uses them more flexibly. Indeed, he used them so flexibly that, in his practice, he declared, "it is possible to not have the criteria but still have fibromyalgia." That may help explain how S. and the other 90 percent of his patients diagnosed as fibromyalgic got their labels. Now, to the extent that clinical medicine is an art and clinicians are allowed artistic license in their work, S.'s diagnosis should perhaps be described not as erroneous, but as unorthodox, idiosyncratic, and largely meaningless. (If people without muscle pain or tender points can be labeled fibromyalgic, what is the meaning of the label?) But because that diagnosis fell so far outside the bounds of commonly accepted professional practice, and because it had such baneful consequences, throughout this book I have called it a misdiagnosis.

A thoughtful article on when to diagnose the disease pointed out the difficulties inherent in diagnosing conditions such as fibromyalgia that are heavily weighted with psychosocial baggage:

> Fibromyalgia is often not an easy disorder for the clinician . . . [because it fits a bio-psychosocial model rather than the more familiar "medical model" of disease] . . . Generally, in clinical practice, we do not know how to identify or measure the nonmedical items (even if we had the time), we find it difficult to understand their role in the illnesses of the specific patients before us, and we often feel powerless to alter them.[6]

The author, who was soon to become one of S.'s "pen pals" (and who is introduced just below), possessed a refreshing humility that S. had never seen in her own doctor. He went on to warn of problems that might arise from misdiagnosis:

> [For patients] whose illnesses appears [sic] to be driven by various psychologic and situational processes[,] it may very well be harmful to "give" such individuals a "diagnosis." Rather, they may do better with counseling . . . Although diagnosing fibromyalgia and thereby labeling patients as "ill" has been criticized as being injurious by causing "a more pervasive illness," this is only true when diagnosis is made without intelligence and concern.[7]

S. was astonished to read these words. The author had described exactly what had happened to her as a result of her doctor's misdiagnosis.

Solving the Neck and Back Pain Mystery

Two of the new symptoms that had emerged during treatment had now been eliminated, but the third, upper back and neck pain, continued to vex S. almost daily. That pain had moderated in the fall but had returned with a vengeance in December, the month after the final meeting with Dr. D. In response to her frequent questions about how this pain had developed, D. had referred offhandedly to a scientific literature on the subject. Tracking down this literature seemed the most direct route to an explanation and, S. hoped, the solution to the problem. Accordingly, S. called Dr. D.'s office and asked his assistant to get the references from him. The next day the assistant called back to say that the doctor had indicated that she should go to a medical library. S. could not believe her ears. Surely there had been some mistake. Telling her to go to a library was like telling her to look for the proverbial needle in a haystack. So she restated the question, asking the assistant to remind the doctor that he had mentioned some specific articles and to tell him she needed only one or two references to start the search. The next day the assistant called back to convey this message: "The doctor says that since you are no longer a patient, there is nothing else he can do for you. Go to the library" (Diary, January 10, 1997).

But S. had already gone to the library, where she had spent hours scanning the Medline computer files only to discover that the question of new pain emerging *after* treatment begins was an arcane subject about which few had written. Not to be deterred by D.'s brush-off, she wrote to three prominent international specialists in the disease. All had been involved in the study that established the ACR criteria for diagnosis. She posed the question this way:

17 January 1997

Dear Dr . . . :

I am doing research on the natural history of fibromyalgia . . . My focus is patients . . . with preexisting arthritis who then develop the symptoms of FMS.

I am looking for published studies that explain why, after the initial sleep and fatigue problems of FMS are brought under control, the pain in various parts of the body, such as the neck and upper back, comes to the fore . . . Why was such pain not evident to the patient before treatment for the sleep problem? And why would it be expressed after the sleep problem was resolved? . . .

One of the specialists responded within days by e-mail; the other two sent long letters with references and enclosures of published articles and patient handouts. S. was immeasurably gratified by their generosity. Two of these experienced researcher-clinicians thought the situation S. described was anomalous and did not know of any published studies on the problem. Frederick Wolfe of the University of Kansas School of Medicine (the pen pal mentioned earlier) registered these concerns: "I have problems with what you wrote. It is not my experience that after sleep and fatigue problems are under control then the pain comes to the fore. There are very few studies on secondary fibromyalgia [that arising from other rheumatological conditions], and none address this issue . . ." (E-mail, 23 January 1997). Adel G. Fam of the University of Toronto Medical School also thought there was something peculiar about S.'s case: "[I]n the clinic setting, fibromyalgia tends to be a chronic syndrome. Most patients who respond in the short term to . . . tricyclic antidepressants . . . often continue to demonstrate: a) the same number of tender points, and b) the same sleep anomaly . . . This is contrary to the situation that you have described in your letter . . ." (Letter, February 2, 1997). These letters seemed to place D.'s views outside the bounds of conventional thinking on fibromyalgia.

In the last letter, from one of the "fathers" of fibromyalgia, S. finally got an answer to her question. This kind gentleman wrote a four-page single-spaced letter to explain one of his pet theories to the curious anthropologist. Here are some excerpts:

Dear Prof. Greenhalgh,

   Perhaps the most important thing about your letter, is that you have asked the question. The answer is not difficult, and in fact very much involves anthropology. The problem has been that almost everything I have written on these issues since the 1960's has vanished from the literature of the past five years . . .

   [M]ost of the patients that I see as a rheumatologist, present with the neck and upper back pain as part of their presenting symptoms. I do see some, however, who primarily emphasise the overwhelming fatigue, and the presence of their neck complaints comes out as a secondary symptom on enquiry. However, the whole study described in the C6–7 Syndrome [an article on pain in discs six and seven of the cervical spine, which supports the neck] arose because I was finding patients such as those you describe, whose symptoms may in fact have become worse during treatment, treatment which included strategies to support the neck during sleep. *It is quite possible that neck support delivered to the mid cervical spine in fact aggravates the process in the lowest part of the cervical spine.* And it is further possible . . . that sedation prevented them from appropriately altering their sleep position, as they fail to be wakened by pain stimuli . . .

   I said that this was relevant to anthropology, and in particular to evolutionary anthropology . . . [F]our-footed mammals do not have collarbones . . . Clavicles appear . . . in monkeys . . . and humans (particularly females) have spectacularly long collarbones . . . The effects on the cervical spine are described in the patient handouts . . .

   With very best regards,

   Yours sincerely,

   Hugh Smythe, MD, FRCPC
   Professor of Medicine, University of Toronto Medical School
   (emphases added)

   What Dr. Smythe suggested was that support provided during treatment—in plain English, the pillow—causes or worsens the neck and upper back pain and that the patient's sensation of pain is cloaked by sleep medications. The problem stems from the length of the collar bone in humans, especially human females. In someone sleeping on her side with a pillow, the combined length of the collar and shoulder bones exceeds the distance from the bed to the jaw. The result is described in his patient handout: "The lower neck is unsupported, sags, and locks, with tight ligaments and crushed bone." Figure 4 illustrates the process.

   Dr. Smythe's solution was to adjust the patient's sleep posture by curving and rolling the upper body forward, placing the lower arm behind the back, and adding pillows under the rib cage, between the knees, and, in difficult cases, under the upper arm as well.

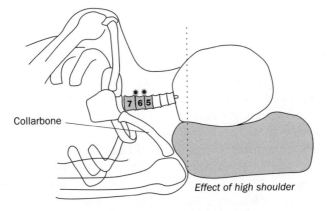

Collarbone

Effect of high shoulder

*During sleep, the unsupported vertebrae
in the lower neck sag, lock, and twist.*

Figure 4. Smythe Patient Handout. ©Hugh Smythe, M.D.

Dr. Smythe's letter and handout made instant sense of S.'s situation. All her life S. had slept on her stomach without a pillow. Dr. D. had badgered her to change to sleeping on her side, using a special pillow with a neck roll. Previous chapters have described the struggles she had with that pillow, which kept her awake more nights than she cared to remember. She proposed to her doctor that the pillow might actually be causing her back and neck pain, but he ridiculed the idea. Dr. Smythe's clinical experience suggested that S. had been right all along. Although many rheumatologists, including Dr. Smythe, believe that sleeping on one's stomach is bad for the neck in other ways, to S. it was clearly better to sleep on her stomach than to get no sleep at all. (She tried Dr. Smythe's three- and four-pillow solutions, with little success.) But the switch back to sleeping on her stomach could not be accomplished overnight. Because her neck had been reconfigured to sleep on her side with a pillow, it took her months of experimentation, and many more nights of lost sleep, to make the shift. When the changeover was finally completed four months later, her upper back and neck pain disappeared and never returned.

Dealing with the Side Effects of the Arthritis Drugs

Although the physical aftereffects of the fibromyalgia episode were now largely behind her, S. was left to deal with the real or imagined side effects of the strong drugs she had been using for arthritis control. The spring of 1997 brought one medical nightmare after the other, as new symptoms kept appearing that seemed suspiciously like the dreaded side effects of the drugs.

For years before moving to California, S. had refused to take Plaquenil, fearing the potential side effects on the retinas of her eyes. Dr. D. had essentially coerced her into taking the drug by striking the fear into her heart that her arthritis was severe and getting more so and by presenting Plaquenil as an integral and unquestionable part of a larger treatment package that would slow the inevitable erosion of her bones. Chapter 9 documented S.'s discovery in the early fall that her eyesight had deteriorated and the fears that discovery induced. Those fears sprang back to life the following spring when she noticed a further, seemingly rapid decline in her near-distance vision. Two visits to the opthamologist confirmed her fears that her near vision was worsening, and fast. Between the baseline eye assessment in April 1996 and May 1997, the near vision in her right eye declined two full points on the Jaegar scale, from 5 to 6 to 7. Was this "aging pure and simple," as Dr. D. had smugly announced, or was the aging of her eyes accelerated by high doses of Plaquenil? Although the Plaquenil toxicity tests indicated no damage, as in most medical matters the science of such tests is not exact. Anxious, S. pursued the matter further. After countless hours in the library reading the literature on Plaquenil toxicity and further discussions with both opthamologists and rheumatologists, the best answer she could come up with was this: no one will ever know.[8]

In December 1997, seven months after our story ends, S. stopped taking Plaquenil. At her eye examination two months later, the near-distance vision in her right eye had improved dramatically to a reading of 3 on the Jaeger scale. This marked restoration of her eyesight confirmed to her and to her opthamologist that the Plaquenil had indeed caused her vision to deteriorate.

During the early spring months S. experienced a striking flushing of her face. It worried her students so much that they sent her home to rest. The flushing persisted, however, prompting S. to visit a dermatologist to see what drug might be interacting with the warm southern California weather to cause it. She got a new diagnosis, but no definitive answer to the question of which drug might be the culprit.

The dermatologist, however, was concerned to learn that she had taken substantial dosages of Methotrexate over the years (a total of 3.2 grams) yet had never had a liver biopsy to check for damage to that organ. He urged her to do so in the strongest possible terms, recommending an article documenting the high probability of some degree of liver damage from such a large cumulative dose of the drug.[9] As he put it, the question was not *whether,* but *how much* damage had been done. S. read the article and, after further discussions with several physicians, decided she had no choice but to undergo the procedure. The weeks before the procedure were filled with terror and dread. After conquering her anxieties about possible complications from the procedure itself—which are far from negligible and include damage to other internal organs—she was overcome by fears that her liver might already be destroyed. After stifling those worries, she succumbed to a morbid dread of what a result of even moderate damage would mean for her arthritis control. If she had to go off the Methotrexate, what would she do? There were few good alternatives. Fortunately, the procedure went reasonably smoothly and showed, on a scale from 1 to 5, only "Grade 1 toxicity," marked by "mild microvesicular steatosis, mild nuclear variability and very minimal portal chronic inflammatory cells" (Dr. Sidney Carpenter Report, June 9, 1997). She could stay on the Methotrexate, at least for a while longer.

An Electronic Exorcism

Although S. devoted much of her time to such biomedical matters, these were not the only strategies she used to rid herself of the evil of the year past. On March 8, 1997, a year to the day after her initial consultation with Dr. D., she staged an electronic exorcism to magically purge him from her life. She invited a close friend who lived in the area to participate in the event held at her home, while encouraging some close friends and relatives who lived elsewhere to join in by e-mail or telephone. The ceremony took the local participants through seven symbolic stages, beginning with the transformation of S. into a "fibromyalgic" and ending with her empowerment and casting off of the label and all its meanings and material effects. The centerpiece of the ritual was a doll-like figure of Dr. D., complete with doctor's coat, curly brown hair, and silly grin. S. and her friend had a grand time sticking pushpins in him and writing imaginative names on his white coat. A key event was the ceremonial dumping of the "poison" drug, Indocin, which S. flushed down the toilet to the flash of a camera.

Building a New Fragmented Self:
Psychosocial Strategies of Growth

The strategies described so far were all aimed at ridding S. of the evils of the recent past. More important for the long run was her search for ways to move forward, to remake her self and her body's place in society, so as to eliminate the psychosocial mechanisms that partly underlay the chronic pain. Equally important was to build a new self, one strong enough to resist the dangerous seductions of someone like Dr. D.

The symptoms that brought S. to Dr. D.'s office in early 1996 were clearly related to the overwhelming stress in her life. The greatest source of tension was her new job. By early 1997 her work stress had been appreciably reduced by the passage of time. S. had rotated off some time-consuming committees. Her courses were now established, freeing her to get back to her own research and writing and, in turn, to make that core part of her identity once more her own. And she had learned, through trial and error, how to get her needs met in the gigantic bureaucracy of her university. The improved situation at work provided a good climate in which to begin therapy on the self.

Taking Dr. K.'s gender theory of chronic pain as her starting point, and extending it along lines suggested by feminist theory and psychoneuroimmunology (the science of mind-body connections), S. fashioned this theory into a working tool to guide her on her quest for self-renewal.[10] Working with a wonderfully sensitive counselor, she set out to constitute a new, stronger self to replace the self that had been virtually extinguished in the encounter with Dr. D. Part of the task was to improve the role of the mind and emotions in her physical well-being. A central goal of therapy was to reduce her bodily pain by lessening the stress in her life and by getting her to stop turning stress and emotions such as anxiety and anger into symptoms. Although a good part of the symptomatology was undoubtedly rooted in biological mechanisms that followed their own logic, the idea was to work hard on the psychosocial issues to see how much physical improvement would result. Much of the distress and harmful emotion was rooted in the larger pattern of compulsive pleasantness and self-silencing, a dynamic learned during a lifetime of gender training. Undoing this dynamic meant learning new skills of assertiveness and self-expression, especially of hostile feelings.

Through the counseling and in many other ways—including, importantly, the writing of this book—S. began to assemble a new self, combining some pieces of the old (the exercise aficionado, for example) with elements that were new (more integrated mind-body relations, a usually symptom-free body, a more harmonious gender identity, keener awareness of the power of professional disciplines, and much more). Since that new self—the I that is writing this book—is a self that is always in process, this story of self-making has no end, but will continue to unfold as time goes by.

During the long ordeal with Dr. D., the profound depression that had descended on S. had led her to close her blinds and seclude herself in her room, shutting potential new friends out of her life and exacerbating the social isolation that often comes with chronic illness. Although these people might have been able to help her by giving her fresh perspectives on her situation or by offering emotional and political support, S. did not want them to see the depths of her despair. As the depression lifted, she emerged from her hiding and began to make new friends, letting them be part of the healing process.

Quitting the Body Job

One day in late May S. woke up to realize that her quest for healing had become almost a full-time job. The previous week she had devoted half a day to exploring the possibility of learning transcendental meditation and another full day to reading up on drug toxicity in the library. And this did not count the time she spent keeping diaries and records, working out, scouring bookstores, seeing her therapist and, most draining of all, worrying constantly about what might be going wrong with her body. She shared her observation with a friend, who joked that she needed a vacation from her body. No, S. said to herself, she needed to quit the body job. And so she quit, just like that. She didn't end all her activities, many of which were helpful and would doubtless be with her for life, but the obsessive need to get rid of the illness, the fear-induced drive to be doing ever more for the suffering body—this is what she quit. And thus it was that, a year and two months after the nightmare started, it finally came to an end.

Part Six | Narrating Illness, Politicizing Pain

CONCLUSION **Re-viewing the Medicine of Chronic Pain**

This case raises troubling questions the reader may well wish to ponder. Who is responsible for this medical tragedy, the doctor, the patient, both of them, or neither of them? Did the doctor do anything wrong, or was he just doing what he was trained to do? Was the patient culpable as well, or was she doing her best, given the codes of gender and science by which she was taught to live? Consideration of such matters is well and good, since this case poses difficult questions of medical ethics for which there are no ready answers. In this conclusion, however, I want to move on to larger issues.

In the preface I posed three sets of questions about the workings of science, gender, and culture in the medical domain. How could scientific medicine, which is supposed to ease bodily pain, end up creating it instead? How do the dynamics of gender complicate an already power-laden doctor-patient relationship, leaving many women (and men) dissatisfied with their medical care? And, finally, how might popular cultures of alternative medicine sometimes compound the problems of the chronically ill? In the problematique, I drew on a number of literatures in the humanities and social sciences to develop the analytic frameworks and arguments I used in the book. The individual chapters then elaborated those arguments ethnographically.

In this conclusion I want to speak more personally to you, the reader. Although this is a scholarly book, it is also, obviously, a deeply personal book. I believe that this tale of senseless suffering will serve a larger purpose if it can help us to understand and undo some of the irrationalities of the medical system we now have. I wrote this book for five groups of readers: patients and potential patients, physicians and medical educators, students of science and medicine in the humanities and social sciences, students of gender and power in American culture, and fellow anthropologists. In the first five sections of this conclusion I write directly to each group of imagined readers to tell you what thoughts I hope you will take away from this book. Although you might read only the sections that apply to you, I hope you will read other sections as well. In the sixth and final section I take a longer historical perspective to suggest why chronic pain conditions like fibromyalgia—which affect a small minority of Americans—should worry us all.

To Patients and Other Ill People: Choose Your Story with Care

Out of this grim experience of medically induced illness has come a deep conviction that we as patients need to revise our understanding of how medicine works. We need to recognize the artful character of the things our doctors tell us. We need to appreciate the choices we have in the stories—both our own and our doctors'—by which we make sense of our ills. Finally, we need to comprehend the crucial consequences of the stories we choose.

Many Stories but No Truth: Dispelling the Myths of Scientific Medicine

Despite the many critiques of medicine, for many of us medicine retains a special mystique. A kind of secular religion, it is haloed by the myths of truth, objectivity, and no harm. I have sought to dispel these myths, because unquestioned belief in them can be dangerous. Following a storytelling approach to science, I have argued that the fundamental work of clinical medicine is to tell a three-part tale about the patient's body (diagnosis-prognosis-treatment), to coax the patient into believing the story, and then to put it into effect to ease the body's ills. Although scientific medicine calls its stories The Truth, by examining how one such story was fabricated, this ethnography has illuminated their artful, artificial character. Viewing Dr. D. as a working scientist, we saw the inherent shakiness of the methods he used to create the scientific "facts" of the case. We observed too the narrow, reductionistic nature of the discourses from which D.'s story was composed. And we witnessed the emotionally coercive character of the verbal tactics by which the doctor converted his patient into a believer in his cause. By taking the processes of story making and telling apart, we were able to see that Dr. D.'s story undoubtedly seemed like the truth to him, because of his adherence to the methods, discourses, and rhetorics of scientific medicine. Once we questioned that framework, the truth of the story outside the narrow context of biomedicine became difficult to sustain.

Dismantling the myths of biomedicine is important because it allows us to look beyond the rhetorics of truth and objectivity to see that medicine's stories are limited in ways that matter. Cultural critics of science such as Sandra Harding and Donna Haraway have argued that, because of the way science is conducted, science's stories are inevitably partial, value laden, and self-interested.[1] Dr. D.'s story was all these things. It was *partial* because it excluded the affective component of the illness from consideration and proceeded to treatment without attending fully to the question of cause. The doctor's treatment program was *value laden* in that it assumed a medical relationship in which the doctor-scientist made all the decisions while the patient-object simply followed orders, regardless of the effects on her body and life. Underlying these arrangements were the hierarchical values of science, which authorized the scientist-expert to dominate nature (of which the patient's body was a part) on the assumption that he knew how to improve its workings. The doctor's diagnosis and prognosis were also *self-interested,* though the doctor remained unaware of this. Although framed as an exclusively scientific endeavor and promoted in the rhetorics of patient benefit, the diagnosis of fibromyalgia, together with the prognosis of lifelong, progressive illness, had the *effect* of increasing the number of rheumatological patients in D.'s practice at a time when rheumatology and other specialized domains of medicine are under threat from managed care. It is not necessary to posit crass material motives to point out that behind the doctor's extravagant propagation of this disease label lie larger struggles of specialists like himself for professional and financial survival in a new medical marketplace dominated by managed care.

Although the doctor presented his story as The Truth of the patient's body, in her search for answers S. encountered two other stories that provided different accounts of the likely causes and best treatments of her symptoms. These were the story of alternative and New Age medicines and the gender theory of chronic pain. Each of these stories was also plausible within its respective frame of reference—holistic theories of health in the former case and social structural theories of the body in society in the latter. Clearly, there is no "right" story of the ill body. There are only different stories, each one true within the discursive frame in which it is told.

Different Stories Have Different Effects

Which story we choose is important, however, for different stories have different effects. As noted many times above, most biomedical stories of acute illness are probably helpful. They name a fixable problem and spec-ify a therapeutic program that will fix it. These stories often work—to everyone's delight. Here is biomedicine at its best. When illness is chronic, however, the consequences of biomedical stories may be harm-ful. Arthur Kleinman has written of the dangers of scientific medicine for the chronically ill patient.[2] Yet the word *dangerous* does not begin to describe the unhinging effects of D.'s biomedical story on the patient studied here.

Today popular cultural discourses on holistic medicine provide the ma-jor alternatives to the stories of biomedicine. Are they good alternatives? The case examined here suggests that some of these narratives may be two-edged swords for the chronically ill. On the positive side, they counter the objectifying discourses of biomedicine with theories of mind-body connections and lessen physician power with self-help programs for the patient. In addition, they supply a multitude of unconventional treatments that appear to be safer than, if not always as efficacious as, the drugs of biomedicine.[3]

At the same time, however, some of these popular discourses carry risks of which those seeking help may not be aware. In the highly com-petitive marketplace of alternative therapies, the ones that have made themselves most visible are not the better established and respected ther-apies like acupuncture and Ayurvedic medicine, but the less proven self-help and New Age approaches that S. consulted. With their seductive promises of self-healing, these are the ones that pose risks. If biomedi-cine reduces illness to the body, some New Age medicines reduce it to the mind and promote "mind-cures" that are no more effective in heal-ing chronic illness than the body-cures of biomedicine. Both New Age and self-help manifestos present only successful cases, conveying false hopes of improvement, when in reality the likelihood of success of a given therapy is unknown. Echoing themes in consumerist culture—we freely choose our lives, it is our fault if we make poor choices—these approaches employ an individualistic discourse that makes the patient responsible both for causing her ailments and for successfully treating them. As Su-san Sontag warned two decades ago, such individualistic discourses pun-ish the patient, who has less control over her body than these discourses imply. S.'s case suggests that they may leave the sick feeling blamed for causing their illness and blamed for failing to remedy it. This blame comes on top of the shame they already feel about having a defective body, a palpable stigma in a culture that worships the perfect body. Paradoxi-cally, these alternative medical discourses may ultimately support biomedicine by deflecting attention from larger structural forces that underlie many of the diseases of late-twentieth-century civilization. They also accept and reinforce the labeling authority of biomedicine by urging ill people to accept their diagnoses and adapt to them, when the better route may be to question them.

Many chronically ill people find themselves going from practitioner to practitioner looking for help. Depending on their tolerance for disappointment, they may wind up spending significant portions of their lives searching for a story that makes sense of their pain. Some never do. The patient in this book was fortunate to find a physician who sketched the outlines of a third, rarely told story of illness that fit her intellectual predilections and seemed to make sense of her life—the gender theory of chronic pain. This story avoided the mind-or-body reductionism of biomedical and some alternative medicines. It located key sources of chronic illness in the larger structures of societal inequality rather than in bodily or personality "flaws" of the individual patient. It pointed the way to a new kind of therapeutic approach—psychological counseling to undo harmful gender socialization and to reduce life stresses—that addressed not just the symptoms, but some of the underlying causes of the problem as well.

Of course, this story too has limitations. It is probably specific to certain race and class groups. It may exaggerate the importance of gender socialization in the genesis of chronic illness. Even if socialization into pleasantness contributes to chronic pain, psychotherapy might not be capable of intervening in so deeply rooted a part of the personality as the tendency to transform social stress into bodily symptom. Indirect and long term by nature, psychological therapies might not always help to alleviate bodily symptoms.

For every one of our bodily ills, there are multiple stories we could tell to make sense of them. If there is one idea that I hope you, the ill or potentially ill reader, will take away from this book, it is that *which story we choose matters*. It matters because our beliefs about our bodies come to shape our bodily reality. Of course, our choices are not free. They are constrained in that the understandings available to us are limited by our social locations of age, class, race, and so forth. But by remaining open to cultural currents, we can broaden the range of stories to which we have access. How can we choose between competing accounts of our pain? Certainly we should opt for the story that best alleviates suffering and most inspires hope. We should prefer the narrative that is the most complete and compelling. Finally, we should adopt the tale that is the most humane. A humane story involves not the domination of an expert, but genuine empowerment of the sick person to effect real change in her life.

To Physicians: A Science That May Endanger Your Chronic Patients' Health

We live in an age of chronic illness, yet our medicine was devised to heal acute ills. This ethnography has shown what can sometimes go wrong when a science of acute illness is applied to chronic pain: medicine can inadvertently produce discomfort and disease rather than reduce them. Moreover, it can damage the patient's self and permit abusive treatment in the name of care. That all this happened in the practice of a physician who deeply cared about his patients' welfare makes it all the more troubling and tragic. If we are to create a better science of medicine to heal our chronic ills, we must resist the temptation to forget about difficult cases such as this one. Instead, we must courageously pursue such cases, seeking out what went wrong and why. The following section lays out my analysis of what went wrong. If it strikes the reader as unkind, I hope he or she will remember that it is motivated by a desire not to pillory the doctor, but to figure out how to prevent such things from happening again.

Anatomy of Iatrogenic Fibromyalgia

The eight-month history of S. and Dr. D. provides a clear case of the medical manufacture of illness. The doctor first diagnosed a disease whose chief symptom—widespread pain—the patient lacked. He then produced in her body a large number of ancillary symptoms to go with the diagnosis. Unknowingly, the physician molded his patient's reality to fit his convictions. A trained specialist in fibromyalgia, the doctor believed that the great majority of rheumatological patients exhibit a set of signs and symptoms that can usefully be understood by the construct of "fibromyalgia." The doctor made this point repeatedly in his examining room and public lectures. One of his patients described his mindset to S. as "everyone with arthritis has fibromyalgia." He believed further that virtually all such patients who consult him will benefit from receiving the label and from coming under his long-term care. His actions made this view clear. Interpreting the diagnostic guidelines idiosyncratically, he diagnosed his new patient as "fibromyalgic" and then proceeded to treat her putative fibromyalgia and preexisting arthritis in his customary fashion. Although neither doctor nor patient realized it at the time, many of those interventions actually created the symptoms of fibromyalgia that the patient initially lacked. (The chief symptom never appeared, however.) The altered sleep posture and new pillow produced pain in the upper back and neck region, a cardinal feature of the disease. Indocin, a drug administered for the patient's arthritis, spawned headaches, mental fogginess, and cognitive dysfunction, all characteristic symptoms of fibromyalgia. Restrictions on exercise led to physical deconditioning, which increased the patient's vulnerability to pain and fatigue, both associated with the disease. The dire diagnosis, poor prognosis, and new symptoms induced a profound depression, another common concomitant of fibromyalgia. Yet so sure was the doctor of his diagnostic and therapeutic skills that he interpreted each new symptom as validation of his diagnosis, missing the connection between his own practices and his patient's pain. Although D. knew very well that Indocin often produces the side effects that S. was experiencing—he reported these risks in the initial consultation—he came to disregard that link as the fibromyalgic interpretation of the new symptoms gained precedence. Unwittingly, the doctor seems to have willed his beliefs into reality, creating a veritable facsimile of the disease he had set out to mitigate.

While this account of an overeager specialist makes sense of what happened, I have argued that such an explanation is inadequate, for it places the blame on D. when ultimate responsibility belongs elsewhere. Certainly D. was part of the problem. His evangelical attitude toward his specialty disorder, combined with his unwillingness to credit anything his patient said, created a climate in which medical misfortune could easily materialize. But D. was only part of the problem. I have contended that medical science itself was deeply implicated in the unfortunate turn this case took. Two aspects of medicine played central roles in the creation of fibromyalgia in a nonfibromyalgic patient: its practice of constructing medical syndromes out of diffuse, nonorganically based symptoms and its overarching cognitive framework. I deal with the cognitive framework here, returning to the nonorganic syndromes in the final section.

Biomedicine purveys a powerful worldview of the causes and cures of bodily ills. This worldview consists of a set of discourses, which are at once enacted in, and concealed by, rhetoric. At the core of this worldview is a mechanistic model of the body as a biological machine separable from the mind and emotions. In the ideal version of this model, the machine-body is knowable only by a trained expert. It is analyzable as a set of pathologies, measurable by quantitative indices of biological processes, and treatable by body-altering drugs or surgical interventions. Most physicians temper these ideals in practice, but the ideals remain the professional standard.

This mechanistic model works reasonably well in fixing acute bodily ills, but it works poorly in treating chronic illness. It operates most poorly in the face of chronic conditions such as fibromyalgia that have no (known) organic basis. In such illnesses, the symptoms are diffuse and difficult to label meaningfully. Their causes lie largely outside the body in a world the patient, not the doctor, knows best. Healing depends on changing the whole person, not just a bodily part. Not surprisingly, when the mechanistic model is applied to chronic illness, the clinical tale the doctor tells is almost always a bad one.

When an ill-fitting story becomes the basis of bodily treatment, many things can go wrong. The ambiguity of the patient's symptoms invites any number of diagnoses, creating space for the doctor's interests and values subtly to color his clinical judgment. The methods of diagnosis and treatment are imperfect, making it easy for slips to occur and remain undetected. The patient is treated as an object of knowledge rather than as a knowing subject, precluding potentially useful feedback from being heard. The doctor is regarded as the sole expert, allowing him to treat the illness in the way he sees fit and to measure his performance by narrow, quantitative criteria that may miss the forest for the trees. These slips and colorations are then linguistically obscured in the rhetoric of truth, objectivity, and beneficence, with the result that neither doctor nor patient can see that things have gone awry. In these ways, the goals of medicine can be perverted, while the perversion remains hidden from sight.

Discursive Damage: The Danger of Diminishing the Patient's Self

The problem is not just one of efficacy—whether medicine works in chronic illness. It is also one of safety—whether the chronically ill patient is actually harmed by the medical encounter. This study has illuminated a wide range of such hazards, from bodily harm to philosophical angst to psychic trauma. In this and the following section I draw attention to two of these injuries that are invisible to practitioners, perceived only by the patients who sustain them. Because patients have no way to articulate their inner wounds in the dominant discourse of truth, objectivity, and beneficence, however, these injuries often remain below the level of consciousness, expressing themselves in vague feelings of discomfort and distress surrounding the medical encounter. In describing these interior injuries as unintentional products of biomedical discourse and rhetoric, I am hoping to find a language in which we can speak about extrabodily patient pain—or suffering. In this endeavor, I carry forward the work of Eric J. Cassell and Arthur Kleinman, who too were deeply concerned about the patient self.[4]

Biomedicine's discourses on the body promise enhancement of life. From the patient's perspective, however, they are fundamentally life negating. These discourses sever the body from the mind and emotions, removing the authority to know and the power to control the body from the person inhabiting it. They then reduce the body to a collection of pathologies, further reduce the pathologies to a set of numbers, and proceed to treat the pathology without fully establishing the cause. When the bodily ills are quickly eased, this violent severing and radical reduction that have taken place in discourse are probably experienced symbolically only and are rapidly put out of mind in the joy of restored health. But when the ills are not made better—as is the case with many chronic illnesses—and the discourse becomes the conceptual basis for long-term treatment, that discourse becomes inscribed in the body in ways that are profoundly life altering. The effect on the object of biomedical intervention is to shrink its humanity, to whittle away its life. It was this deflation of her self that took S. to the edge of madness. Her case was extreme—made so by a doctor who took these discourses in an unusually literal way—but it reveals the inner damage that can inadvertently be done when a person is reduced to a mere object of scientific knowledge and intervention.

Rhetorical Excess: The Danger of Verbal and Emotional Abuse

The rhetorics of biomedicine are also dangerous because they may justify verbal abuse in the name of patient benefit. The term *abuse* may strike readers as overly harsh, since the practitioner's intentions are better than good. Unfortunately, good intentions can be carried out in abusive ways. What is abuse? Following Beverly Engel, author of *The Emotionally Abused Woman*, we can define abuse as "behavior that is designed to control and subjugate another human being through the use of fear, humiliation, and verbal or physical assaults." Whether physical or emotional, abuse is almost always damaging because "it systematically wears away at the victim's self-confidence, sense of self-worth, trust in her perceptions, and self-concept."[5] While any medical relationship can contain abusive elements, because of prior gender socialization, abuse is more likely when the doctor is male and the patient female.

This case well illustrates the dangers of abuse. Dr. D.'s style was regrettably abusive. In the interests of rheumatological care, he sought to control his patient, to get her first to believe his story of her ills and then to follow his orders for their treatment. When the patient resisted these orders, the doctor became verbally abusive. Earlier chapters analyzed these conversational deployments as rhetoric—and that is how they functioned *cognitively* to bolster the conceptual apparatus of biomedicine. But these same tactics also performed the *emotional* function of intimidating and frightening the patient, in that way silencing her into submission. When we consider their emotional impact, the doctor's threats, accusations, and sarcasms can only be described as verbal assaults. His trivializations of the patient's suffering and his expectation that she should massively alter her life for the sake of his therapeutic program constituted abusive treatment.

The doctor's verbal batterings had the predictable effects. The patient lost confidence in herself. With the deepening of her sense of ontological and epistemic invalidation—the feeling that she and her knowledge had been voided out of existence—her ability to separate her own perceptions from her doctor's wore thin. In turn she became deeply dependent on the very person who was intimidating and berating her. As is typical in such situations, she did not and could not see what was happening as abuse. To the contrary, she accepted the blame for all her problems, crediting her doctor with everything that went right.

Many readers will resist—if not angrily reject—the idea that physicians can, and in rare cases routinely do, abuse their patients. Indeed, such practices are almost impossible to witness, since deeply ingrained beliefs in physician autonomy protect the privacy of the doctor-patient relationship and all that goes on within it. Difficult though it is to see, it is crucial to look once again at this problem, which was first raised by women's health advocates in the 1970s. The issue of patient abuse must be confronted, because it erodes the patient's self-esteem and ability to cope, undermining the doctor's efforts and inflicting psychological damage that may last well beyond the end of the doctor-patient relationship. When a patient is in long-term care with an abusive practitioner, the physician's emotional abuse may even become an additional source of chronic pain. Dr. D.'s experience with S. shows how easy it is to slip from a respectful attitude toward a patient into an abusive one when the patient balks at following the doctor's carefully worked out plans. D.'s conduct shows too how easy it is to subtly coerce an intimidated and fearful patient into being treated in ways she regards as dangerous—like being "tolerized" to toxic drugs. Quiet coercion may serve the doctor's interests in gaining compliance, but it is poor practice, for it is medically unsafe, it is unethical, and it is inhumane.

A Better Science of Medicine for an Age of Chronic Illness

Despite my sharp critique of scientific medicine, my position is neither antiscientific nor antibiomedical. Quite the contrary, I have great respect for both science and biomedicine. But I believe strongly that the tools of scientific medicine should not be monopolized by physicians and medical researchers. (And, with the spread of internet-based medicine, increasingly they are not.) In the story I have told, the systematic collection and analysis of data *by the patient* played a vital role in the constitution of medical knowledge. These numbers helped to save the patient's life by exposing the downward trend in her physical and mental health and by galvanizing her into seeking a second opinion. Later, the patient's rigorous pursuit of alternative hypotheses enabled her to track down the causes of the symptoms she had acquired and to eliminate them from her life. As a practicing social scientist, the patient may have been an unusually careful observer, record keeper, and hypothesis tester. But most patients are probably good empiricists who, if invited to participate, could make a valuable contribution to their medical care.

Within biomedicine itself, there are exceptional practitioners who acknowledge the patient as a suffering person as well as a diseased body. For example, the "biopsychosocial" model articulated by George L. Engel in the 1970s decried the reductionism of the biomedical model and its deleterious effects on the healing powers of the physician.[6] Engel urged colleagues to broaden their conceptual framework to include the social, psychological, and behavioral concomitants of illness and to extend the scientific method to include these factors in the treatment of disease in their patients. Clinicians concerned about humanizing an increasingly technology-intensive medicine may want to return to Engels's writings for insights, now unfortunately marginalized by the seemingly rapid progress of biomedical knowledge. Despite Engels's attempts to broaden his colleagues' strictly biological or organic representation of illness, however, from a social scientist's perspective, Engel still fails to approach the broader question of how science and illness are themselves social constructs.[7] Physicians will need to join forces with social scientists to search for the richer, more complex models needed to conceptualize illness and to practice medicine in a manner that recognizes the shaping role of society on biology and the scientific method.

This issue of the scope of inquiry carries particular import in the identification and alleviation of medical mistakes. Since the episode detailed in this book came to an end, news of some egregious medical mistakes, coupled with some startling new statistics, have transformed the relatively neglected topic of medical error into a major public concern. A National Academy of Sciences report issued in late 1999 suggested that the American health-care system, long considered the best in the world, actually kills tens of thousands of patients a year.[8] Alarmed by the magnitude of the problem, government and business have begun to establish mechanisms to reduce the number of iatrogenic injuries.[9] While this is a welcome development, the analysis offered here suggests that this new concern about mistakes may not go far enough. Reformers have focused on relatively conspicuous errors in treatment modalities such as medication and surgery, passing over less visible slips in the fundamental tasks of medicine: the creation of medical "facts" such as diagnoses and prognoses. Though less often fatal, such errors may be more common than the technical mistakes that are the object of concern today. The current conversation is also limited in its exclusive focus on the bodily injuries caused by medicine. Damage to the patient's inner world, which may be more pervasive and cause more suffering than physical harm, has not been identified as a problem worthy of professional or public attention. Finally, current strategies to reduce the extent of error emphasize a "systems approach" that designs safety into the systems of health-care delivery. Although inefficiencies in the organization of health care undoubtedly cause countless mistakes, this book has suggested that the roots of many errors lie deeper, in the conceptual models that structure biomedical knowledge. The academy's call to arms presents an opportunity to address a much wider set of problems surrounding medical error. If we are serious about diminishing medically induced suffering, we must begin by expanding our cultural and political conversations about what counts as a mistake, what kinds of injuries matter, and what parts of biomedicine are open to critique and reform.

The aim of the critique developed here has been not to find fault, but to find ways to create a better practice and better science of clinical medicine. To the larger debates on medical reform, this case contributes a sense of what better practice and science might mean from the chronically ill patient's point of view. Since the great bulk of medical services are now devoted to the treatment of chronic conditions, enhancing the care of the chronically ill is a matter of some importance, not only to the sufferers themselves, but to the health-care system as a whole.[10] This case suggests that better practice means practice that treats the patient not as an object of the medical gaze but as a subject who is knowledgeable about important aspects of her health and capable of making informed and good decisions about her treatment. Better practice is not authoritarian but democratic, enlisting the patient's help in a collaborative quest for healing. Better science is inclusive rather than exclusive, embraces the mind and heart as well as the body, and looks for the sources of pain not only in the body physical but in the body politic as well. Finally, better science acknowledges the presence of human error and the imprint of personal values and interests on medicine. It abandons the claims of Truth and Objectivity, professing instead to be a partial and particularistic science that inevitably bears the mark of the physician-scientist practicing it. A partial and situated science is locatable and thus accountable for what it does.

To Students of Science and Medicine: Why the Scienceness of Medicine Matters

For many years, anthropologists and sociologists of medicine maintained a respectful distinction between the sociocultural and cognitive aspects of biomedicine, focusing on the social and cultural while placing scientific knowledge itself beyond the scope of the social science enterprise. The emergence of the social studies of science has dissolved this distinction between the social and the intellectual, revealing the cognitive dimension of science to be cultural through and through.[11] "The facts" are no longer simply unquestionable truths, but social and cultural creations. Working in this emerging borderland connecting technoscience studies and the medical social sciences, in this ethnography I have focused on the scienceness of biomedical constructs, language, and practice. Though biomedicine is indubitably a profession, as an earlier generation of sociologists has shown, this more recent focus on its scientific core has enabled powerful new insights into how it works and how it gains such power over individual lives.[12]

Clinical Medicine as Laboratory Science:
The Making of a Scientific Fact

The medical social sciences have studied many aspects of biomedical ideology and practice, but the heart of the medical enterprise—the making and implementing of clinical decisions—has rarely been problematized for social research. Following in the footsteps of ethnographers of science, I conducted an ethnographic study of medicine, using the metaphor of laboratory science to inform my observations of clinical work.[13] By attending closely to the most mundane of matters—raw materials, technical instruments, history-taking procedures, examination practices, and so forth—I have shown that the solving of medical problems closely resembles the solving of scientific problems. Even the analytic procedures the doctor followed—the narrowing of the domain of interest, the constitution of an "N of 1," the collection and analysis of quantitative data, the systematic testing of hypotheses, the methodical experimentation on the patient body—were strikingly parallel to those employed in the "real" sciences. Evidently there is more science to clinical medicine than we social scientists had thought.

In the public imaginary, science and scientific medicine are serious pursuits devoted to discovering the truths of nature and describing them in the form of hard, objective "scientific facts." By closely observing the creation of one influential medical fact—a diagnosis of fibromyalgia—I have shown that "the facts" of medicine are not discovered but humanly created. The fact studied began with something in nature—a suffering body—but that suffering had to be humanly transformed before it could be born as a scientific fact. During that process of transformation, the fact-in-the-making was touched by a number of "soft" and subjective things: unstable definitions of the disease, contested diagnostic procedures, and the gut beliefs and values of the practitioner. The diagnosis he produced was not simply a truth he had uncovered, but a construction he had coaxed into being. As such, it bore the fingerprints of its maker and of the procedures by which it had been created.

After the fact was formed, the soft, subjective process by which it had been created was then concealed by a rhetoric of hard, objective scienticity. Inspired by David Locke's work on error and error-camouflaging rhetoric in science, I searched for evidence of such persuasional work in the doctor's medical practice.[14] That evidence was not hard to find, for the doctor was an inspired rhetorician who peppered his clinical conversation with the rhetorics of scientific rationality, reification of the only possibly real, domination over nature, and medical infallibility. Although I have devoted special attention to the doctor's colorful linguistic tactics, language was only one of the media through which he deployed the rhetoric of science. The doctor's rhetorical work at large took the character of an elaborate performance in which many aspects of his self-presentation and professional practice contributed to the dramatic effect. The serious and somber demeanor, the authority of the white coat, the blandness of the overall appearance, the attention to the most minute bodily detail, the collection of a huge number of numbers, the impenetrability of the clinical reporting, the grammatical carelessness of the clinical writing, the duration of the appointments, the size of the bills—these and countless other features of the medical encounter that are rarely noted were all crucial aspects of the practitioner's unconscious efforts to underscore the scientific robustness of his work. They also served to make the constructedness of his facts disappear from view. By stripping away the seriousness of the scientific endeavor and exposing its performative character, I have attempted to show not that medical science is duplicitous or bad, but that it is human. Appearances notwithstanding, the science of medicine embodies the values, beliefs, and interests of its makers.

Science and Subjectivity: Spoiled Identities, Shrunken Lives

Although medicine claims to be a discipline of the body, this ethnography has highlighted its ability to effect massive interventions in our lives as a whole. As Cassell suggested twenty years ago, it does so by altering our identities, what he called our "personhood."[15] When we are given diagnostic labels, we are assigned new, medicalized subjectivities—the diabetic, the tuberculotic, the fibromyalgic. Although innocent, even helpful, from the doctor's point of view, these labels have the potential to spoil our identities, in Goffman's well-chosen phrase.[16] And the spoilage can be instantaneous. Dr. D. had only to utter three words—"you have fibromyalgia"—and his patient's sense of her self and its possibilities was forever changed. When the disease is chronic—for life—the spoilage can be permanent too. Once thrust upon us, the new identity is hard to cast off or give back: "No, I am *not* a diabetic, a tuberculotic, a fibromyalgic!" Dispensed by a man or woman of medicine, the label is backed by the cultural authority and social power of biomedicine and, behind that, science itself. Who are we, mere individuals, to challenge the accumulated wisdom of Science?

This ethnography has shown how a biomedically "spoiled" identity can precipitate a cycle of decline that ends in the undoing of a life. How can the subject position "fibromyalgic" be so destructive? People with fibromyalgia-like conditions know, for they must resist, accommodate, or otherwise come to terms with that identity every day. Here I can only suggest a few of the ways in which that subjectivity can undermine a life, using the patients described in the research literature as my point of reference. First, a "fibromyalgic" is a lifelong patient. To be a protracted patient is to be a part-person—a body only—and a relatively powerless person in an ongoing interaction with a highly significant other. In the words of one woman who deplored her dependence on doctors and drugs, becoming a fibromyalgic was like "being given a life sentence."[17] A "fibromyalgic" is also a person whose body is out of control for no discernible reason. Living with daily pain, fatigue, and sleep deprivation, the fibromyalgic has a hard time carrying on a normal life. Some are engulfed by panic and fear.[18] A "fibromyalgic" is also a subject with no known future; to the extent that it is known, it is known to be filled with pain and disability. To be a fibromyalgic is to be forced to pare back one's life plans. For obvious reasons, for many this is a depressing prospect. Finally a "fibromyalgic" is a subject who disciplines the self, surveilling her life closely, eliminating activities that exacerbate pain, and adhering to a rigid routine.[19] To be a fibromyalgic is to lead a restricted life. As one sufferer put it, it is to be "imprisoned" by one's illness.[20]

While the effects of this new identity will vary from person to person, in S.'s case it obliterated the self she had spent decades creating. The effect was particularly damaging because of her long history of internal struggles to hold onto her belief that she was "normal" despite an occasionally debilitating arthritic condition. The new bodily identity put "normalcy" beyond reach, pushing her over the edge. As her "fibromyalgic" identity replaced her earlier, "basically healthy" body identity, she fell into a deep despair and began slicing off pieces of her life in a desperate attempt to bring the "fibromyalgic" symptoms under control. When this did not work, she edged dangerously close to the edge of a psychological abyss. Had she gone further and taken her life, the death of the body would have been a fitting metaphor for the already accomplished death of the self.

Do medicalized identities always have such destructive consequences? Of course not. Medical identities can be both welcome and helpful. Especially when the illness is acute and curable, a person is likely to appreciate such a label, which is temporary in any case. Even in chronic illness, a medicalized identity, which by definition is long term, can be a source of relief when it names and legitimizes one's suffering. Many people in chronic pain find the "fibromyalgia" appellation helpful. But there are also cases in which the medicalization of one's sense of self is harmful. The effects may be particularly insidious when the labels refer to chronic illnesses with no organic component. Such labels are hard to resist, because no definitive tests exist that can disconfirm them. Sue E. Estroff's work with psychiatric patients shows how people subject to long-term treatment by mental health workers literally *become their diagnoses.*[21] In this book I have shown how a similar process can occur in chronic illnesses of the body. Once we are labeled, it is hard to resist metamorphosing into our labels, letting what is known about the disease, its symptoms, and likely course infiltrate our sense of who we are and can be. As pharmacological treatment proceeds, our bodies are biochemically altered to "match" our new identities. Through this process, the psychological and physical are aligned with each other and with the disease entity we have acquired. Biomedicine's institutional power is awesome, but its discursive power to medicalize our subjectivities is even more so. This kind of power is frightening because it is invisible and unlocatable—it seems to be everywhere and nowhere at the same time—and thus difficult to pin down and protest.

To Students of Gender and Power: Theorizing Patient Identity and Micropolitics

Medical sociology has illuminated the asymmetrical character of the doctor-patient relationship and the real limits on women's resistance to biomedical power, especially in interactions with male physicians.[22] Building on these important insights, and on the trenchant critiques of the women's health movement, in this ethnography I have sought in-depth answers to the question of why women usually comply with, and how they sometimes resist, biomedical power. To understand these micropolitical dimensions of the medical encounter, we need to theorize women's agency and how it is psychologically managed and socially enacted.

Drawing on work in women's psychology and feminist theory, I have developed a theory of gender identity to ground an understanding of women's agency in the biomedical encounter. Identity is important because it forms the basis for political action. Working from poststruc-turalist theories of subjectivity, I have argued that women's identity is multiple, often contradictory, and always in flux. Identities are discur-sive constructions, constituted out of the discourses on femininity avail-able in the larger culture. The case examined here illuminates the work-ings of two such identities in the medical interaction.

The Relational Self Goes to the Doctor

In her struggles to obtain the best care possible from a controlling provider, the patient studied here assembled and enacted two radically different gender identities. Each had different relational, emotional, and political entailments. Scripted from the dominant discourses on femi-ninity in mainstream (white, middle-class, heterosexual) culture, the first, or "feminine" identity was none other than the self-in-relationship de-scribed in the influential work of psychologists Carol Gilligan, Lyn Mikel Brown, and Dana Jack.[23] This self was a compliant self that sought to secure good care by creating an artificially warm and fuzzy relationship with the doctor. This relationship was built on a distorted ethic of care in which the patient concerned herself more with her doctor's happi-ness than with her own physical and emotional well-being. Creating such a warped relationship required the patient to forge a falsely pleasant outer self while silencing her worries and suppressing her anger. While this relationship-first strategy worked to secure her doctor's attentions, it had devastating consequences for the patient. It left her thinking she was attracted to her doctor, when that attraction was only the confused emotional concomitant of a bloated and inappropriate ethic of care. The relationship-first approach was also costly, for it left the patient unable to communicate her concerns and unprotected against her doctor's mis-takes. It also rendered her vulnerable to verbal and emotional abuse and susceptible to depression stemming from the abnegation of her self. These psychodynamics of patienthood—which, conversations with many women suggest, may be quite common—validate and extend the sociological notion of limited resistance by showing that women are not only victims of biomedical oppression, but also that they actively pro-mote their own powerlessness by enacting routines of femininity the cul-ture defines as ideal. Psychologically harmful in many contexts, these self-silencing, other-centered routines of femininity may be particularly harmful in the medical context, where the health of the body is also at stake.

The Resistant Self Challenges Biomedical Power

Although we are subject to the power of our culture's dominant discourses, the theory of patient identity holds that we are also capable of resisting domination. We can oppose repression because we are self-creating subjects who can reject the reigning discourses, fashioning new identities for ourselves out of culturally marginal discourses. The patient's second gendered self was a resistant, "feminist" self scripted out of the discourses of feminism. Although this self was submerged when the compliant, "feminine" self held sway, it spawned invisible tactics of subversion and forms of political struggle that provided crucial emotional and intellectual tools of resistance to physician power in the end. It was this resistant "feminist" self that finally found its way to open anger and revolt. Such rebellion against medical authority revises the conventional picture of the woman patient by showing that women can challenge biomedical power and succeed. Even in this society, where the cards are heavily stacked against them, women can be (ambiguous) victors as well as victims. Patient insurrection alters the current image of white middle-class women as especially accepting of biomedical authority by showing that these women have multiple, often contradictory identities that can produce acceptance in one context and rejection in another. Like the identities that undergird them, the politics are contradictory and always in flux. While retaining the notion of difference as something social—marked by race, class, and other socially given attributes—this ethnography suggests the value of taking difference to another, intrapersonal, level as well. In other words, difference lies within as well as without; medical subjects are more complex than we thought. When we split the individual up into her many different selves, the issue of who resists power, when, and how becomes much more complex.

The Difference That Class Makes

I have repeatedly stressed the limitation of my analysis to white, middle-class, heterosexual women. To make this point more forcefully, I want briefly to elaborate on the difference that one of these dimensions—class—made in the case examined here. In her important book, *Cancer in the Community*, medical anthropologist Martha Balshem points to the centrality of professional authority—the judging of others by professional, education-based, standards—in modern society.[24] She argues, cogently I believe, that we live with the sense of a great divide between the judges and the judged. Being a judge equates with social success, while being judged means failure. Enjoying privileged access to resources and education, the middle class plays the "authority game" of trying to be, or at least to affiliate with, the judges. The working class, denied access to society's resources, serves as the prime model of the judged. Balshem's book goes on to explore the dynamics of class and medical authority in a working-class Philadelphia neighborhood that suffers from high rates of cancer. Excluded from power at many levels and blamed by the medical community for their "cancerous lifestyle," neighborhood residents reacted to the professional authority of scientific medicine by displaying a vibrant working-class culture that actively critiqued and resisted scientific authority. This culture was marked by denial of the scientific view of cancer causation, distrust of medical authority, and defiance of medical advice.

Inhabiting the heart of Balshem's book is the captivating figure of Jennifer, a middle-aged white woman whose husband has recently died of cancer. Jennifer's story is of her struggle to persuade her husband's physician to change his medical records so that smoking and drinking are not listed as the causes of his cancer and death. The contrast between the working-class politics of a character like Jennifer and the middle-class politics of a figure like S. could not be more striking. S. saw her relations with her doctor in terms of gender because her class and racial (and heterosexual) advantages remained invisible to her. But Jennifer's case shows how deeply S.'s actions were shaped by her privileged middle-class location. With little control over her life and little education, Jennifer rightly viewed herself as one of the judged. She angrily confronted medical authority on the assumption that institutionalized medicine was arrogant and controlling and would not only deny her reality, but blame her husband's working-class lifestyle, rather than his unhealthy environment, for his cancer. Jennifer saw what S. could not: that physicians routinely make mistakes, often put their own interests before the well-being of their patients, and enjoy excessive and illegitimate power to control knowledge about illness and the body. Jennifer's subordinate location in the class hierarchy endowed her with a keen vision of how power works.

The middle-class S., with her lifetime of access to all that society offers, her advanced education, and her comfortable insider's sense that the world was her oyster, clearly saw herself as one of the appointed. Her comment—"he had an M.D., I had a Ph.D; to me that made us equal"—reveals that she considered herself a winner of the authority game, a judge in her own right. After a brief verbal tussle with her doctor, she agreed to be pleasant and to comply with medical authority on the assumption that the doctor could be trusted to use his knowledge to make her better. Not perceiving the inequalities that Jennifer saw, this middle-class professor readily succumbed to the medical gaze.

When S. discovered that the myths of biomedical truth, objectivity, and beneficence were just that, she too mounted a direct challenge to medical authority, staging a meeting in which she demanded truth and accountability from her doctor. Both challenges failed: neither doctor was willing to change his ways or even admit he had made mistakes. But the two protesters must not be considered equal in their defeat, for the middle-class challenger had the means to secure not only better health care and better health but also closure on her battles with biomedical authority. S., for example, had the intellectual skills necessary to discern how her doctor had erred and the professional authority as an anthropologist to publicly critique biomedicine in this book. She got the emotional resolution she needed by writing this book. Jennifer had no way to obtain closure on the cause of her husband's death. Instead, she was left with the wound of unresolved emotions that, years later, was still painfully open. In the end, the hidden privileges of class gave S. an enormous edge.

To Anthropologists at Large: Auto-Ethnography and Other Productive Genres

The cultural upheavals of the late twentieth century have provoked growing self-reflexivity and self-narrativization in anthropological writing.[25] In this book I have experimented with two new reflexive genres to throw light on political and experiential aspects of medicine that traditional forms of scholarly writing, with their emphasis on distanced objectivity, tend to obscure. Appropriating autobiographical materials for ethnographic purposes, I have written an auto-ethnography of a medical encounter in the form of a feminist crime story. In the preface I explained why the auto-ethnography was a productive genre for my analytical and political purposes. Here I highlight the new insights that I hope this genre has produced. Wishing to draw the reader into my tale of botched care and secret passion, in the preface I only hinted at my intention also to write a medical mystery story. Now that the whodunit has been unraveled, I want to explain why I found this an attractive genre in which to pursue my goals as a feminist ethnographer. I begin with the auto-

ethnographic form, which has some precedent in anthropology, then turn
to the crime story, which does not.

Auto-Ethnography and Anthropological In-sight

From native ethnography to ethnic, feminist, and auto-ethnography, in
recent years anthropologists have been writing parts of themselves into
their studies of culture.[26] In this book I have taken the "auto" to an extreme by making an autobiographical experience the central focus of the
work. This genre has been intellectually and politically empowering, enabling me to pursue goals that would be difficult to achieve using conventional forms of writing. Let me mention just a few of the things I hope
to have accomplished.

First, privileged access to all the private writings of the patient, as well
as the historical memory needed to interpret them correctly, have given
me the opportunity to flesh out large domains of the patient experience
that have not previously come to light. These newly illuminated dimensions of patienthood range from the emotional to the philosophical, relational, and political. In a way probably not possible in conventional,
third-person writing, "the patient" has come to life. (Unfortunately, I have
not been able to bring the doctor to life in the same way.)

Auto-ethnography also provides a promising vehicle by which to em-
pathically grasp and meaningfully represent suffering, a new topic of anthropological concern.[27] In lingering on the emotions so rawly exposed
in the patient's diary, I have sought to provide an "experience-near" portrait of medically induced suffering.[28] By breaking down the traditional
distinction between researcher-subject and researched-object, such an account avoids the objectification of the sufferer and the dehumanization
of suffering that tend to vex more conventional forms of medical anthropology writing.[29]

Through a kind of "vulnerable writing" that is writable only by the
vulnerable observer him or herself, I have sought to deflate the myth of
the heroic anthropologist by showing that emotions such as grief and
bodily conditions such as pain can, and perhaps frequently do, shape the
production of anthropological knowledge.[30] By subjecting ourselves to
such close scrutiny, we can see how anthropological knowledges are situated not only socially—reflecting our locations of class, race, gender,
and so on—but also personally—reflecting our bodily and emotional
states. Acknowledging these influences forces us to pare back our claims
to produce "objective truth." Instead, we produce positioned truths, par-

tial perspectives that are not only honest—too honest, some will surely say—but also locatable and hence responsible for their claims.

The auto-ethnographic genre has also permitted me to pursue critical political goals. I have argued that biomedicine exerts its power over our lives largely by colonizing our selves, remaking our identities in new, medicalized terms. Auto-ethnography provides a way to resist biomedical power through the renarrativization of the self.[31] Through a dual process of de- and renarrativization—first exposing the process by which colonization has occurred and then claiming the right to other, nonmedicalized identities—the writing of auto-ethnography becomes an act of resistance. This political act is not a trivial pursuit—"mere" identity politics—for to reclaim one's identity is to reclaim one's life.

The Feminist Crime Story:
Woman as Crime Victim/Detective/Perpetrator

In crime fiction, the central hermeneutic is discovery: a crime has been committed, and a detective, usually a private eye, sets out to find out how. Traditionally, crime fiction has been a masculine and conservative genre, in which the mythic male hero uncovers the source of the crime, restoring society to the safe and stable status quo. From Agatha Christie onward, however, women writers have exploited the genre for new and transgressive purposes. In her lively study, *Murder by the Book*, Sally R. Munt traces how women have developed the genre's potential as protest literature. They have done so by feminizing and deheroizing the private eye, abandoning the triumphal ending, and radicalizing the politics of the genre, among other ways.[32] This book belongs to that tradition of women's writing. Yet it diverges from it in using a fictional form to write a story based on fact. Some readers may worry about this blurring of genres, this whiff of fiction that I have associated with my facts. To these readers I would reply that the use of a fictional form to tell a factual story is fully appropriate—indeed, perhaps, even inevitable. This is so because "the facts" always come to us in the form of stories, stories so powerful that *they determine what counts as fact*. After all, even classic ethnography was shaped by a narrative device—the heroic anthropologist, the culturally Other native—that counted some things as anthropological and worth recording, while discounting others and eliminating them from anthropological history.[33]

In writing this book I have poured the jumble of facts surrounding S.'s encounter with Dr. D. into the mold of a crime story. Focusing on the virtual murder/near suicide of the patient, I made the central problem a set of interlinked questions: Who ruined the patient's health? Who killed her soul, bringing her to the brink of taking her own life? The central character, S., was an ambiguous heroine at best. The unwitting possessor of multiple and contradictory identities, she was the victim who, uncovering her victimhood, turned into the private eye. In her investigative quest, the book's central narrative device, she discovered that the villain of the piece was not so much her individual doctor as the larger biomedical system of which he was a part. Probing further, she unearthed the disconcerting fact that the nefarious institutions included the culture of femininity, which she herself embodied. In making this discovery, she acquired a new identity—that of perpetrator of crimes against the self—further compromising any heroic status. The story ended not with the triumphant bringing to justice of the guilty parties, but with the victim scrappily struggling to restore her health and recover her sanity in a disease-inducing, crazy-making world. Justice was not done, but injustice was named.

Nontraditional genres like the crime story can be appropriated to serve important anthropological ends. These genres are appealing because they permit the writer to make difficult or sensitive points in subtle and suggestive ways. In this book I have used the crime form to press a number of intellectual and political points. By advancing the crime metaphor, I have tried to expose serious injustices that occur regularly in medical practice yet rarely come to light. In showing how the patient's "femininity," a product of a patriarchal culture, was implicated in the "crime," my aim has been to put patriarchy itself on trial. In doing so, I wanted to remind readers of the continued importance of feminist analysis in a world still stratified by gender, race, class, and other dimensions of social difference. By bringing in patriarchy, I also wanted to awaken memories of the need for change not just in individuals—today's answer to all problems—but in the larger structures of society. By associating the patient/private eye with the figure of the detective in crime fiction, I have placed the patient in a culturally honored class of moral watchdogs who pursue an alternative sense of justice outside the formal institutions of power. With this device I meant to suggest that medical justice can be done only when the patient is given a moral voice. By making S.'s unraveling of the "crime" the central story line, I have tried to evoke in the reader fantasies of justice in which the sources of oppression in our society can be incriminated in words if not in action. Finally, by turning S.'s story into a document for public consumption, I have sought to suggest that the problems of doctor-induced illness and medical devastation of the patient's inner world are not personal problems, but political problems that can be resolved only through public debate and collective action.

A New "Women's Disease" for the Twenty-First Century?

Although I have told the story of only one "fibromyalgic," my larger concern about fibromyalgia and other nonorganic chronic pain syndromes stems from the relatively uncritical acceptance of these biomedical constructs in the culture at large. A foray into the popular culture of illness shows that fibromyalgia, one of the newest of these conditions, is a "hot" disease today. Like chronic fatigue syndrome before it, fibromyalgia is becoming culturally contagious, in Showalter's apt phrase, spread by stories in myriad sites of cultural communication, from newspapers and magazines to TV talk shows, patient support groups, internet chatrooms, and more.[34] As stories about the disease proliferate, more and more people are seeing it as the cause of their pain and turning to rheumatologists and other physicians for help.

Women (and a few men) are embracing their new identities as "fibromyalgics," but are there hidden dangers attending the medicalization of their pain? For those who want to look, hints of possible problems are not hard to find. The gaps in expert knowledge—the absence of known cause, effective treatment, and clearly defined biological basis—might well give one pause. But there is more. We have seen that fibromyalgia is highly controversial among biomedical specialists. Although few doubt the existence of a painful clinical condition, many question whether this pain is best understood by the construct of "fibromyalgia." Many have worried about the problem of tautology in the definition of the disease. With fibromyalgia, Milton L. Cohen and John L. Quintner complain in *The Lancet*, "the evidence on which the construct is based [i.e., the tender points] is taken as proof of [the construct's] veracity."[35] In other words, the cause is not distinguished from the effect. The sharpest debate has revolved around the question of diagnosis, in particular, its cardinal feature, the tender points. To skeptics the tender points suffer not only from the problems of measurement and physician bias described in chapter 12. In the critics' view, the tender points are virtually meaningless, since their physiology remains unexplained and—more damaging still—they fail to correlate with any symptoms.[36] Moreover, as we also saw in chapter 12, neither the chief symptom nor the ancillary symptoms are specific to fibromyalgia. Fibromyalgia suffers from the same problem as all syndromes: "variable combinations of features are put forward as an entity, which then implies [false] pathogenetic homogeneity."[37] "[F]ibromyalgia has become a proposition so broad," Quinter and Cohen write in The Lancet in 1999, "that it includes all possibilities. Despite this objection, fibromyalgia seems to be an entrenched diagnostic label—at least in rheumatological circles—but it is a label so easily abused as to have become meaningless."[38]

Most people in chronic pain long for a diagnosis.[39] With the passage of time many become desperate for one. Getting a name for their problem helps them make sense of it. The medical label gives their suffering social legitimacy and suggests therapies for pain relief. Yet given the conceptual problems with the fibromyalgia construct and the room for physician creativity in the procedures for diagnosing it, it behooves us to ask: Who is helped by the dispensing of the label, which, even proponents believe, is now "out of control"?[40] A visit to the doctor takes the patient from symptoms to diagnosis to treatment, bypassing the causes of the disease. While the emphasis on pain alleviation is appropriate and laudable, might not something be lost when the sources of pain drop from sight? Are women empowered or disempowered by allowing scientific medicine to name and manage these ill-defined ailments? A look backward into history suggests some disturbing answers.

The Medicalization of Women's Pain: A History Lesson

Readers who know Charlotte Perkins Gilman's harrowing short story, "The Yellow Wall-paper" (published in 1892), will have noted the astonishing parallels between that tale and the case presented in these pages.[41] "The Yellow Wall-paper" was a fictionalized account of Gilman's real, life-threatening encounter with S. Weir Mitchell, a doctor whose style was more Machiavellian by far than that of Dr. D.[42] Because the commonalities between the two individual cases hint at larger parallels between the historical eras in which they lived, it is useful to briefly relate the real story of Gilman's "neurasthenia" and its "cure." Gilman left an autobiography, enabling me to tell much of her story in her own words.

Charlotte Perkins Gilman was a leading social critic and theorist of the large-scale movement for women's rights that emerged in the late nineteenth century. As a young woman, she saw traditional notions of woman's proper place as confining and decided to devote herself to a "steady lifetime of social study and service."[43] Soon after her marriage, Charlotte fell into a deep depression. After the birth of her daughter she grew fatigued and despondent, feeling "a constant dragging weariness . . . Absolute incapacity. Absolute misery."[44] Deeply concerned about her illness, Gilman traveled to Philadelphia to consult Dr. S. Weir Mitchell, the leading nerve specialist of the day. Finding no physical abnormality, the good doctor diagnosed her with neurasthenia and sent her off to undergo his famous rest cure. After a month of bed rest, rich foods, and massage, the doctor sent Charlotte home with the prescription: "Live as domestic a life as possible. Have your child with you all the time . . . Have but two hours' intellectual life a day. And never touch pen, brush or pencil as long as you live."[45]

Gilman followed Mitchell's directions for three months. Confined to bed and deprived of the social and intellectual stimulation that had made her thrive, she descended into a dark fog of distress and disability. As she describes it, "[I] came so near the borderline of utter mental ruin that I could see over."[46] Finally, in a moment of clear vision, she was able to "us[e] the remnants of intelligence that remained" to see that the doctor's cure was part of the problem.[47] She cast the specialist's advice aside and began a life of lecturing, writing, and activism on political and social issues of the day.

Social science students of medicine have long worried about the dangers of the growing medicalization of social life.[48] Because of the masculinist nature of biomedicine, however, those dangers are particularly great for women. Despite the growing interest in fibromyalgia, none of the emerging literatures on the subject—biomedical, patient self-help, or patient testimonial—acknowledges these dangers. Feminist health scholars and activists have amply documented the risks that women face when every phase of their reproductive cycle is managed by the high-tech world of scientific medicine.[49] At the same time, they have neglected parallel problems of gender and power in the rheumatological domain. Yet chronic pain is a women's health issue too. Women are the primary sufferers not only of arthritis, the major rheumatic disease, but also of most of the chronic pain syndromes.[50] Women outnumber men in chronic fatigue syndrome, irritable bowel syndrome, chronic headache conditions, and fibromyalgia, among many other conditions.[51] The large numbers of women affected by these conditions should also recommend the domain of musculoskeletal health to the attention of women's health specialists. In the mid-1990s, 29 percent of women aged forty-five to sixty-four, 50 percent aged sixty-five to seventy-four, and 62 percent aged seventy-five and older were afflicted by arthritis.[52] As the baby boom generation ages, rheumatic disease will complicate the lives of ever larger proportions of American women. The final and perhaps most compelling reason for feminist concern is that the medicalization of chronic pain poses dangers that rival those attending the medicalization of childbirth and menopause. I return to these dangers shortly.

This neglect of the medicalization of chronic pain should worry us, for the parallels between the late-nineteenth and late-twentieth centuries suggest that history is repeating itself. In both eras, large numbers of aspiring middle-class women found their lives cut short when they experienced vague but debilitating symptoms, turned to scientific medicine for help, and found themselves sent home with disease labels and treatment plans that rarely made them better and sometimes made them worse.[53] Read politically, the historical record suggests that the late-twentieth-century proliferation of female-dominant pain syndromes is part of a larger, historically rooted extension of biomedical power over women's lives. Since the rise of scientific medicine in the nineteenth century, there has been a long history of nonorganic "women's diseases" that have been named, diagnosed, and treated by masculinist medical science. Hysteria and neurasthenia are the best known, but there have been many more. In their widely acclaimed book, *For Her Own Good: 150 Years of Expert Advice to Women*, Barbara Ehrenreich and Deidre English argue that women were harmed when they lost control over their bodies to doctors and other scientific experts in the nineteenth century.[54] Ironically, women themselves actively participated in their own acquiescence to the experts. Craving the attention the specialists devoted to their problems and believing in the religion of science, women sought out the medicalization of their pain. Yet allowing physicians to name and manage their pain was costly, for it led to the devaluation of women's traditional knowledge of the body and the destruction of their healing networks. Without the resources that once protected them, women were left vulnerable to the application of unproven theories and unhelpful, sometimes brutally repressive, treatments to their bodies.[55]

Medicalization Poses Dangers to Women—and to Men

I worry that fibromyalgia, an invention of the last two decades, is becoming the latest in this long line of female disorders treated by masculinist medical science. To be sure, medicine offers valuable services to people in inexplicable pain. Even if they cannot alleviate the pain, sympathetic doctors can provide psychological solace, social support, and bodily relief from some symptoms. Yet today, too, the medicalization of chronic pain may ultimately harm women. It is not that physicians *intend* to cause harm; quite the contrary, most are deeply committed to easing their patients' pain. But they are caught in a larger system of power—analyzed in this book—that produces this perverse effect *against the will* of any participant. The case of S. provides graphic testimony to the dangers that may attend the medicalization of women's pain *by a well-meaning physician*. A more disturbing case is that of a Boston-area woman who, in August 1996, became Dr. Jack Kevorkian's thirty-fifth known assisted-suicide case. Her chief medical complaints were fibromyalgia and chronic fatigue syndrome—hardly fatal conditions.[56]

Beyond these individual cases, there are at least five sets of reasons that the medicalization of chronic pain may generally be less helpful to women than physicians and patients now recognize. Some of these problems vex male patients as well. First, by turning their pain over to a physician to manage, men and women lose control over their bodies to biomedical practitioners whose underlying, though generally unconscious, interests may differ from theirs. The case of S. shows how a physician's unconscious but nonetheless real professional and material interests in promoting his specialty disease can conflict with and override a patient's interest in becoming disease free. The growing presence of managed care in today's health-care market may be exacerbating this problem. Although the doctor featured here refused to subscribe to any managed plan, the spread of managed medicine clearly threatened his patient load, necessitating the use of muscular means to recruit and retain patients. This constant threat to the viability of his practice put pressure on him to tell clinical tales that kept his patients coming back. His stories of a debilitating, progressive illness called "fibromyalgia" had precisely that effect. For her part, the patient's history of "managed rheumatology" convinced her that this maverick doctor, who spent hours with each patient (and charged for it), was a gift from heaven. In her need for understanding and help, so unavailable in managed practices, she heard the doctor's story as The Truth, missing the possibility that that truth might be tainted by his personal interests. In this case, the managed-care environment both encouraged the clinical production of "fibromyalgia" and discouraged the "fibromyalgic" from seeing the clash of interests her diagnosis embodied.

A second problem with the medicalization of pain is that it may needlessly diminish men's and women's lives. The medical construction of their problems as "fibromyalgia," a potentially disabling, lifelong condition, may rob patients of the hope that they will get better and convince them to give up their dreams for work, family, and service to society to devote themselves to a career of full-time patienthood. As biomedical critics have argued and I have documented at length in this ethnography, the labeling itself may have iatrogenic consequences.[57]

The medicalization of pain is also detrimental to women specifically because it places them within a masculinist biomedical order in which the patient's knowledge of her body and life is silenced in discourses of objectification that make the doctor the expert on the patient's body. The void created by the patient's silence is often filled with the conservative gender values of the practitioner, and the sexism and gender inequality are then erased in rhetorics of patient benefit. Dr. D. did not articulate his views about woman's proper role in the openly sexist ways that were acceptable in the late nineteenth century, but those views, aired in a public lecture, were every bit as conventional as S. Weir Mitchell's. D.'s treatment program for his "fibromyalgics" reflected those gender assumptions. His management plan assumed a female patient who made a career of tending her body, rested much and exercised little, and depended on her doctor to monitor and manage her putative disease. Had the doctor's program been fully implemented, the patient studied here would have been turned into a latter-day, self-preoccupied, stay-home-and-rest Victorian neurasthenic. What is at stake in these battles over the claiming and naming of a new disease is not only women's health, although that is important enough. What is at stake is also the *political question* of what roles women will be allowed to play in a "postfeminist" era in which the backlash against feminism is threatening the gains that women have made in recent decades.[58]

The medicalization of suffering may also harm women because it exposes them to a sexual politics in the clinical encounter in which their dual subordination in the hierarchies of gender and science places them at risk of verbal and emotional abuse. As argued at length in the chapters on "Doing Gender," this political dynamic is insidious because women may silence their critical voices, contributing to their own victimization.

Finally, the medicalization of chronic pain ultimately hurts both men and women, but women in particular, because it focuses their attention on disease *management,* discouraging inquiry into the *sources* of their pain. As S.'s case suggests, when the causes of pain remain unidentified, the treatment may be misguided at best. While the causes of chronic pain are multiple and poorly understood, in the case of fibromyalgia they appear to include disturbing rates of sexual and physical abuse and rising levels of life stress. Although gender abuse is not a conventional variable in biomedical research, to its credit, the research community has recently begun to address the connection between abuse and musculoskeletal pain. This new research, which we encountered briefly in chapter 6, shows that women fibromyalgics exhibit higher levels of physical and sexual abuse than groups of controls and that prolonged or intense abuse is associated with a larger number and greater severity of symptoms.[59] A history of physical and especially sexual abuse is common not only in "fibro-myalgics" but also in women with ailments such as irritable bowel syndrome, chronic headache, chronic pelvic pain, chronic back pain, and eating disorders—all more prevalent among women.[60] Following standard scientific practice, most of the research literature treats gender and abuse as decontextualized variables lacking in social and political content. Not constrained by the requirements of quantitative research, a few culturally sensitive clinicians have begun to understand this complex of abuse and pain as a product of a larger culture that devalues and silences women. In her courageous book, *Lost Voices: Women, Chronic Pain, and Abuse,* physician Nellie A. Radomsky chronicles her slow and painful realization that the chronic pain her patients exhibit is a language of those who can speak in no other way. Her reflexive analysis of her own field suggests that medicine tends to contribute to women's problems by mimicking the dynamics of abuse and disempowerment that women face in the wider society.[61]

Although the connections between abuse and chronic pain are better studied, stress can also be expressed in the idiom of symptoms. While men also symptomize stress, women may be particularly vulnerable to somatizing the difficulties in their lives because of differences in the ways they cognitively appraise, psychologically cope with, and biologically respond to stress.[62] If this is so, the sharp escalation of demands placed on women in recent decades—what stress researchers would call a steep increase in "exposure to stress"—might be a crucial piece of the puzzle of the pervasiveness of chronic pain among some groups of American women today. Because women's public roles have multiplied, while their private responsibilities have changed little, "the stress of being a woman," psychologist Georgia Witkin writes in her popular book, *The Female Stress Syndrome,* "is going up."[63] Today, with "mommy tracks" and glass ceilings, biological clocks and single mothers, high divorce rates and two-career couples, it may be, as Witkin says, that "having it all . . . means [having] all the symptoms of stress."[64]

The medicalization of chronic pain diverts attention from its structural sources, treating as individual malady a set of problems whose roots lie ultimately in the larger structures of the culture and society. Students of health in the social sciences need to join forces with concerned biomedical researchers and clinicians to identify those larger social and cultural forces that are interacting with individual biology to produce today's proliferation of chronic pain syndromes and the culturally epidemic quality of their spread. If the structural sources could be addressed directly, the dynamic of somatization of stress and abuse could be stopped at its point of origin, and physicians would no longer have to spend their time trying to treat conditions for which they can do little in any case.

Although today chronic pain syndromes are treated as biomedical problems, they also need to be viewed as cultural problems, that is, as somatic responses to a larger set of difficulties that women face in a culture that still devalues the feminine. We need to learn more about the associations among silence, abuse, stress, and pain. We need to know more about how these connections vary by race, class, and sexuality, a subject I was unable to pursue in this auto-ethnography. When large groups of women are at risk of turning the pain imposed on them by the culture back upon themselves, the cost in terms of suffering bodies, diminished lives, and wasted potential is staggering. Surely it is time to name this problem that still has no name and to make this bodily pain that is so personal, political.

Speaking of Pain

*On Stories, Cultural Recuperations,
and Political Interventions*

In *The Culture of Pain,* David B. Morris shows that throughout human history, pain has been a mysterious experience that has taken on multiple meanings depending on the personal biographies and cultural contexts of the sufferers.[1] In our day, however, those variegated interpretations have been stripped away by the dominant biomedical understanding of pain as a matter of nerves and neurotransmitters. The biomedicalization of pain has brought not only loss of cultural riches, but also human peril, for the paradigms of scientific medicine have all too often silenced the ill, diminished the person in the painful body, and even failed to ease the physical discomfort.

What is the alternative to medicalization? In this book I have joined the growing chorus of voices contending that the alternative is to restore the meanings that have been lost by recovering the voices that have been silenced: the voices of the ill themselves. In this age of narrative florescence and political quiescence, it may be that individual and communal storytelling is one of the most viable routes to cultural and political change. The sociologist Arthur W. Frank, a venerable storyteller himself, has described the many ends that storytelling by the ill serves.[2] In this brief epilogue I want to share some of Frank's thoughts and add a few of my own.

Storytelling does important cultural work. For individuals, narrativizing their pain is a way to give meaning to suffering and, as Frank writes, to learn what one's own voice sounds like, perhaps for the very first time.[3] On a communal level, when we tell stories we create communities, groups of people who are tied together by common accountings of human experience. Whether narrated orally, written down, or simply enacted in daily life, by telling our stories we also make resources available for others. Our stories empower listeners not only to spin their own yarns but also to learn from our "mistakes," enabling them to live their lives differently. I hope this book might have such an effect. In exposing so brutally the follies of S. and D., I hope I have convinced readers that there must never again be another patient like S. or another physician like Dr. D. More than simply understanding, I hope they will use this troubling tale as a springboard for creating new and better forms of patient and physician practice.

Creating narratives is also a means to political awareness and political action. For individuals, storytelling is a way to resist the medical construction of one's identity, the transformation of the person one always thought one was into "patient with diagnosis." Crafting our personal narratives is a way to keep our lives our own, to protect all or part of our identities from threat or assault. Recounting our stories can also serve more overtly political ends when those tales directly challenge biomedical stories, take them apart, or document their damaging effects. Our illness stories can also serve to call a medical mistake an injustice; when they do, the stories serve as political interventions. As such stories pile up, one on top of the other, they work to create communities of potential political actors. Just as the civil rights and women's movements—to name just two—emerged from shared stories, illness communities are now forming to demand and to help devise better approaches to the care of illnesses such as AIDS and breast cancer. Perhaps publication of this book, coming on top of other stories of chronic pain, will incite more people to recount their pain-full histories, encourage them to join forces, and turn chronic pain into the next focus for organized political activity. If I have accomplished nothing else with this book, I hope I have persuaded readers that the care of chronic pain needs public attention and political reform.

Notes

Works cited in the notes by author and year of publication receive full citation in the bibliography.

Preface

1. By *epidemic* I refer to the culturally contagious nature of chronic pain syndromes, which are spread by stories in the media and other sites of cultural communication (Showalter 1997). This notion will be elaborated below. On the number of Americans with chronic conditions, Hoffman, Rice, and Sung (1996) found that in 1987, 46 percent of the noninstitutionalized population, or 88 and one-half million persons, had one or more chronic diseases or impairments. This statistic does not include people who are institutionalized. Adding the 1.5 million people in nursing and personal-care homes raises the number of chronically ill or impaired to 90 million. Chronic illness is not confined to the elderly. In 1987, 25 percent of those seventeen and younger, 35 percent of people eighteen to forty-four, 68 percent of those aged forty-five to sixty-four, and 88 percent of people sixty-five and older were chronically ill or impaired. The authors projected that the number of Americans with chronic conditions would continue to rise, reaching 100 million in 1995 and 148 million by 2030.

These statistics are based on data from the household survey component of the 1987 National Medical Expenditure Survey. Detailed information on health conditions was provided by survey respondents. Professional coders then classified those conditions by ICD-9 (International Classification of Diseases, 9th Revision) code. The study underestimates the proportion of people with chronic conditions because conditions that did not cause disability or health service use during the survey period were not counted.

This book deals with chronic diseases, but not impairments. A chronic disease is one that is not self-limiting, but rather creates persistent and recurring health consequences lasting for years rather than months or days (Hoffman, Rice, and Sung 1996, p. 1474).

2. According to data gathered by the U.S. National Center for Health Statistics, in 1995 the leading sources of chronic pain and disability were arthritis (32.7 million), physical deformity (31.8 million), hypertension (30.0 million), hay fever (25.7 million), hearing impairment (22.5 million), heart disease (21.1 million), asthma (14.9 million), chronic bronchitis (14.5 million), and migraine headache (11.9 million). See United States Department of Commerce (1998, p.149). These figures cover the civilian noninstitutional population.

3. See especially Foucault (1975). Scholars such as Armstrong (1984) and Arney and Bergen (1984) have detected a shift, beginning around 1950, from the clinical gaze to a new, more patient-centered mode of medical perception in

which the encounter is one between two subjects rather than between subject and object of medical science. Baszanger argues, persuasively I think, that most medical practice today remains based on the older "clinical gaze." Instead of a radical break, her research suggests that there has been a growing heterogeneity in which different modes of medical perception coexist at the same time and even in the same practice. See Baszanger (1998, esp. pp. 3–7, 183–88).

4. Schaefer (1997, p. 567).

5. Wolfe et al. (1990). For the subjective experience of these symptoms, see Schaefer (1995; 1997); Soderberg, Lundman, and Norberg (1999); Mannerkopi, Kroksmark, and Ekdahl (1999).

6. Schaefer (1995, p. 96).

7. Tierney et al. (1996, p. 764), Wilson et al. (1991, p. 1487), and many others note its nonprogressive nature.

8. Research on the causes of fibromyalgia has exploded in the last few years, with some pursuing the organic bases of the symptoms and others exploring their psychosocial roots. On organic mechanisms see, for example, Buskila et al. (1997); Bennett (1999); Leal-Cerro et al. (1999); Neeck and Riedel (1999); Schwarz et al. (1999). Psychosocial pathways are traced in Aaron et al. (1997); Walker et al. (1997); Goldberg, Pachas, and Keith (1999); Winfield (1999).

9. For more on treatment options and efficacy, see Levanthal (1999); Rossy et al. (1999).

10. Wolfe et al. (1995).

11. Wolfe et al. (1995).

12. Smythe and Modolfsky (1977).

13. Bennett (1987). Some proponents have (mis)represented this as an American Medical Association endorsement of the syndrome. See, for example, Starlanyl and Copeland (1996, p. 8).

14. Wolfe et al. (1990).

15. Outspoken skeptics include Cohen and Quintner (1993); Bohr (1995); Shorter (1995); Quintner and Cohen (1999). Hadler (1997) provides a critical history of this "'committee' of advocates" and its efforts to promote the fibromyalgia construct.

16. Schaefer (1995).

17. On the social lives of commodities, see Appadurai (1986).

18. I had hoped to use Dr. D.'s handwritten notes taken during appointments with S. as a source of information on his interpretation of her ills. Unfortunately, the notes that I acquired from the doctor turned out to be so illegible that neither I nor a physician I consulted could make any sense of them.

Problematique

1. A partial history of the machine metaphor is offered by Osherson and AmaraSingham (1981). A useful review of its broad implications can be found in Lupton (1994, pp. 59–61).

2. Foucault (1975). The original French for "the gaze" is *le regard*, signaling both perception and an active manner of seeing. For more on the importance

of perception—the gaze—to modern medicine, see, for example, Armstrong (1983; 1984; 1995; 1997); Scott (1987); Good (1994, pp. 65–87).

3. Because the vast majority (roughly 80 percent in 1995 [Weisman 1998, p. 143]) of medical doctors are male, and the maleness of medicine is an important part of my story, in this general discussion of medicine I use the masculine pronoun for physicians. When discussing patients, I alternate between the masculine and feminine pronoun. Women accounted for 40 percent of medical students in 1993 and are projected to represent 29 percent of all physicians by 2010 (Weisman 1998, p. 143). The implications of this shift for medical practice, however, are far from clear, for women doctors are trained in the same biomedical, pathology-oriented curriculum as are men doctors. While female physicians present themselves as more communicative and supportive, whether they are more attuned to the whole patient or to the patient's expressed needs remains open to question. Patient outcomes appear to vary little with the gender of the doctor. For more on this subject see Fisher (1995), Lorber (1997), Weisman (1998, pp. 142–53).

4. Foucault (1975, p. 89).

5. Foucault (1975, p. 97).

6. Foucault (1975, p. 84).

7. See especially Mishler (1984), who argues that the "voice of medicine" and the "voice of the lifeworld" spoken by the patient are not only different but in conflict. A compelling phenomenological account of the differing perspectives of doctor and patient is Toombs (1992).

8. Many have written about the disruptions caused by illness, but fewer have reflected on the disturbances created by the experience of care itself. Thoughtful treatments of this latter subject include Cassell (1982; 1991), who reflects on the disruptions to the patient's identity (in his terms, "the person"); Kleinman (1988), who explores the cultural meanings of diagnoses; Young (1997), who traces the narrative reconstruction of the disembodied self; Wendell (1996), who ruminates on the philosophical implications of chronic illness; and Toombs (1992), who traces the dehumanizing effects of medicine's objectification of the body. Of these, only the latter two speak in the voice of the patient.

9. Arthur Kleinman, a harsh critic of conventional medicine, argues that biomedicine must be indicted for reducing the treatment of chronic illness to a technical quest for symptom control, a process that disables the healer and disempowers the chronically ill. See Kleinman (1988, pp. 6–10). For a lively history of medicine's conquest of acute infectious disease and failings in the area of chronic illness, see Golub (1997).

10. Hoffman, Rice, and Sung (1996). See note 2 of the Preface for some statistics.

11. Kleinman (1988, pp. 56–57). The sociologist Anselm L. Strauss was an early contributor to this line of thought. See, for example, Strauss and Glaser (1975); Strauss and Corbin (1988).

12. Locke (1992). Many others, including cultural and feminist critics of science, have also challenged conventional equations of science with impartial, value-free objectivity. An especially cogent analysis is Sandra Harding's *The Science*

Question in Feminism (1986). Locke's work provides a useful entry into these critiques, because he starts from the vantage point of the working scientist. This enables him not only to see the full range of procedural, theoretical, conceptual, and linguistic difficulties that might lead the scientist to make mistakes but also to convey a sense of the uncertainty and worry that consequently attend the scientific project. Locke's work is also helpful because it systematically explores the linguistic and especially the rhetorical aspects of the scientific enterprise that have received less attention elsewhere. These two emphases in Locke's work—mistake making and mistake-masking rhetoric—are central to the ethnography presented in the following chapters. Locke's account neglects issues of power and gender, which are central in all scientific practice, including the practice of the medical scientist described in these pages. I treat these issues in the following section of the problematique.

13. Locke (1992, p. 28).

14. Undoubtedly the best-known narrative account of a research science is Haraway's (1989) work on primatology.

15. Sacks (1986). Narrative approaches to the work of medical practitioners are developed in Brody (1994); Epstein (1995, esp. pp. 25–75); Mattingly (1998). A sampling of such studies in the periodical literature includes Charon (1986; 1989); Sacks (1986); Stoeckle and Billings (1987); Donnelly (1989); Leder (1990); Monroe et al. (1992); P. Brown (1993); Jones (1994). Storytelling approaches have also been widely applied to patients' experiences of illness. For work on illness narratives see, for example, Brody (1987); Kleinman (1988); Clark and Mishler (1992); Hawkins (1993); Oakley (1993); Epstein (1994); Frank (1995; 1997a; 1997b); Saris (1995); Hyden (1997). There are also numerous studies featuring the narratives of patients with specific illnesses.

16. A major exception is Baszanger (1998). Earlier sociological research on the structure, content, and sequential ordering of the medical interview certainly dealt with physician rhetoric in the sense of persuasive talk (see, for example, Mishler [1984]; West [1984]; Fisher [1986; 1995]; Todd [1989]; Waitzkin [1991]). The assumptions about power that underlay that work, however, differ from those of Locke and scholars working in a Foucauldian tradition, with important consequences for the content and function of rhetoric. Exaggerating the differences, one could say that in the earlier conversational analyses, power was generally construed as possessed and repressive; the doctor-patient relationship was depicted as hierarchical; and physician rhetoric was portrayed as enhancing the power of physician over patient. In the work of Locke and Foucauldian scholars, power tends to be positive and socially dispersed, the interaction is more collaborative, and physician rhetoric heightens the influence of scientific "truth" over the thinking of physician and patient alike. The content of the rhetoric of interest differs as well. Although my study falls in the latter tradition, the earlier work has greatly enhanced my understanding of doctor-patient interactions.

17. Traditionally there were two sources of medical knowledge and legitimation, "clinical expertise" or "experience," and "clinical science," better known as medicine-as-art and medicine-as-science. Physicians have varied in their allegiance to one or the other. In recent decades there has been a movement to make

clinical medicine more scientific, that is, more rational, explicit, quantitative, and formal, through the introduction of patient-care guidelines, decision-support techniques, and other "scientific" methods. This process is traced by D. Gordon (1988a) and Berg (1995). The scientific basis of medicine is stressed during the first two years of medical school. It is then that medical students learn to "think . . . of [them]selves as scientists." See Good and Good (1993, p. 89 and elsewhere).

18. For an overview of these new intersections in sociology see Casper and Berg (1995). New work along the borders of medical anthropology and technoscience studies is reviewed in Franklin (1995) and Casper and Koenig (1996). Clarke and Olesen (1999) revision women's health through the lenses of cultural studies, technoscience studies, and feminist theory.

19. Early yet still useful discussions of the social construction of illness are Freidson (1970) and Mishler (1981a). More recent writings include P. Brown's work on diagnosis (1989; 1995) and Berg's on the patient record (1996) and medical disposals (1992). Brown (1995) usefully reviews three different versions of social constructionism in medical sociology. Fineman's work (1991) shows how other aspects of medical work, such as the notion of patient "noncompliance," are also clinically constructed.

20. Young (1995).

21. Studies of the clinical construction of illness are extremely rare. Barrett's (1988) account of the "documentary construction" of schizophrenia is the only study of this sort that I have been able to locate.

22. I thank Sandra Harding for discussion of these points.

23. See, for example, Knorr-Cetina (1981; 1983); Latour (1987); Latour and Woolgar (1979); Traweek (1988); Oudshoorn (1994). Berg (1992) applies the science-as-practice perspective to the work of medical decision making. His approach is very similar to the one I take here.

24. Baszanger (1998, esp. pp. 8–10, 145–89).

25. See especially Foucault (1975; 1978; 1979); C. Gordon (1980). Foucault's work on medicine is limited by its inattention to the gendered nature of biomedical power, the dynamics of resistance, the negotiation of power in the doctor-patient relationship, and the emotional and experiential dimensions of medicine. I seek to overcome these limitations by drawing on other work within the rapidly growing body of Foucauldian scholarship in the medical social sciences that highlights these features of clinical medicine. A partial list of book-length studies of this sort includes Armstrong (1983); Silverman (1987); Lock and Gordon (1988); Turner (1992; 1995); Fox (1994); Jones and Porter (1994); Lupton (1994); Atkinson (1995); Petersen and Bunton (1997); Lock and Kaufert (1998).

26. Of course, organized medicine played a big part in fostering its own rise to power. For the details, see Starr (1982).

27. On "do-able" problems see Fujimura (1987; 1996); Berg (1992). This discussion is not meant to suggest that patients are simply cultural dupes of scientific medicine. Clinician success in performing these tasks requires negotiation with patients, who use the medical interview to pursue their own goals.

28. The classic theory of disease on which scientific medicine is based is laid out with special clarity in Cassell (1991, pp. 3–16, 81–93).

29. See, for example, Mishler (1981b).

30. Analyses of medical interviews that use discourse in this sense include Mishler (1984); West (1984); Fisher (1986; 1995); Fisher and Todd (1986); Todd (1989); Waitzkin (1991).

31. Studies of doctor-patient communications taking a Foucauldian perspective include Armstrong (1983); Silverman (1987); Lupton (1994); Atkinson (1995).

32. On Foucauldian discourse more generally, see Dreyfus and Rabinow (1982).

33. A shared institutional and legal setting also induces similar physician work styles.

34. Seminal contributions include Mishler (1981b); D. Gordon (1988b); Kirmayer (1988). Freidson's description of the "clinical mentality" of the doctor (1970, pp. 158–184) still makes fascinating reading.

35. Illness symptoms are what the patient feels; disease signs are what the physician detects.

36. These points were inspired by discussions with Sandra Harding.

37. Baszanger's (1992) discussion of chronic pain as a "problematic reality" highlights the problems that physicians face in trying to make biomedical sense out of it. Kleinman et al. (1992, p. 9) argue that biomedical paradigms of chronic pain are "so inadequate as to virtually assure inaccurate diagnoses and unsuccessful treatment." The difficulties of diagnosing chronic pain syndromes are also treated in Ware (1992); Cooper (1997); Hyden and Sachs (1998). For more on anthropological perspectives on chronic pain, see, for example, Jackson (1992; 2000); other contributions in Good et al. (1992); Heurtin-Roberts and Becker (1993).

38. See, for example, Kleinman (1988); Charmaz (1991).

39. Kleinman (1988, pp. 8–10).

40. See, for example, Davis (1960); Gorovitz and MacIntyre (1976); Illich (1976); Bosk (1979); Light (1979); Fox (1980); Atkinson (1984); Mizrahi (1984); Paget (1988); Adamson (1997). Other sources of physician mistakes include human or technical error in the systems that produce diagnostic tests and medical records, as well as fatigue, haste, and fear.

41. Gorovitz and MacIntyre (1976, p. 63). These same authors write, "It is, one suspects, only recently that the statistical chances rose above 50 percent that a randomly chosen patient with a randomly chosen disease who encountered a randomly chosen physician would benefit from the encounter" (p. 63). Illich goes further to argue, "The medical establishment has become a major threat to health." (1976, p. 3). At least one-third of the states have systems for the mandatory reporting of "serious injury" due to hospital-based error. However, serious underreporting, due in part to what regulators call a "culture of defensiveness and secretiveness" on the part of practitioners, is believed to plague all the programs. For details see Kohn, Corrigan, and Donaldson (1999); Altman (1999); Kilborn (1999).

42. Kohn, Corrigan, and Donaldson (1999). These numbers underestimate the extent of medical error, since they exclude injuries not leading to death and patients treated in settings other than hospitals. A recent study supports the

alarmist view. A meta-analysis of studies of adverse drug reactions in hospitalized patients suggests that in 1994 2.2 million patients experienced serious drug reactions. A further 106,000 patients died from a drug reaction, making such reactions between the fourth and sixth leading cause of death. These figures *exclude* adverse reactions due to errors in prescription and administration. Were such errors to be included, the figure would rise substantially. See Lazarou et al. (1998). The existing literature on the prevalence of medical error, virtually all dealing with hospital settings, is reviewed in Kohn, Corrigan, and Donaldson (1999, pp. 22–41).

Medical sociologists have taken the high probability of error as a starting point for analyzing the ways in which physicians "manage" medical mistakes and deflect accountability. Some of the early work along these lines helps to make sense of the actions of the doctor described in these pages. Mizrahi (1984) stresses the mechanisms of denial, discounting, and distancing as well as the insistence that only medical staff—and certainly not patients—have the right to decide what is a medical mistake. Light (1979) explores how physicians' professional education prepares them to control uncertainty by training them to adhere to one school of thought; to treat patients in domineering ways (using esoteric language, withholding information, and so forth); to define competence in terms of use of correct technique rather than improvement in the patient's condition; and to rely on a system of individual autonomy in which oversight by others is negligible. All these mechanisms were operative in the case examined below.

43. This point was inspired by Kleinman, who argues that practitioners listen to patients' accounts of their problems in light of their own particular interests, which include, among others, advancing a career. He worries that this "enormous problem in clinical practice" is simply not addressed by the profession. See Kleinman (1988, pp. 52–53).

44. Paget (1988, p. 17).

45. The difficulties of admitting mistakes and the emotional consequences of that denial for the physician are eloquently explored by David Hilfiker (1984). The extent to which physicians acknowledge uncertainty and error seems to vary from specialty to specialty and individual to individual. For discussion of these issues, see Bosk (1979) and other references cited in note 40. I am grateful to Kay White Drew, Arthur Kleinman, and Arthur Rubel, who are all physicians, for reminding me of the complexity of this issue.

46. Cassell (1985, pp. 140–43). As Milligan and More (1994) emphasize in *The Empathic Practitioner,* medicine seeks certainty and control, making empathy difficult. Instead of humility, the physician responds with a rhetoric of scientific control.

47. On the use of metaphor in medicine see, for example, Martin (1987; 1991); Gogel and Terry (1987); Carter (1989); Stein (1990). Lupton (1994, pp. 50–78) provides an illuminating overview of metaphoric representations of medicine and illness in professional discourse and popular culture. Baszanger (1998) offers a fascinating account of physician rhetoric deployed in pain clinics.

48. Keller (1985, p. 126). See also her later study, *Secrets of Life, Secrets of Death* (1992).

49. Locke (1992, p. 90). On reification, or biologization, in the medical encounter and its functions of ideological reproduction, see Taussig (1980).

50. Locke (1992, p. 93).

51. On the emotional oscillations of chronic illness see Charmaz (1983; 1991) and Kleinman (1988, esp. pp. 45–48). Depression is common in people with chronic fatigue syndrome, lupus, and many other chronic conditions. See, for example, Ware (1992); German et al. (1997); Jackson (2000). For more on the existential dilemmas of chronic patients and their vulnerability to their doctors' judgments, see Reid, Ewan, and Lowy (1991); Garro (1992; 1994); Ware (1992); Cooper (1997); Jackson (2000).

52. The social isolation of the chronically ill person is described with particular force in Charmaz (1983, pp. 176–81). See also Kutner (1987, p. 52) and German et al. (1997).

53. The process by which medical students are reconstituted as fledgling physicians is traced in a fascinating series of papers by Byron J. Good and Mary-Jo DelVecchio Good. See Good and Good (1993); Good (1994, pp. 65–87).

54. Conventional medical wisdom holds that physicians have the right to make decisions on behalf of their patients, even without their full understanding or consent, on the assumption that they know what is best for the patients. This is called "benevolent paternalism." Ethical issues surrounding medical paternalism are fleshed out in Sherwin (1992, pp. 137–57), among many other places.

55. A physician's lament about the expectations of perfection inculcated in medical school and the resulting sense of sin surrounding the topic of physician error can be found in Hilfiker (1984). The literature on medical mistakes, cited in note 40, documents the myriad means physicians learn in medical school to keep from acknowledging, even to themselves, that they have made mistakes. Things are changing, but slowly. In one study, cited in Wu et al. (1997), patients or their families were told of serious medical mistakes in fewer than a quarter of the cases. In the last few years some physicians have begun to urge their colleagues on ethical grounds to disclose their mistakes to patients. An exemplary plea for openness is Wu et al. (1997). These appeals for greater honesty have drawn mixed reviews from the medical community, insurance companies, and lawyers. For more see Grady (1997).

56. Cassell (1982; also 1991). The feminist theorist Susan J. Brison (1997) develops a related argument about the bodily nature of the self, and the annihilating effects on the self of bodily traumas such as rape. I argue that under certain conditions, the receipt of poor medical care is a traumatic, self-destroying experience.

57. On the assaults to the sense of self suffered by the chronically ill, see Charmaz (1983; 1987; 1991); Bury (1982); Williams (1984); Conrad (1987); Corbin and Strauss (1987); Kutner (1987); Jackson (2000, pp. 141-68).

58. Goffman (1963). See also Frank (1997a) and Waitzkin (1991, pp. 189, 299–300, n. 8), who draw on Althusser's notion of interpellation to argue that diagnosis "hails" a new subject, effectively imposing on the ill person the new identity of patient-with-disease.

59. For a philosophical disquisition on some of these epistemological traumas see Wendell (1996).

60. Kleinman (1988, p. 22).

61. Boston Women's Health Book Collective (1973, p. 1).

62. In the early years of the women's health movement, researcher-activists focused on the problems women faced as patients. See, for example, Boston Women's Health Book Collective (1973); Corea (1985); Dreifus (1977); Scully (1994). Later work, seeking to disrupt the image of women as passive victims of biomedical oppression, stressed the ways in which certain categories of women collaborated with the medical community in the medicalization of their problems. See, for example, Riessman (1983); Figert (1996). More recently the focus has shifted from problems in the doctor-patient relationship to issues of androcentric bias in clinical research, career opportunities for women in medicine, and diversity in women's health needs. Useful overviews of these current concerns can be found in Dan (1994); Fee and Krieger (1994); Rosser (1994); Laurence and Weinhouse (1994); Auerbach and Figert (1995); Doyal (1995); Lorber (1997); Ruzek, Olesen, and Clarke (1997). Recent work in the politics of women's health is showcased in Sherwin (1998). Today, scholarship on women's health is "revisioning" the domain of concern by merging feminist, cultural, and technoscience perspectives. An exemplary text is Clarke and Olesen (1999). For histories of the women's health movement see Ruzek (1978); Zimmerman (1987); Doyal (1994); Norsigian (1996); Weisman (1998, pp. 37-93). I am indebted to Adele E. Clarke for guiding me through this literature.

63. Sociological research shows that when the doctor is male and patient female, the doctor interrupts the patient more, the prognoses are worse, there is greater expectation that the patient will adhere to traditional gender roles, and the physician's explanations less often answer the patient's questions. See Stevens (1996) for more.

64. Common forms of verbal abuse include withholding information, doomsaying (poor diagnoses and prognoses), defensive dismissal of women's input, sexist comments, and even sexual harassment. See Stevens (1996) for details. Although Stevens's research was with lesbian patients, this kind of treatment is not confined to lesbians. While "domination" is the typical model for doctor-patient relationships, Stevens notes the existence of another, "solidarity," model in which the doctor uses his or her power in ways that are compassionate, competent, and empowering for the patient.

65. Fisher (1986); Todd (1989).

66. An excellent review of research on patient reactions to their doctors can be found in Lupton (1994, pp. 113–17). The diversity of patient responses is stressed in Mitchinson (1998).

67. Fisher (1986); Todd (1989).

68. Baszanger (1998, p. 294). Baszanger shows that patients' proclivity to agree or disagree with their doctor's treatment proposals, far from reflecting "patient power," depends heavily on the conceptual model the physician is using. See Baszanger (1998, pp. 235–96). In her in-depth study of a small number of doctor-patient interactions, Fisher shows that women often conversationally resist their doctor's diagnoses, theories, treatment plans, and/or implicit ideological messages in such ways as trying to insert information into the discussion or broadening the topic. But their struggles to influence their doctors' treatment of

their cases virtually never succeed. See Fisher (1995, esp. pp. 182-88). Davis's (1988) earlier research produced similar findings.

69. When patient complaints go unheard, care suffers in numerous ways: needed information is not provided, important tests are not conducted, useful medications are not prescribed, and so forth. The medical costs of miscommunication are documented in Todd (1989) and Fisher (1986; 1995), among other places.

70. Martin (1987); Rapp (1999). Resistance to biomedical power has been a growing area of anthropological interest. A short list of such studies includes Davis-Floyd (1992); Ginsburg and Rapp (1995); Davis-Floyd and Sargent (1997); Lock and Kaufert (1998).

71. Lock and Kaufert (1998). The extraordinary case of "Joan" documented and analyzed by Mark Nichter (1998) shows that individual agency can extend to the self-initiation of medicalization. In Joan's case, the insistence on the medical nature of her illness was motivated not only by psychological factors but also by the social mission of inducing the medical community to respect patients at the margins.

72. See esp. Martin (1987); Rapp (1990; 1999, esp. pp. 136-42, 168-72); Davis-Floyd (1992).

73. The sociosexual dimension of the doctor-patient relationship has been brought out, albeit with different intent, in recent work on sexual misconduct by clinicians. See, for example, Redleaf with Baird (1998). Also relevant here are psychodynamic perspectives that highlight the influence of unconscious psychological factors on physicians' approaches to patient care. See esp. Balint (1957); Stein (1985).

74. These, of course, are simplifications. For a broad overview of sociological perspectives on the doctor-patient encounter, see Lupton (1994, pp. 105-30). Baszanger's (1998) more recent notion of "regimes of physician-patient relations," while giving the patient a more active, agentic role in a relationship traditionally construed as doctor dominant, nevertheless continues to place medical decision making at the core of the relationship. Here I highlight a relationship that was created ultimately to ensure quality medical care but whose character was first and foremost social, or even "sociosexual."

75. See Campo (1997) for a gay physician's perspective.

76. A recent paper by Deborah Lupton (1996) discusses the emotional needs, dependencies, and ambivalences patients take into their medical encounters. This paper, which reflects a growing interest among medical sociologists in the emotional dimensions of health, does not address questions of gender or sexuality in the doctor-patient relationship. On emotions and health more generally, see, for example, Olesen (1990); James and Gabe (1996).

77. Major scholarly forums on this work were published in *Signs* in 1986 and *Feminism and Psychology* in 1994. The earlier discussion focused on Gilligan (1982), the latter on Brown and Gilligan (1992). See Kerber et al. (1986) and Wilkinson (1994). Tronto (1987) and Tavris (1993) provide more interesting commentary. What is politically problematic about this body of work for many feminists is its tendency to treat the feminine "relational self" and "ethic of care" (these terms are explained below in the text) as traits that are essential

to women rather than structurally induced by the larger systems of gender inequality in which they are embedded. The theoretical problems many see with this work surround the notion of identity. These are discussed below.

78. See esp. Hekman (1995).

79. See Foucault (e.g., 1971; 1978; 1979); Butler (1990); Haraway (1991), among many others. My discussion of this large literature relies heavily on Hekman (1995), who creatively connects Gilligan's work to this larger body of feminist writing on selfhood; and Weedon (1997). Selfhood continues to be a lively area of feminist theorizing. In recent work notions of fragmentation, embodiment, difference, relationality, emotion, and narrative—all central to the ethnography presented below—are central to the philosophical explorations of the self.

80. See Hekman (1995, pp. 71–112). In a fine exegesis of relational, postmodern, and feminist theories of subjectivity, she both traces the intellectual lineage of "the discursive self" and shows how it implies morality, agency, and resistance, or political action.

81. Hekman (1995, p. 82).

82. See, for example, Greeno and Maccoby (1986); Luria (1986); Gremmen (1994); Tavris (1994).

83. This critique is advanced by Stack (1986); Tronto (1987); and Lykes (1994), among others. Recent empirical research suggests that, unlike the middle-class white girls studied by Brown and Gilligan (1992), poor minority girls do not lose their voices in adolescence. African-American women silence themselves in adulthood, but, in contrast to the white women studied by Jack (1993), they do not grow depressed as a result. These results are reported in Robinson and Ward (1991); Way (1995); and Carr, Gilroy, and Sherman (1996).

84. See especially Taylor, Gilligan, and Sullivan (1995) and L. Brown (1998).

85. The critique of the unitary and stable nature of identity (or "voice") in the work of Gilligan, Brown, and Jack is developed by K. Davis (1994) and Hekman (1995, esp. pp. 74–76), among others. L. Brown's (1994) early response has been followed up by a major study emphasizing the complex and contradictory nature of girls' subjectivity. See L. Brown (1998).

86. The classic article on "doing gender" is West and Zimmerman (1987). See also Fenstermaker, West, and Zimmerman (1991). West (1993) extends the gender-as-accomplishment perspective to physician-patient relationships. More recently West and Fenstermaker (1995) have extended the approach to race and class, prompting wide debate. For the controversy see Collins et al. (1995). This discussion was prompted by stimulating conversations with Valerie Jenness.

87. Hekman (1995, p. 84).

88. Hekman (1995, p. 111).

89. Gilligan (1982).

90. Brown and Gilligan (1992); see also Gilligan, Lyons, and Hanmer (1990). Later works explore psychosocial development and the politics of anger and resistance among girls of working-class and ethnically diverse backgrounds. See Taylor, Gilligan, and Sullivan (1995) and L. Brown (1998). Mary Pipher's (1994) clinical work, presented in her best-selling book, *Reviving Ophelia*, documents the persistence if not intensification of these patterns of socialization in adolescents today.

91. See, for example, Davis (1994); Gremmen (1994); Kitzinger (1994); Hekman (1995).

92. L. Brown (1994, p. 388).

93. Jack (1993).

94. I thank Arthur Rubel for discussion on this point.

95. Lupton (1996, esp. pp. 166–67).

96. Lupton (1996, esp. p. 169).

97. The notion of "mind rehearsals" of anger, introduced by Jack (1993), is elaborated in chapter 5.

98. Mahoney (1996, pp. 605, 622).

99. Mahoney (1996, pp. 621–22).

100. Sontag (1990). Sontag's otherwise stimulating essay has been criticized for advocating stripping metaphorical meanings from constructions of illness. Most believe that doing so is neither feasible nor desirable.

101. Leichter (1997, p. 359); also Conrad (1994); Lupton (1995); Petersen and Lupton (1996, pp. 61–88); Brandt and Rozin (1997); Lock (1998).

102. Showalter (1997).

103. The work of psychoneuroimmunology has documented the mutual influences of mind on body and body on mind. An excellent and highly accessible review of the field's findings can be found in Martin (1997).

104. Showalter (1997, p. 8).

105. Showalter (1997, pp. 206, 207).

106. See Finerman and Bennett (1995).

107. See, for example, DiGiacomo (1992); Finerman and Bennett (1995); and the works cited in note 101.

108. The phrase "longing for organicity" belongs to the historian of medicine Edward Shorter. He explains thus: "Few patients wish to receive a psychiatric diagnosis . . . This is partly because patients fear the mystery and hopelessness that cling to the action of the mind. In addition, anything of a psychiatric nature continues to be stigmatized in our society. Patients find an organic diagnosis far more acceptable socially and have sought them out throughout history." See Shorter (1995, p. 233).

109. These labels come from Weintraub (1995, p. 343); and Shorter (1995, p. 230).

110. See, for example, Garro (1992; 1994); Ware (1992); Cooper (1997); Jackson (2000).

111. Hawkins (1993, pp. 9, 125–57).

112. Recent illness memoirs that I find particularly affecting include Alice Wexler's family story of Huntington's disease (1995); Kay Redfield Jamison's testimonial of her struggle with manic depression (1996); Kat Duff's account of her struggles with chronic fatigue syndrome (1993); Susanna Kaysen's account of mental illness (1993); Tracy Thomson's "reckoning with depression" (1995); and Arthur W. Frank's reflections on cancer (1991). The poet Audre Lorde's cancer journals (1980) and the sociologist Marianne A. Paget's "reflections on cancer and an abbreviated life" (1993) explore different genres of illness autobiography. In anthropology, Robert Murphy's (1990) account of his final odyssey

with a tumor of the spinal chord is unlikely ever to be surpassed for its reflexive and ethnographic insight into the world of the very ill.

113. A wide-ranging review of recent medical ethnographies can be found in Kleinman (1995, pp. 193–256). Ethnographic work in medical sociology is illuminatingly reviewed in Charmaz and Olesen (1997).

114. In anthropology, the term *auto-ethnography* historically has been used in two senses: as an ethnography of one's own culture or as autobiographical writing with ethnographic interest. The distinction between the two is now breaking down. A useful definition of auto-ethnography is a form of social narrative that places the self within its social context. For more, see Reed-Danahay (1997a).

115. On "writing culture" in anthropology, see Clifford and Marcus (1986) and Behar and Gordon (1995).

116. I thank Susan M. DiGiacomo for prompting my thoughts in this section.

117. These ideas were stimulated by Susan M. DiGiacomo.

118. In some sections of the book, especially parts IV and V, the argument develops chronologically, but the temporal narrative does not displace the thematic concerns.

119. Kleinman and Kleinman (1991); DiGiacomo (1992). See also Kleinman, Das, and Lock (1997) on "social suffering."

120. A masterful account of the discipline's critique of classic ethnography is Rosaldo (1989).

121. Linda Layne's (1996) account of her struggles as a parent of a child in neonatal intensive care is the first first-person account ever to appear in the *Medical Anthropology Quarterly*, the journal of the Society for Medical Anthropology. Another precedent is Susan M. DiGiacomo's (1987; 1995) analysis of her cancer experiences.

122. Harding (1991, esp. pp. 138–63); Haraway (1991).

123. I thank Arthur Kleinman for reminding me of these shortcomings of the genre.

124. See especially Behar and Gordon (1995). This book illuminates the dilemmas women anthropologists have encountered in using personal testimony for ethnographic purposes.

125. Behar (1996); Behar and Gordon (1995). The term *vulnerable writing* comes from Behar (1996). Perhaps the first ethnography to acknowledge the importance of emotions in the creation of anthropological knowledge was Jean Briggs's *Never in Anger* (1970).

126. Jaggar (1989).

127. Jaggar (1989).

128. Jaggar (1989).

Chapter 1. The Initial Consultation: The Making of a "Fibromyalgic"

1. Dr. D. subscribed to the "gate control theory of pain" elaborated in an important article published in *Science* in 1965. See Melzack and Wall (1965).

For the historical background, theoretical context, and therapeutic implications of the gate control theory, which provides the scientific basis of work conducted in many pain clinics, see Baszanger (1998, esp. pp. 19–140).

2. Wolfe et al. (1990).

3. In his critique of biomedicine's neglect and delegitimation of personal suffering, Kleinman (1995, pp. 68–92) has shown that "subjective" knowledge and lay interpretations of illness are sometimes more valid and useful in assessing disease process than the "objective" measures of biomedicine.

Chapter 2. Medicating the "Fibromyalgic"–Arthritic Body

1. The term *epistemic invalidation* comes from Wendell (1996). The term *ontological invalidation* is mine.

Chapter 3. Producing the Good Patient

1. Dr. D.'s working definition of "the good patient" conforms closely to that of American physicians generally. Howard F. Stein describes the unofficial, moralistic taxonomy of patients used by many physicians: "Good patients are those diagnosed with bona fide organic disease . . . Good patients are those who respond quickly to physicians' efforts to alleviate their suffering, who accept and understand the physician's model, and who submit to and enthusiastically comply with the physician's treatment recommendation. Good patients obey the physician's 'rule of silence' in not disagreeing with or contradicting the physician and take up little of the physician's time . . . The good patient is one who affirms the self-image of the 'good doctor' and makes the physician feel successful, competent, in control, powerful, a 'winner' in the battle against disease" (Stein 1990, p. 98).

2. Such financial arrangements are increasingly common among today's physician-entrepreneurs. They are in part a response to the decline in physician incomes caused by the spread of managed care. In cardiology, investigative reporters for the *New York Times* found, specialists without financial conflicts of interest "stand out like a sore thumb" (Eichenwald and Kolata 1999).

3. On the nonprogressive character of fibromyalgia, see Tierney et al. (1996, p. 764); Wilson et al. (1991, p. 1487). In making this remark, Dr. D. might have been thinking of the "gate control theory of pain," which holds that pain continues to spread until the "pain pathways" are closed. He articulated this view in the March 8 appointment. Even if he had that pain theory in mind, the claim that fibromyalgia is progressive was misleading at best.

Chapter 4. A Most Pleasant Patient

1. See in particular Gilligan (1982).

2. See Brown and Gilligan (1992); Gilligan, Lyons, and Hanmer (1990).

3. Jack (1993).

4. Boston Women's Health Book Collective (1973).

5. De Beauvoir (1962).

6. The gender training she received is much like that described by Wini Breines in her book, *Young, White and Miserable: Growing Up Female in the Fifties* (1992).

7. I am indebted to Kathy Radke for retrieving this poem for me from her collection of childhood treasures.

Chapter 5. Silent Rebellion and Rage

1. See, for example, Boston Women's Health Book Collective (1973); Corea (1985); Scully (1994). An excellent overview of these critiques is provided by Ruzek (1978).

2. The term *mind rehearsal* was used by Dana Jack to describe the imaginary scenes in which depressed women dare to speak their anger and confront their partners with the harm done them in the relationship. These mind rehearsals fail to resolve the problem while siphoning off enough anger to allow women to stay in intolerable relationships. Jack argues that these imaginary rebellions are ineffective forms of resistance in the short run, but that in the long run they may dissolve the tie enough to prepare women to leave unhealthy relationships. See Jack (1993, pp. 49–54).

Chapter 6. A Depression Worse Than the Disease

1. The following discussion of Dr. D.'s lecture is based on S.'s notes. The quotations come from a tape of the lecture the author later purchased from the sponsoring organization.

2. Kennedy and Felson (1996).

3. Kennedy and Felson (1996, pp. 682).

4. Ledingham, Doherty, and Doherty (1993).

5. Henricksson (1994).

6. See, for example, Wolfe et al. (1995); Boisset-Pioro, Esdaile, and Fitzcharles (1995). Some researchers associate the mood disorders with care-seeking rather than the illness per se. See Aaron et al. (1996).

7. Aaron et al. (1996).

8. Boisset-Pioro, Esdaile, and Fitzcharles (1995); Taylor, Trotter, and Csuka (1995); Aaron et al. (1996); also Hudson and Pope (1995).

9. Taylor, Trotter, and Csuka (1995).

Chapter 8. "Accept It!" Alternative Medicines Offer Medicine for the Mind

1. I thank Kay White Drew for illuminating discussions of alternatives to conventional medicine.

2. Weil (1995).

3. Weil (1995, p. 7).

4. Weil (1995, pp. 194–209).

5. Weil (1995, p. 201).

6. Weil (1995, p. 103).

7. Weil (1995, p. 88).

8. Weil (1995, pp. 248–52).
9. Kabat-Zinn (1990).
10. Kabat-Zinn (1990, p. 5).
11. Kabat-Zinn (1990, p. 11).
12. Kabat-Zinn (1990, p. 11).
13. Kabat-Zinn (1990, pp. 33–40).
14. Kabat-Zinn (1990, p. 39).
15. Kabat-Zinn (1990, p. 66).
16. Kabat-Zinn (1990, p. 280).
17. Kabat-Zinn (1990, p. 168).
18. Kabat-Zinn (1990, p. 168).
19. Gawain (1995).
20. Gawain (1995, p. 18).
21. Gawain (1995, pp. 17, 25–26).
22. Gawain (1995, pp. 93–94).
23. Gawain (1995, p. 98).
24. Gawain (1995, p. 87).
25. Gawain (1995, pp. 87–88).
26. Gawain (1995, p. 48).
27. Gawain (1995, p. 152).
28. Gawain (1995, p. 93).
29. Weil (1995, pp. 112–13). Gawain also maintained that people should not feel guilty for being ill (1995, p. 96), but the passage cited above leaves her work open to that interpretation.

Chapter 10. A Second Opinion: The Unmaking of a "Fibromyalgic"

1. I thank Arthur Rubel for his queries on this point.

Chapter 11. The Final Meeting: A Tale of Decline and a Denial

1. Another patient S. talked to later described Dr. D. as "paranoid about being sued."

2. Although I have no direct evidence of changes in the doctor's practice, a public lecture on fibromyalgia that he gave six months after the final meeting suggests that, if anything, his certitude about the widespread prevalence of his specialty disease and the correctness of his approach to it had grown stronger. This information comes from a tape of a lecture delivered in May 1997. The tape was purchased from the sponsoring group.

3. Interestingly, physicians in other specialties with whom S. talked about the experience with Dr. D. reacted more strongly. One even suggested that she file a complaint with the state board of medicine.

Chapter 12. Out from under the Medical Gaze

1. Wolfe (1994, p. 494).
2. Wolfe et al. (1990, p. 163).

3. Wolfe et al. (1990).

4. All figures calculated from Wolfe et al. (1990, p. 165).

5. Figures calculated from Wolfe et al. (1990, p. 167).

6. Wolfe (1994, p. 485).

7. Wolfe (1994, p. 499).

8. On Plaquenil toxicity see, for example, Aylward (1993); Mazzuca et al. (1994); Potter (1993).

9. Roenigk et al. (1988). She also consulted Boffa et al. (1995); Tobkes and Nord (1995); and Hassan (1996), among many others.

10. An excellent introduction to the findings of psychoneuroimmunology is Martin (1997).

Conclusion: Re-viewing the Medicine of Chronic Pain

1. See especially Harding (1991); Haraway (1991).

2. Kleinman (1988).

3. A useful compendium of these treatments is Burton Goldberg Group (1994). With a very few exceptions, the efficacy and safety of these alternative therapies have not been put to scientific test. Today there is a growing awareness of the potential dangers of inappropriate use of herbal supplements.

4. See especially Cassell (1982) and Kleinman (1988).

5. B. Engel (1990, p. 10).

6. See especially G. Engel (1977a; 1977b; 1987; 1997) and the festschrift devoted to his work in *Psychosomatic Medicine* (Joynt 1980). An exemplary application of a biopsychosocial model to chronic pain syndromes is Barsky and Borus (1999).

7. A trenchant critique from a social-scientific point of view is Armstrong (1987).

8. Kohn, Corrigan, and Donaldson (1999).

9. See, for example, Altman (1999); Kilborn (1999); Pear (1999).

10. In the late 1980s, 83 percent of prescription drug use, 80 percent of hospital days, and 66 percent of physician visits were devoted to the care of the 46 percent of the population that suffers from chronic conditions. See Hoffman, Rice, and Sung (1996) for details.

11. For overviews of this work see Berg (1992); Casper and Berg (1995); Casper and Koenig (1996).

12. A key text on medicine as a profession is Freidson (1970).

13. Particularly influential were Knorr-Cetina (1981; 1983); Latour (1987); Latour and Woolgar (1979).

14. Locke (1992).

15. Cassell (1982).

16. Goffman (1963).

17. Schaefer (1995, p. 100)

18. Schaefer (1995, pp. 97–98).

19. Schaefer (1997, p. 568).

20. Schaefer (1995, p. 97).

21. Estroff (1981, esp. pp. 213–39; 1993).

22. See especially Fisher (1986; 1995); Todd (1989); and Waitzkin (1991).

23. Especially Gilligan (1982); Brown and Gilligan (1992); and Jack (1993).

24. Balshem (1993). I am grateful to Susan M. DiGiacomo for bringing this book to my attention and for provoking me to see the class dimension of S.'s politics.

25. For discussions of these trends see Strathern (1987); Denzin (1989); Lavie, Narayan, and Rosaldo (1993); van Maanen (1995); Ochs and Capps (1996).

26. Contributions in native and/or ethnic ethnography include Herzfeld (1997); Motzafi-Haller (1997); Warren (1997); in feminist ethnography, Behar and Gordon (1995); in auto-ethnography, Ellis and Bochner (1996); Reed-Danahay (1997).

27. Kleinman and Kleinman (1991); see also Kleinman, Das, and Lock (1997) on "social suffering."

28. Cf. Kleinman and Kleinman (1991).

29. This argument has been developed most fully, perhaps, in Kleinman and Kleinman (1991) and DiGiacomo (1992).

30. The term *vulnerable writing* is Behar's. See Behar (1996).

31. On self-making through narrativizing, see esp. Ochs and Capps (1996). On the narrative reconstitution of the self that has been destroyed by bodily trauma, see Brison (1997).

32. Munt (1994).

33. One of the best accounts of these narrative devices is Rosaldo (1989). Another influential critique of classic ethnography was Clifford and Marcus (1986).

34. Showalter (1997).

35. Cohen and Quintner (1993, p. 906).

36. See Cohen and Quintner (1993); Bohr (1995); Shorter (1995); Kavanaugh (1996), among others. Proponents of the syndrome now acknowledge that the boundary between fibromyalgia and non-fibromyalgia is not discrete. See esp. Wolfe (1997a).

37. Cohen and Quintner (1993, p. 906). Similar arguments are developed by Russell (1995); Hadler (1997); and Quintner and Cohen (1999).

38. Quintner and Cohen (1999, p. 1092). Hadler (1997, p. 1250) goes further, calling fibromyalgia "a belief system held by a cadre of clinicians and communicated to any patient sufficiently wretched to be receptive." He argues that the construct is counterproductive: instead of helping the patient, it promotes a life of somatizing.

39. On the desire for a diagnosis among patients with chronic pain syndromes similar to fibromyalgia, see, for example, Reid, Ewan, and Lowy (1991); Ware (1992); Garro (1992; 1994); Cooper (1997); German et al. (1997); Hyden and Sachs (1998).

40. Wolfe (1997b, p. 1247).

41. Gilman's story is reprinted in Knight (1994, pp. 39–53), as well as many other places. I encountered it only after the episode charted in this book had come to an end.

42. Mitchell's rest cure required patients to relinquish control over their lives

and care to the physician. Physically and socially isolated, they were put to bed, fattened, and then reeducated to appreciate the virtues of patience, resignation, and self-restraint. For more see Bassuk (1986).

43. Knight (1994, pp. 11–12).

44. Gilman (1935, p. 91).

45. Gilman (1935, p. 96).

46. Gilman 1913 in Lane (1980, p. 20).

47. Gilman 1913 in Lane (1980, p. 20).

48. Key references include Zola (1972; 1975); Freidson (1970); Conrad and Schneider (1980); Riessman (1983); Conrad (1992).

49. The literature on the dangers of the medicalization of reproduction is vast and multidisciplinary. Recent collections of work in anthropology include Ginsburg and Rapp (1995); Davis-Floyd and Sargent (1997); Franklin and Ragone (1997).

50. Women under sixty-five are 1.6 times more likely to have arthritis than men of their age. That number falls to 1.4 in the seventy-five-plus group and 1.3 in the sixty-five-to-seventy-four age group. These numbers are based on the non-institutionalized civilian population. See United States Department of Commerce (1998, p. 149).

51. Radomsky (1995, pp. 43–48).

52. United States Department of Commerce (1998, p. 149).

53. On the plight of middle-class women in the late nineteenth century, see Ehrenreich and English (1978); Vertinsky (1990).

54. Ehrenreich and English (1978).

55. Ehrenreich and English (1978, pp. 29–126). De Marneffe (1996) and Theriot (1996) show that women patients were active participants in the medicalization of their problems.

56. "Clash in Detroit" (1996).

57. Wolfe (1994); Bohr (1995); Barsky and Borus (1999).

58. On the "backlash" against the women's movement, see Faludi (1991).

59. Boisset-Pioro, Esdaile, and Fitzcharles (1995); Taylor, Trotter, and Csuka (1995); Walker et al. (1997); Goldberg, Pachas, and Keith (1999). Boisset-Pioro et al. found significant differences between fibromyalgic patients and controls in lifetime sexual abuse (17 vs. 6 percent), physical abuse (18 vs. 4 percent), and childhood sexual abuse (37 vs. 22 percent), among other things. In these studies, between 50 and 65 percent of women with fibromyalgia report histories of sexual abuse (Taylor et al. 1995); 53 to 65 percent have histories of sexual or physical abuse (Boisset-Pioro et al. 1995; Alexander et al. 1998; Goldberg, Pachas, and Keith 1999). On sexual abuse and chronic pelvic pain see Walling et al. (1994); Walker et al. (1995).

60. This literature is reviewed in Boisset-Pioro, Esdaile, and Fitzcharles (1995); Hudson and Pope (1995); Radomsky (1995, pp. 55–64).

61. Radomsky (1995, esp. pp. 55–64).

62. Carroll and Niven (1993); Lovallo (1997).

63. Witkin (1991, p. 85).

64. Witkin (1991, p. 121).

**Epilogue: Speaking of Pain—On Stories,
Cultural Recuperations, and Political Interventions**

1. Morris (1991).
2. Frank (1995; 1997a; 1997b).
3. Frank (1997a, p. 32).

References

I. Patient Materials

Medical Diary
MANL (Make-a-New-Life) Book
S. G. Well-Being Charts
Transition File
Various Letters, E-mails, and Handwritten Notes

II. Works in the Humanities and Social Sciences

Abel, Emily K., and Margaret K. Nelson, eds. 1990. *Circles of Care: Work and Identity in Women's Lives.* Albany: State University of New York Press.

Adamson, Christopher. 1997. "Existential and Clinical Uncertainty in the Medical Encounter: An Idiographic Account of an Illness Trajectory Defined by Inflammatory Bowel Disease and Avascular Necrosis." *Sociology of Health and Illness* 19 (2): 133–59.

Appadurai, Arjun, ed. 1986. *The Social Life of Things: Commodities in Cultural Perspective.* Cambridge: Cambridge University Press.

Armstrong, David. 1983. *Political Anatomy of the Body: Medical Knowledge in Britain in the Twentieth Century.* Cambridge: Cambridge University Press.

———. 1984. "The Patient's View." *Social Science and Medicine* 18 (9): 737–44.

———. 1987. "Theoretical Tensions in Biopsychosocial Medicine." *Social Science and Medicine* 25 (11): 1213–18.

———. 1995. "The Rise of Surveillance Medicine." *Sociology of Health and Illness* 17 (3): 393–404.

———. 1997. "Foucault and the Sociology of Health and Illness: A Prismatic Reading." In *Foucault, Health and Medicine,* ed. Alan Petersen and Robin Bunton, pp. 15–30. London: Routledge.

Arney, William Ray, and Bernard J. Bergen. 1984. *Medicine and the Management of the Living: Taming the Last Great Beast.* Chicago: University of Chicago Press.

Atkinson, Paul. 1984. "Training for Certainty." *Social Science and Medicine* 19 (9): 949–56.

———. 1995. *Medical Talk and Medical Work: The Liturgy of the Clinic.* London: Sage.

Auerbach, Judith D., and Anne E. Figert. 1995. "Women's Health Research: Public Policy and Sociology." *Journal of Health and Social Behavior,* Extra issue, 115–31.

Balint, Michael. 1957. *The Doctor, His Patient, and the Illness.* New York: International Universities Press.

Balshem, Martha. 1993. *Cancer in the Community: Class and Medical Authority.* Washington, DC: Smithsonian Institution Press.

Barrett, Robert J. 1988. "Clinical Writing and the Documentary Construction of Schizophrenia." *Culture, Medicine and Psychiatry* 12 (3): 265–99.

Bassuk, Ellen L. 1986. "The Rest Cure: Repetition or Resolution of Victorian Women's Conflicts?" In *The Feminine Body in Western Culture: Contemporary Perspectives,* ed. Susan Rubin Suleiman, pp. 139–51. Cambridge: Harvard University Press.

Baszanger, Isabelle. 1992. "Deciphering Chronic Pain." *Sociology of Health and Illness* 14 (2): 181–215.

———. 1998. *Inventing Pain Medicine: From the Laboratory to the Clinic.* New Brunswick, NJ: Rutgers University Press.

Behar, Ruth. 1996. *The Vulnerable Observer: Anthropology That Breaks Your Heart.* Boston: Beacon.

Behar, Ruth, and Deborah A. Gordon, eds. 1995. *Women Writing Culture.* Berkeley: University of California Press.

Berg, Marc. 1992. "The Construction of Medical Disposals: Medical Sociology and Medical Problem Solving in Clinical Practice." *Sociology of Health and Illness* 14 (2): 151–80.

———. 1995. "Turning a Practice into a Science: Reconceptualizing Postwar Medical Practice." *Social Studies of Science* 25 (3): 437–76.

———. 1996. "Practices of Reading and Writing: The Constitutive Role of the Patient Record in Medical Work." *Sociology of Health and Illness* 18 (4): 499–524.

Bosk, Charles L. 1979. *Forgive and Remember: Managing Medical Failure.* Chicago: University of Chicago Press.

Boston Women's Health Book Collective. 1973. *Our Bodies, Ourselves: A Book by and for Women.* New York: Simon and Schuster, 1971. Reprint, New York: Simon and Schuster.

Brandt, Allan M., and Paul Rozin, eds. 1997. *Morality and Health.* New York: Routledge.

Breines, Wini. 1992. *Young, White, and Miserable: Growing Up Female in the Fifties.* Boston: Beacon.

Briggs, Jean. 1970. *Never in Anger: Portrait of an Eskimo Family.* Cambridge: Harvard University Press.

Brison, Susan J. 1997. "Outliving Oneself: Trauma, Memory, and Personal Identity." In *Feminists Rethink the Self,* ed. Diana Tietjens Meyers, pp. 12–39. Boulder: Westview.

Brody, Howard. 1987. *Stories of Sickness.* New Haven: Yale University Press.

———. 1994. "'My Story Is Broken; Can You Help Me Fix It?' Medical Ethics and the Joint Construction of Narrative." *Literature and Medicine* 13 (1): 79–92.

Brown, Lyn Mikel. 1994. "Standing in the Crossfire: A Response to Tavris,

Gremmen, Lykes, Davis and Contratto." *Feminism and Psychology* 4 (3): 382–98.

———. 1998. *Raising Their Voices: The Politics of Girls' Anger.* Cambridge: Harvard University Press.

Brown, Lyn Mikel, and Carol Gilligan. 1992. *Meeting at the Crossroads: Women's Psychology and Girls' Development.* Cambridge: Harvard University Press.

Brown, Phil. 1989. "The Name Game: Toward a Sociology of Diagnosis." *Journal of Mind and Behavior* 11 (3, 4): 385–406.

———. 1993. "Psychiatric Intake as a Mystery Story." *Culture, Medicine and Psychiatry* 17 (2): 255–80.

———. 1995. "Naming and Framing: The Social Construction of Diagnosis and Illness." *Journal of Health and Social Behavior,* Extra issue, 34–52.

Bury, M. 1982. "Chronic Illness as Biographical Disruption." *Sociology of Health and Illness* 5: 168–95.

Butler, Judith. 1990. *Gender Trouble: Gender and the Subversion of Identity.* New York: Routledge.

Campo, Rafael. 1997. *The Poetry of Healing: A Doctor's Education in Empathy, Identity, and Desire.* New York: W. W. Norton.

Carr, Judith G., Faith D. Gilroy, and Martin F. Sherman. 1996. "Silencing the Self and Depression Among Women." *Psychology of Women Quarterly* 20 (3): 375–92.

Carter, Albert Howard III. 1989. "Metaphors in the Physician-Patient Relationship." *Soundings* 72 (1): 153–64.

Casper, Monica J., and Marc Berg. 1995. "Constructivist Perspectives on Medical Work: Medical Practices and Science and Technology Studies." *Science, Technology, and Human Values* 20 (4): 395–407.

Casper, Monica J., and Barbara A. Koenig. 1996. "Reconfiguring Nature and Culture: Intersections of Medical Anthropology and Technoscience Studies." *Medical Anthropology Quarterly* 10 (4): 523–36.

Charmaz, Kathy. 1983. "Loss of Self: A Fundamental Form of Suffering in the Chronically Ill." *Sociology of Health and Illness* 5 (2): 168–95.

———. 1987. "Struggling for a Self: Identity Levels of the Chronically Ill." In *The Experience and Management of Chronic Illness.* Research in the Sociology of Health Care, vol. 6, ed. Julius A. Roth and Peter Conrad, pp. 283–321. Greenwich, CT: JAI Press.

———. 1991. *Good Days, Bad Days: The Self in Chronic Illness and Time.* New Brunswick, NJ: Rutgers University Press.

Charmaz, Kathy, and Virginia Olesen. 1997. "Ethnographic Research in Medical Sociology: Its Foci and Distinctive Contributions." *Sociological Methods and Research* 25 (4): 452–94.

Charon, Rita. 1986. "To Render the Lives of Patients." *Literature and Medicine* 5: 58–74.

———. 1989. "Doctor-Patient/Reader-Writer: Learning to Find the Text." *Soundings* 71 (1): 137–51.

Clark, Jack A., and Elliott G. Mishler. 1992. "Attending to Patients' Stories: Reframing the Clinical Task." *Sociology of Health and Illness* 14 (3): 344–72.

Clarke, Adele E., and Virginia L. Olesen, eds. 1999. *Revisioning Women, Health, and Healing: Feminist, Cultural, and Technoscience Perspectives*. New York: Routledge.

"Clash in Detroit over How Ill a Kevorkian Client Really Was." 1996. *New York Times*, 20 August.

Clifford, James, and George E. Marcus, eds. 1986. *Writing Culture: The Poetics and Politics of Ethnography*. Berkeley: University of California Press.

Collins, Patricia Hill, Lionel A. Maldonado, Dana Y. Takagi, Barrie Thorne, Lynn Weber, and Howard Winant. 1995. "Symposium on West and Fenstermaker's 'Doing Difference.'" *Gender and Society* 9 (4): 491–513.

Conrad, Peter. 1987. "The Experience of Illness: Recent and New Directions." In *The Experience and Management of Chronic Illness*. Research in the Sociology of Health Care, vol. 6, ed. Julius A. Roth and Peter Conrad, pp. 1–31. Greenwich, CT: JAI Press.

———. 1992. "Medicalization and Social Control." *Annual Review of Sociology* 18: 209–32.

———. 1994. "Wellness as Virtue: Morality and the Pursuit of Health." *Culture, Medicine and Psychiatry* 18 (3): 385–401.

Conrad, Peter, and J. Schneider. 1980. *Deviance and Medicalization: From Badness to Sickness*. St. Louis: C. V. Mosby.

Cooper, Lesley. 1997. "Myalgic Encephalomyelitis and the Medical Encounter." *Sociology of Health and Illness* 19 (2): 186–207.

Corbin, Juliet, and Anselm L. Strauss. 1987. "Accompaniments of Chronic Illness: Changes in Body, Self, Biography, and Biographical Time." In *The Experience and Management of Chronic Illness*. Research in the Sociology of Health Care, vol. 6, ed. Julius A. Roth and Peter Conrad, pp. 249–81. Greenwich, CT: JAI Press.

Corea, Gena. 1985. *The Hidden Malpractice: How American Medicine Mistreats Women*. New York: Morrow, 1977. Rev. ed., New York: Harper & Row.

Dan, Alice J., ed. 1994. *Reframing Women's Health: Multidisciplinary Research and Practice*. Thousand Oaks, CA: Sage.

Davis, Fred. 1960. "Uncertainty in Medical Prognosis, Clinical and Functional." *American Journal of Sociology* 66 (1): 41–47.

Davis, Kathy. 1988. *Power Under the Microscope*. Dordrecht: Foris.

———. 1994. "What's in a Voice? Methods and Metaphors." *Feminism and Psychology* 4 (3): 353–61.

Davis-Floyd, Robbie E. 1992. *Birth as an American Rite of Passage*. Berkeley: University of California Press.

Davis-Floyd, Robbie E., and Carolyn F. Sargent, eds. 1997. *Childbirth and Authoritative Knowledge: Cross-Cultural Perspectives*. Berkeley: University of California Press.

de Beauvoir, Simone. 1962. *The Prime of Life*. Cleveland: World.

de Marneffe, Daphne. 1996. "Looking and Listening: The Construction of Clinical Knowledge in Charcot and Freud." In *Gender and Scientific Authority*, ed. Barbara Laslett, Sally Gregory Kohlstedt, Helen Longino, and Evelynn Hammonds, pp. 241–81. Chicago: University of Chicago Press.

Denzin, Norman. 1989. *Interpretive Biography*. Newbury Park, CA: Sage.

DiGiacomo, Susan M. 1987. "Biomedicine as a Cultural System: An Anthropologist in the Kingdom of the Sick." In *Encounters with Biomedicine: Case Studies in Medical Anthropology*, ed. Hans A. Baer, pp. 315–46. New York: Gordon and Breach.

———. 1992. "Metaphor as Illness: Postmodern Dilemmas in the Representation of Body, Mind and Disorder." *Medical Anthropology* 14 (1): 109–37.

———. 1995. "A Narrative Deconstruction of 'Diagnostic Delay.'" *Second Opinion* 20 (4): 21–35.

Dreifus, Claudia, ed. 1977. *Seizing Our Bodies: The Politics of Women's Health*. New York: Random House.

Dreyfus, Hubert L., and Paul Rabinow. 1982. *Michel Foucault: Beyond Structuralism and Hermeneutics*. 2d ed. Chicago: University of Chicago Press.

Doyal, Lesley. 1994. "Women, Health, and the Sexual Division of Labor: A Case Study of the Women's Health Movement in Britain." In *Women's Health, Politics, and Power: Essays on Sex/Gender, Medicine, and Public Health*, ed. Elizabeth Fee and Nancy Krieger, pp. 61–76. Amityville, NY: Baywood.

———. 1995. *What Makes Women Sick: Gender and the Political Economy of Health*. New Brunswick, NJ: Rutgers University Press.

Duff, Kat. 1993. *The Alchemy of Illness*. New York: Pantheon.

Ehrenreich, Barbara, and Deirdre English. 1978. *For Her Own Good: 150 Years of the Experts' Advice to Women*. Garden City, NY: Anchor/Doubleday.

Ellis, Carolyn, and Arthur P. Bochner. 1996. *Composing Ethnography: Alternative Forms of Qualitative Writing*. Walnut Creek, CA: AltaMira.

Engel, Beverly. 1990. *The Emotionally Abused Woman*. New York: Fawcett Columbine.

Epstein, Julia. 1995. *Altered Conditions: Disease, Medicine, and Storytelling*. New York: Routledge.

Estroff, Sue E. 1981. *Making It Crazy: An Ethnography of Psychiatric Clients in an American Community*. Berkeley: University of California Press.

———. 1993. "Identity, Disability, and Schizophrenia: The Problem of Chronicity." In *Knowledge, Power and Practice: The Anthropology of Medicine and Everyday Life*, ed. Shirley Lindenbaum and Margaret Lock, pp. 247–86. Berkeley: University of California Press.

Faludi, Susan. 1991. *Backlash: The Undeclared War Against American Women*. New York: Doubleday.

Fee, Elizabeth, and Nancy Krieger, eds. 1994. *Women's Health, Politics, and Power: Essays on Sex/Gender, Medicine, and Public Health*. Amityville, NY: Baywood.

Fenstermaker, Sarah, Candace West, and Don H. Zimmerman. 1991. "Gender Inequality: New Conceptual Terrain." In *Gender, Family, and Economy: The Triple Overlap*, ed. Rae Lesser Blumberg, pp. 289–307. Newbury Park, CA: Sage.

Figert, Anne E. 1996. *Women and the Ownership of PMS: The Structuring of a Psychiatric Disorder*. New York: Aldine de Gruyter.

Fineman, Norman. 1991. "The Social Construction of Noncompliance: A Study of Health Care and Social Service Providers in Everyday Practice." *Sociology of Health and Illness* 13 (3): 354–74.

Finerman, Ruthbeth, and Linda A. Bennett. 1995. "Guilt, Blame and Shame: Responsibility in Health and Sickness." *Social Science and Medicine* 40 (1): 1–3.

Finkler, Kaja. 1994. *Women in Pain: Gender and Morbidity in Mexico.* Philadelphia: University of Pennsylvania Press.

Fisher, Sue. 1986. *In the Patient's Best Interest: Women and the Politics of Medical Decisions.* New Brunswick, NJ: Rutgers University Press.

———. 1995. *Nursing Wounds: Nurse Practitioners, Doctors, Women Patients and the Negotiation of Meaning.* New Brunswick, NJ: Rutgers University Press.

Fisher, Sue, and Alexandra Dundas Todd, eds. 1986. *Discourse and Institutional Authority: Medicine, Education, and Law.* Norwood, NJ: Ablex.

Foucault, Michel. 1971. *The Order of Things: An Archaeology of the Human Sciences.* New York: Random House.

———. 1975. *The Birth of the Clinic: An Archaeology of Medical Perception.* New York: Vintage.

———. 1978. *The History of Sexuality.* Vol. 1, *An Introduction.* New York: Random House.

———. 1979. *Discipline and Punish: The Birth of the Prison.* New York: Random House.

Fox, Nicholas J. 1994. *Postmodernism, Sociology and Health.* Toronto: University of Toronto Press.

Fox, Renee C. 1980. "The Evolution of Medical Uncertainty." *Milbank Memorial Fund Quarterly* 58 (1): 1–49.

Frank, Arthur W. 1991. *At the Will of the Body: Reflections on Illness.* Boston: Houghton Mifflin.

———. 1995. *The Wounded Storyteller: Body, Illness, and Ethics.* Chicago: University of Chicago Press.

———. 1997a. "Enacting Illness Stories: When, What, and Why." In *Stories and Their Limits: Narrative Approaches to Bioethics,* ed. Hilde Lindemann Nelson, pp. 31–49. New York: Routledge.

———. 1997b. "Illness as Moral Occasion: Restoring Agency to Ill People." *Health* 1 (2): 131–48.

Franklin, Sarah. 1995. "Science as Culture, Cultures of Science." *Annual Review of Anthropology* 24: 163–84.

Franklin, Sarah, and Helena Ragone, eds. 1997. *Reproducing Reproduction.* Philadelphia: University of Pennsylvania Press.

Freidson, Eliot. 1970. *Profession of Medicine: A Study in the Sociology of Applied Knowledge.* New York: Harper & Row.

Freund, Peter E. S. 1982. *The Civilized Body: Social Domination, Control, and Health.* Philadelphia: Temple University Press.

Fujimura, Joan H. 1987. "Constructing 'Do-able' Problems in Cancer Research: Articulating Alignment." *Social Studies of Science* 17 (2): 257–93.

———. 1996. *Crafting Science: A Sociohistory of the Quest for the Genetics of Cancer.* Cambridge: Harvard University Press.

Garro, Linda C. 1992. "Chronic Illness and the Construction of Narratives." In *Pain as Human Experience: An Anthropological Perspective,* ed. Mary-Jo Good et al., pp. 100–37. Berkeley: University of California Press.

———. 1994. "Narrative Representations of Chronic Illness Experience: Cultural Models of Illness, Mind, and Body in Stories Concerning the Temporo-mandibular Joint (TMJ)." *Social Science and Medicine* 38 (6): 775–88.

German, Danielle, Kendra Hatfield-Timajchy, and Megan Reynolds. 1997. "'Get Well or Die': The Dilemma of Chronic Systemic Lupus Erythematosis." Department of Anthropology, Emory University.

Gilligan, Carol. 1982. *In a Different Voice: Psychological Theory and Women's Development*. Cambridge: Harvard University Press.

Gilligan, Carol, Nona P. Lyons, and Trudy J. Hanmer, ed. 1990. *Making Connections: The Relational Worlds of Adolescent Girls at Emma Willard School*. Cambridge: Harvard University Press.

Gilman, Charlotte Perkins. 1935. *The Living of Charlotte Perkins Gilman: An Autobiography*. New York: D. Appleton-Century.

Ginsburg, Faye, and Rayna Rapp, eds. 1995. *Conceiving the New World Order: The Global Politics of Reproduction*. Berkeley: University of California Press.

Goffman, Erving. 1963. *Stigma: Notes of the Management of Spoiled Identity*. Englewood Cliffs, NJ: Prentice-Hall.

Gogel, Edward L., and James S. Terry. 1987. "Medicine as Interpretation: The Uses of Literary Metaphors and Methods." *Journal of Medicine and Philosophy* 12 (3): 205–17.

Golub, Edward S. 1997. *The Limits of Medicine: How Science Shapes Our Hope for the Cure*. New York: Times Books, 1994. Reprint, Chicago: University of Chicago Press.

Good, Byron J. 1994. *Medicine, Rationality, and Experience: An Anthropological Perspective*. Cambridge: Cambridge University Press.

Good, Byron J., and Mary-Jo DelVecchio Good. 1993. "'Learning Medicine': The Constructing of Medical Knowledge at Harvard Medical School." In *Knowledge, Power and Practice: The Anthropology of Medicine and Everyday Life*, ed. Shirley Lindenbaum and Margaret Lock, pp. 81–107. Berkeley: University of California Press.

Good, Mary-Jo DelVecchio, Paul E. Brodwin, Byron J. Good, and Arthur Kleinman, eds. 1992. *Pain as Human Experience: An Anthropological Perspective*. Berkeley: University of California Press.

Gordon, Colin, ed. 1980. *Power/Knowledge: Selected Interviews and Other Writings by Michel Foucault, 1972–1977*. New York: Pantheon.

Gordon, Deborah R. 1988a. "Clinical Science and Clinical Expertise: Changing Boundaries Between Art and Science in Medicine." In *Biomedicine Examined*, ed. Margaret Lock and Deborah Gordon, pp. 257–95. Dordrecht: Kluwer Academic Publishers.

———. 1988b. "Tenacious Assumptions in Western Medicine." In *Biomedicine Examined*, ed. Margaret Lock and Deborah Gordon, pp. 19–56. Dordrecht: Kluwer Academic Publishers.

Gorovitz, Samuel, and Alasdair MacIntyre. 1976. "Toward a Theory of Medical Fallibility." *Journal of Medicine and Philosophy* 1 (1): 51–71.

Greeno, Catherine G., and Eleanor E. Maccoby. 1986. "How Different Is the 'Different Voice'?" *Signs* 11 (2): 310–16.

Gremmen, Ine. 1994. "Struggling at the Crossroads." *Feminism and Psychology* 4 (3): 362–66.

Haraway, Donna. 1986. "Primatology Is Politics by Other Means." In *Feminist Approaches to Science,* ed. Ruth Bleier, pp. 77–118. New York: Pergamon.

———. 1989. *Primate Visions: Gender, Race, and Nature in the World of Modern Science.* New York: Routledge.

———. 1991. "Situated Knowledges: The Science Question in Feminism and the Privilege of Partial Perspective." In *Simians, Cyborgs, and Women: The Reinvention of Nature.* New York: Routledge. First published in 1988, *Feminist Studies* 14 (3): 575–99.

Harding, Sandra. 1986. *The Science Question in Feminism.* Ithaca: Cornell University Press.

———. 1991. *Whose Science? Whose Knowledge? Thinking from Women's Lives.* Ithaca: Cornell University Press.

Hawkins, Anne Hunsaker. 1993. *Reconstructing Illness: Studies in Pathography.* West Lafayette, IN: Purdue University Press.

Hekman, Susan J. 1995. *Moral Voices, Moral Selves: Carol Gilligan and Feminist Moral Theory.* University Park: Pennsylvania State University Press.

Herzfeld, Michael. 1997. *Portrait of a Greek Imagination: An Ethnographic Biography of Andreas Nenedakis.* Chicago: University of Chicago Press.

Heurtin-Roberts, M., and Gay Becker. 1993. "Anthropological Perspectives on Chronic Illness." *Social Science and Medicine* 37 (3): 281–83.

Hyden, Lars-Christer. 1997. "Illness and Narrative." *Sociology of Health and Illness* 19 (1): 48–69.

Hyden, Lars-Christer, and Lisbeth Sachs. 1998. "Suffering, Hope and Diagnosis: On the Negotiation of Chronic Fatigue Syndrome." *Health* 2 (2): 175–93.

Illich, Ivan. 1976. *Medical Nemesis: The Expropriation of Health.* New York: Pantheon.

Jack, Dana. 1993. *Silencing the Self: Women and Depression.* Cambridge: Harvard University Press, 1991. Reprint, New York: HarperPerennial.

Jackson, Jean E. 1992. "'After a While No One Believes You': Real and Unreal Pain." In *Pain as Human Experience: An Anthropological Perspective,* ed. Mary-Jo Good et al., pp. 138–168. Berkeley: University of California Press.

———. 2000 *"Camp Pain": Talking with Chronic Pain Patients.* Philadelphia: University of Pennsylvania Press.

Jaggar, Alison M. 1989. "Love and Knowledge: Emotion in Feminist Epistemology." in *Gender/Body/Knowledge: Feminist Reconstructions of Being and Knowing,* ed. Alison M. Jaggar and Susan R. Bordo, pp. 145–71. New Brunswick, NJ: Rutgers University Press.

James, Veronica, and Jonathan Gabe, eds. 1996. *Health and the Sociology of Emotions.* Oxford: Blackwell.

Jamison, Kay Redfield. 1996. *An Unquiet Mind.* New York: Knopf.

Jones, Anne Hudson. 1994. "Reading Patients—Cautions and Concerns." *Literature and Medicine* 13 (2): 190–200.

Jones, Colin, and Roy Porter, eds. 1994. *Reassessing Foucault: Power, Medicine and the Body.* London: Routledge.

Kaysen, Susanna. 1993. *Girl, Interrupted.* New York: Random House.

Keller, Evelyn Fox. 1985. *Reflections on Gender and Science.* New Haven: Yale University Press.

————. 1992. *Secrets of Life, Secrets of Death: Essays on Language, Gender and Science.* New Haven: Yale University Press.

Kerber, Linda K., Catherine G. Greeno, Eleanor E. Maccoby, Zella Luria, Carol B. Stack, and Carol Gilligan. 1986. "On *In a Different Voice:* An Interdisciplinary Forum." *Signs* 11 (2): 304–33.

Kirmayer, Laurence J. 1988. "Mind and Body as Metaphors: Hidden Values in Biomedicine." In *Biomedicine Examined,* ed. Margaret Lock and Deborah Gordon, pp. 57–93. Dordrecht: Kluwer Academic Publishers.

Kitzinger, Celia. 1994. "The Spoken Word: Listening to a Different Voice. Celia Kitzinger Interviews Carol Gilligan." *Feminism and Psychology* 4 (3): 408–19.

Kleinman, Arthur. 1988. *The Illness Narratives: Suffering, Healing, and the Human Condition.* New York: Basic.

————. 1992. "Pain and Resistance: The Delegitimation and Relegitimation of Local Worlds." In *Pain as Human Experience: An Anthropological Perspective,* ed. Mary-Jo Good et al., pp. 169–97. Berkeley: University of California Press.

————. 1995. *Writing at the Margin: Discourse Between Anthropology and Medicine.* Berkeley: University of California Press.

Kleinman, Arthur, and Joan Kleinman. 1991. "Suffering and Its Professional Transformation: Toward an Ethnography of Interpersonal Experience." *Culture, Medicine and Psychiatry* 15 (3): 275–301.

Kleinman, Arthur, Paul E. Brodwin, Byron J. Good, and Mary-Jo DelVecchio Good. 1992. "Pain as Human Experience: An Introduction," In *Pain as Human Experience: An Anthropological Perspective,* ed. Mary-Jo Good et al., pp. 1–28. Berkeley: University of California Press.

Kleinman, Arthur, Veena Das, and Margaret Lock, eds. 1997. *Social Suffering.* Berkeley: University of California Press.

Knight, Denise D., ed. 1994. *"The Yellow Wall-Paper" and Selected Stories of Charlotte Perkins Gilman.* Newark: University of Delaware Press.

Knorr-Cetina, Karin D. 1981. *The Manufacture of Knowledge.* Oxford: Pergamon.

————. 1983. "The Ethnographic Study of Scientific Work: Towards a Constructivist Interpretation of Science." In *Science Observed,* ed. Karin D. Knorr-Cetina and Michael Mulkay. London: Sage.

Kutner, Nancy G. 1987. "Social Worlds and Identity in End-Stage Renal Disease (ESRD)." In *The Experience and Management of Chronic Illness.* Research in the Sociology of Health Care, vol. 6, ed. Julius A. Roth and Peter Conrad, pp. 33–72. Greenwich, CT: JAI Press.

Lane, Ann J., ed. 1980. *The Charlotte Perkins Gilman Reader.* New York: Pantheon.

Latour, Bruno. 1987. *Science in Action: How to Follow Scientists and Engineers Through Society.* Cambridge: Harvard University Press.

Latour, Bruno, and Steve Woolgar. 1979. *Laboratory Life: The Social Construction of Scientific Facts.* Beverly Hills: Sage.

Laurence, Leslie, and Beth Weinhouse. 1994. *Outrageous Practices: The Alarming Truth About How Medicine Mistreats Women.* New York: Fawcett Columbine.

Lavie, Smadar, Kirin Narayan, and Renato Rosaldo, eds. 1993. *Creativity/Anthropology.* Ithaca: Cornell University Press.

Layne, Linda L. 1996. " 'How's the Baby Doing?' Struggling with Narratives of Progress in a Neonatal Intensive Care Unit." *Medical Anthropology Quarterly* 10 (4): 624–56.

Leder, Drew. 1990. "Clinical Interpretation: The Hermeneutics of Medicine." *Theoretical Medicine* 11 (1): 9–24.

Leichter, Howard M. 1997. "Lifestyle Correctness and the New Secular Morality." In *Morality and Health,* ed. Allan M. Brandt and Paul Rozin, pp. 359–78. New York: Routledge.

Light, Donald, Jr. 1979. "Uncertainty and Control in Professional Training." *Journal of Health and Social Behavior* 20 (3): 310–22.

Lindenbaum, Shirley, and Margaret Lock, eds. 1993. *Knowledge, Power and Practice: The Anthropology of Medicine and Everyday Life.* Berkeley: University of California Press.

Lock, Margaret. 1998. "Situating Women in the Politics of Health." In *The Politics of Women's Health: Exploring Agency and Autonomy,* ed. Susan Sherwin, pp. 48-63. Philadelphia: Temple University Press.

Lock, Margaret, and Deborah Gordon, eds. 1998. *Biomedicine Examined.* Dordrecht: Kluwer Academic Publishers.

Lock, Margaret, and Patricia A. Kaufert, eds. 1998. *Pragmatic Women and Body Politics.* Cambridge: Cambridge University Press.

Locke, David. 1992. *Science as Writing.* New Haven: Yale University Press.

Lorber, Judith. 1997. *Gender and the Social Construction of Illness.* Thousand Oaks, CA: Sage.

Lorde, Audre. 1980. *The Cancer Journals.* Argyle, NY: Spinsters, Ink.

Lupton, Deborah. 1994. *Medicine as Culture: Illness, Disease and the Body in Western Societies.* London: Sage.

———. 1995. *The Imperative of Health: Public Health and the Regulated Body.* London: Sage.

———. 1996. "Your Life in Their Hands: Trust in the Medical Encounter." In *Health and the Sociology of Emotions,* ed. Veronica James and Jonathan Gabe, pp. 157–72.Oxford: Blackwell.

Luria, Zella. 1986. "A Methodological Critique." *Signs* 11 (2): 316–21.

Lykes, M. Brinton. 1994. "Whose Meeting at Which Crossroads? A Response to Brown and Gilligan." *Feminism and Psychology* 4 (3): 345–49.

Mahoney, Maureen A. 1996. "The Problem of Silence in Feminist Psychology." *Feminist Studies* 22 (3): 603–25.

Martin, Emily. 1987. *The Woman in the Body.* Boston: Beacon.

———. 1991. "The Egg and the Sperm: How Science Has Constructed a Romance Based on Stereotypical Male-Female Roles." *Signs* 16 (3): 485–502.

Mattingly, Cheryl. 1998. *Healing Dramas and Clinical Plots: The Narrative Structure of Experience.* Cambridge: Cambridge University Press.

McCullough, Laurence B. 1989. "The Abstract Character and Transforming Power of Medical Language." *Soundings* 72 (1): 111–25.

Milligan, Maureen A., and Ellen Singer More. 1994. "Introduction." In *The Empathic Practitioner: Empathy, Gender, and Medicine,* ed. E. S. More and M. A. Milligan, pp. 1–15. New Brunswick, NJ: Rutgers University Press.

Mishler, Elliott G. 1981a. "The Social Construction of Illness." In *Social Con-*

texts of Health, Illness, and Patient Care, ed. Mishler et al., pp. 141–68. Cambridge: Cambridge University Press.

———. 1981b. "Viewpoint: Critical Perspectives on the Biomedical Model." In *Social Contexts of Health, Illness, and Patient Care,* ed. Mishler et al., pp. 1–23. Cambridge: Cambridge University Press.

———. 1984. *The Discourse of Medicine: Dialectics of Medical Interviews.* Norwood, NJ: Ablex.

Mishler, Elliott G., Lorna R. AmaraSingham, Stuart T. Hauser, Samuel D. Osherson, Nancy E. Waxler, and Ramsay Liem. 1981. *Social Contexts of Health, Illness, and Patient Care.* Cambridge: Cambridge University Press.

Mitchinson, Wendy. 1988. "Agency, Diversity, and Constraints: Women and Their Physicians, Canada, 1850–1950." In *The Politics of Women's Health: Exploring Agency and Autonomy,* ed. Susan Sherwin, pp. 122–49. Philadelphia: Temple University Press.

Mizrahi, Terry. 1984. "Managing Medical Mistakes: Ideology, Insularity and Accountability among Internists-in-Training." *Social Science and Medicine* 19 (2): 135–46.

Monroe, William Frank, Warren Lee Holleman, and Marsha Cline Holleman. 1992. "'Is There a Person in This Case?'" *Literature and Medicine* 11 (1): 45–63.

Morris, David B. 1991. *The Culture of Pain.* Berkeley: University of California Press.

Motzafi-Haller, Pnina. 1997. "Writing Birthright: On Native Anthropologists and the Politics of Representation." In *Auto/Ethnography: Rewriting the Self and the Social,* ed. Deborah E. Reed-Danahay, pp. 195–222. Oxford: Berg.

Munt, Sally R. 1994. *Murder by the Book? Feminism and the Crime Novel.* London: Routledge.

Murphy, Robert. 1990. *The Body Silent.* New York: Henry Holt, 1987. Reprint, New York: W. W. Norton.

Nichter, Mark. 1998. "The Mission within the Madness: Self-Initiated Medicalization as Expression of Agency." In *Pragmatic Women and Body Politics,* ed. Margaret Lock and Patricia A. Kaufert, pp. 327–53. Cambridge: Cambridge University Press.

Norsigian, Judy. 1996. "The Women's Health Movement in the United States." In *Man-made Medicine: Women's Health, Public Policy, and Reform,* ed. Kary L. Moss, pp. 79–88. Durham, NC: Duke University Press.

Oakley, Ann. 1993. "Review Article: Telling Stories: Auto/Biography and the Sociology of Health and Illness." *Sociology of Health and Illness* 15 (3): 414–18.

Ochs, Elinor, and Lisa Capps. 1996. "Narrating a Self." *Annual Review of Anthropology* 25: 19–43.

Olesen, Virginia L. 1990. "The Neglected Emotions: A Challenge to Medical Sociology." *Medical Sociology News* 15: 10–15.

Ong, L. M. L., J. C. J. M. de Haes, A. M. Hoos, and F. B. Lammes. 1995. "Doctor-Patient Communication: A Review of the Literature." *Social Science and Medicine* 40 (7): 903–18.

Osherson, Samuel, and Lorna AmaraSingham. 1981. "The Machine Metaphor

in Medicine." In *Social Contexts of Health, Illness, and Patient Care,* ed. Elliott G. Mishler et al., pp. 218–49. Cambridge: Cambridge University Press.

Oudshoorn, Nelly. 1994. *Beyond the Natural Body: An Archaeology of Sex Hor-
mones.* London: Routledge.

Paget, Marianne A. 1988. *The Unity of Mistakes: A Phenomenological Interpretation of Medical Work.* Philadelphia: Temple University Press.

———. 1993. *A Complex Sorrow: Reflections on Cancer and an Abbreviated
Life,* ed. Marjorie L. DeVault. Philadelphia: Temple University Press.

Petersen, Alan, and Robin Bunton, eds. 1997. *Foucault, Health and Medicine.*
London: Routledge.

Petersen, Alan, and Deborah Lupton. 1996. *The New Public Health: Health and
Self in the Age of Risk.* London: Sage.

Pipher, Mary. 1994. *Reviving Ophelia: Saving the Selves of Adolescent Girls.* New
York: Ballantine.

Rapp, Rayna. 1990. "Constructing Amniocentesis: Maternal and Medical Discourses." In *Uncertain Terms: Negotiating Gender in American Culture,* ed.
Faye Ginsburg and Anna Lowenhaupt Tsing, pp. 28–42. Boston: Beacon.

———. 1999. *Testing Women, Testing the Fetus: The Social Impact of Amniocentesis in America.* New York: Routledge.

Reed-Danahay, Deborah E., ed. 1997a. *Auto/Ethnography: Rewriting the Self
and the Social.* Oxford: Berg.

———. 1997b. "Introduction," in *Auto/Ethnography: Rewriting the Self and the
Social,* ed. Reed-Danahay, pp. 1–17. Oxford: Berg.

Reid, Janice, Christine Ewan, and Eva Lowy. 1991. "Pilgrimage of Pain: The Illness Experience of Women with Repetition Strain Injury and the Search for
Credibility." *Social Science and Medicine* 32 (5): 601–12.

Riessman, Catherine Kohler. 1983. "Women and Medicalization: A New Perspective." *Social Policy* 14 (1): 3–18.

Robinson, Tracy, and Janie W. Ward. 1991. "A Belief in Self Far Greater Than
Anyone's Disbelief: Cultivating Resistance Among African-American Female
Adolescents." In *Women, Girls and Psychotherapy: Reframing Resistance,* ed.
Carol Gilligan, Annie Rogers, and Deborah Tolman, pp. 87–110. New York:
Harrington.

Rosaldo, Renato. 1989. *Culture and Truth.* Boston: Beacon.

Rosser, Sue V. 1994. *Women's Health—Missing from U.S. Medicine.* Bloomington: Indiana University Press.

Roth, Julius A., and Peter Conrad, eds. 1987. *The Experience and Management
of Chronic Illness.* Research in the Sociology of Health Care, vol. 6. Greenwich, CT: JAI Press.

Ruzek, Sheryl Burt. 1978. *The Women's Health Movement: Feminist Alternatives to Medical Control.* New York: Praeger.

Ruzek, Sheryl Burt, Virginia L. Olesen, and Adele E. Clarke, eds. 1997. *Women's
Health: Complexities and Differences.* Columbus: Ohio State University Press.

Sacks, Oliver. 1986. "Clinical Tales." *Literature and Medicine* 5: 16–23.

Saris, A. Jamie. 1995. "Telling Stories: Life Histories, Illness Narratives, and Institutional Landscapes." *Culture, Psychiatry and Medicine* 19 (1): 39–72.

Scott, Charles E. 1987. "The Power of Medicine, The Power of Ethics." *Journal of Medicine and Philosophy* 12 (4): 335–50.

Scully, Diana. 1994. *Men Who Control Women's Health: The Miseducation of Obstetrician-Gynecologists.* New York: Houghton Mifflin, 1980. Reprint, New York: Teachers College Press.

Sharf, Barbara F. 1990. "Physician-Patient Communication as Interpersonal Rhetoric: A Narrative Approach." *Health Communication* 2 (4): 217–31.

Sherwin, Susan. 1992. *No Longer Patient: Feminist Ethics and Health Care.* Philadelphia: Temple University Press.

———. ed. 1998. *The Politics of Women's Health: Exploring Agency and Autonomy.* Philadelphia: Temple University Press.

Showalter, Elaine. 1997. *Hystories: Hysterical Epidemics and Modern Culture.* New York: Columbia University Press.

Silverman, David. 1987. *Communication and Medical Practice: Social Relations in the Clinic.* London: Sage.

Sontag, Susan. 1990. *Illness as Metaphor and AIDS and Its Metaphors.* New York, Farrar, Straus and Giroux, 1978. Reprint, New York: Doubleday.

Stack, Carol B. 1986. "The Culture of Gender: Women and Men of Color." *Signs* 11 (2): 321–24.

Starr, Paul. 1982. *The Social Transformation of American Medicine.* New York: Basic.

Stein, Howard F. 1985. *The Psychodynamics of Medical Practice: Unconscious Factors in Patient Care.* Berkeley: University of California Press.

———. 1990. *American Medicine as Culture.* Boulder: Westview.

Stevens, Patricia E. 1996. "Lesbians and Doctors: Experiences of Solidarity and Domination in Health Care Settings." *Gender and Society* 10 (1): 24–41.

Strathern, Marilyn. 1987. "The Limits of Auto-Anthropology." In *Anthropology at Home,* ed. Anthony Jackson, pp. 16–37. London: Tavistock.

Strauss, Anselm L., and Juliet M. Corbin. 1988. *Shaping a New Health Care System: The Explosion of Chronic Illness as a Catalyst for Change.* San Francisco: Jossey-Bass.

Strauss, Anselm L., and B. Glaser. 1975. *Chronic Illness and the Quality of Life.* St. Louis: Mosby.

Taussig, Michael T. 1980. "Reification and the Consciousness of the Patient." *Social Science and Medicine* 14B: 3–13.

Tavris, Carol. 1993. "The Mismeasure of Woman." *Feminism and Psychology* 3 (2): 149–68.

———. 1994. "Reply to Brown and Gilligan." *Feminism and Psychology* 4 (3): 350–52.

Taylor, Jill McLean, Carol Gilligan, and Amy M. Sullivan. 1995. *Between Voice and Silence: Women and Girls, Race and Relationship.* Cambridge: Harvard University Press.

Theriot, Nancy M. 1996. "Women's Voices in Nineteenth-Century Medical Discourse: A Step toward Deconstructing Science." In *Gender and Scientific Authority,* ed. Barbara Laslett, Sally Gregory Kohlstedt, Helen Longino, and Evelynn Hammonds, pp. 124–154. Chicago: University of Chicago Press.

Thompson, Tracy. 1995. *The Beast: A Reckoning with Depression*. New York: G. P. Putnam's Sons.

Todd, Alexandra Dundas. 1989. *Intimate Adversaries: Cultural Conflict Between Doctors and Women Patients*. Philadelphia: University of Pennsylvania Press.

Toombs, S. Kay. 1992. *The Meaning of Illness: A Phenomenological Account of the Different Perspectives of Physician and Patient*. Dordrecht: Kluwer Academic Publishers.

Traweek, Sharon. 1988. *Beamtimes and Lifetimes: The World of High Energy Physicists*. Cambridge: Harvard University Press.

Tronto, Joan C. 1987. "Beyond Gender Difference to a Theory of Care." *Signs* 12 (4): 644–63.

Turner, Bryan S. 1992. *Regulating Bodies: Essays in Medical Sociology*. London: Routledge.

———. 1995. *Medical Power and Social Knowledge*. Rev. ed. London: Sage.

van Maanen, John. 1995. "An End to Innocence: The Ethnography of Ethnography." In *Representation in Ethnography*, ed. J. Van Maanen, pp. 1–35. Thousand Oaks, CA: Sage.

Vertinsky, Patricia. 1990. *The Eternally Wounded Woman: Women, Doctors, and Exercise in the Late Nineteenth Century*. Manchester: Manchester University Press.

Waitzkin, Howard. 1991. *The Politics of Medical Encounters: How Patients and Doctors Deal with Social Problems*. New Haven: Yale University Press.

Ware, Norma C. 1992. "Suffering and the Social Construction of Illness: The Delegitimation of Illness Experience in Chronic Fatigue Syndrome." *Medical Anthropology Quarterly* 6 (4): 347–61.

Warren, Kay B. 1997. "Narrating Cultural Resurgence: Genre and Self-Representation for Pan-Mayan Writers." In *Auto/Ethnography: Rewriting the Self and the Social*, ed. Deborah E. Reed-Danahay, pp. 21–46. Oxford: Berg.

Way, N. 1995. "'Can't You See the Courage, the Strength That I Have?' Listening to Urban Adolescent Girls Speak About their Relationships." *Psychology of Women Quarterly* 19 (1): 107–28.

Wear, Delese, and Lois LaCivita Nixon. 1994. *Literary Anatomies: Women's Bodies and Health in Literature*. Albany: State University of New York Press.

Weedon, Chris. 1997. *Feminist Practice and Poststructuralist Theory*. 2d ed. Oxford: Blackwell.

Weisman, Carol S. 1998. *Women's Health Care: Activist Traditions and Institutional Change*. Baltimore: Johns Hopkins University Press.

Wendell, Susan. 1996. *The Rejected Body: Feminist Philosophical Reflections on Disability*. New York: Routledge.

West, Candace. 1984. *Routine Complications: Troubles with Talk Between Doctors and Patients*. Bloomington: Indiana University Press.

———. 1993. "Reconceptualizing Gender in Physician-Patient Relationships." *Social Science and Medicine* 36 (1): 57–66.

West, Candace, and Sarah Fenstermaker. 1995. "Doing Difference." *Gender and Society* 9 (1): 8–37.

West, Candace, and Don H. Zimmerman. 1987. "Doing Gender." *Gender and Society* 1 (2): 125–51.

Wexler, Alice. 1995. *Mapping Fate: A Memoir of Family, Risk, and Genetic Research.* New York: Random House.

Wilkinson, Sue, ed. 1994. "Critical Connections: The Harvard Project on Women's Psychology and Girls' Development." *Feminism and Psychology* 4 (3): 343–424.

Williams, G. 1984. "The Genesis of Chronic Illness: Narrative Reconstruction." *Sociology of Health and Illness* 6: 175–200.

Witkin, Georgia. 1991. *The Female Stress Syndrome: How to Become Stresswise in the '90s.* New York: Newmarket.

Young, Allan. 1995. *The Harmony of Illusions: Inventing Post-Traumatic Stress Disorder.* Princeton: Princeton University Press.

Young, Katherine. 1997. *Presence in the Flesh: The Body in Medicine.* Cambridge: Harvard University Press.

Zimmerman, Mary K. 1987. "The Women's Health Movement: A Critique of Medical Enterprise and the Position of Women." In *Analyzing Gender: A Handbook of Social Science Research,* ed. Beth B. Hess and Myra Marx Ferree, pp. 442–72. Newbury Park, CA: Sage.

Zola, Irving K. 1972. "Medicine as an Institution of Social Control." *Sociological Review* 20: 487–504.

———. 1975. "In the Name of Health and Illness: On the Socio-Political Consequences of Medical Influence." *Social Science and Medicine* 8 (1): 83–87.

III. Biomedical Literature, Works on Alternative and New Age Medicine, and News Reports on Developments in Medical Practice

Aaron, Leslie A., et al. 1996. "Psychiatric Diagnoses in Patients with Fibromyalgia Are Related to Health Care–Seeking Behavior Rather Than to Illness." *Arthritis and Rheumatism* 39 (3): 436–45.

Alexander, Ronald W., et al. 1998. "Sexual and Physical Abuse in Women with Fibromyalgia: Association with Outpatient Health Care Utilization and Pain Medication Usage." *Arthritis Care and Research* 11 (2): 102–15.

Altman, Lawrence K. 1999. "Policing Health Care." *New York Times,* 1 December.

Aylward, James M. 1993. "Hydroxychloroquine and Chloroquine: Assessing the Risk of Retinal Toxicity." *Journal of the American Optometric Association* 64 (11): 787–97.

Barsky, Arthur J., and Jonathan F. Borus. 1999. "Functional Somatic Syndromes." *Annals of Internal Medicine* 130 (11): 910–21.

Bennett, Robert M. 1987. "Editorial. Fibromyalgia." *Journal of the American Medical Association* 257 (20): 2802–3.

———. 1999. "Emerging Concepts in the Neurobiology of Chronic Pain: Evidence of Abnormal Sensory Processing in Fibromyalgia." *Mayo Clinic Proceedings* 74 (4): 385–98.

Berkow, Robert, editor-in-chief. 1997. *The Merck Manual of Medical Information,* Home Edition. Whitehouse Station, NJ: Merck Research Laboratories.

Boffa, M. J., R. J. Chalmers, N. Y. Haboubi, M. Shomaf, and D. M. Mitchell. 1995. "Sequential Liver Biopsies During Long-term Methotrexate Treatment for Psoriasis: A Reappraisal." *British Journal of Dermatology* 133 (5): 774–78.

Bohr, Thomas W. 1995. "Fibromyalgia Syndrome and Myofascial Pain Syndrome: Do They Exist?" *Neurologic Clinics* 13 (2): 365–84.

Boisset-Pioro, Mathilde H., John M. Esdaile, and Mary-Ann Fitzcharles. 1995. "Sexual and Physical Abuse in Women with Fibromyalgia Syndrome." *Arthritis and Rheumatism* 38 (2): 235–41.

Burton Goldberg Group, comp. 1994. *Alternative Medicine: The Definitive Guide.* Fife, WA: Future Medicine Publishing.

Buskila, Dan, Lily Neumann, Genady Vaisberg, Daphna Alkalay, and Frederick Wolfe. 1997. "Increased Rates of Fibromyalgia Following Cervical Spine Injury." *Arthritis and Rheumatism* 40 (3): 446–52.

Carroll, Douglas, and Catherine A. Niven. 1993. "Gender, Health, and Stress." In *The Health Psychology of Women*, ed. Catherine A. Niven and Douglas Carroll, pp. 1–12. Langhorne, PA: Harwood Academic.

Cassell, Eric J. 1982. "The Nature of Suffering and the Goals of Medicine." *New England Journal of Medicine* 306 (11): 639–45.

———. 1985. *The Healer's Art.* Cambridge, MA: MIT Press.

———. 1991. *The Nature of Suffering and the Goals of Medicine.* New York: Oxford University Press.

Cohen, Milton L., and John L. Quintner. 1993. "Fibromyalgia Syndrome, a Problem of Tautology." *Lancet* 342 (8876): 906–9.

Donnelly, William J. 1986. "Medical Language as Symptom: Doctor Talk in Teaching Hospitals." *Perspectives in Biology and Medicine* 30 (1): 81–94.

———. 1989. "Righting the Medical Record: Transforming Chronicle into Story." *Soundings* 72 (1): 127–35.

Eichenwald, Kurt, and Gina Kolata. 1999. "When Physicians Double as Businessmen." *New York Times,* November 30.

Eisenberg, Carola. 1997. "Medicine Is No Longer a Man's Profession, or, When the Men's Club Goes Coed It's Time to Change the Regs." In *The Social Medicine Reader*, ed. Gail E. Henderson, Nancy M. P. King, Ronald P. Strauss, Sue E. Estroff, and Larry R. Churchill, pp. 266–70. Durham, NC: Duke University Press. First published in *New England Journal of Medicine* 321 (22): 1542–44.

Engel, George L. 1977a. "The Need for a New Medical Model." *Science* 196 (428b): 129–36.

———. 1977b. "The Care of the Patient: Art or Science?" *Johns Hopkins Medical Journal* 140: 222–32.

———. 1987. "Physician-Scientists and Scientific Physicians: Resolving the Humanism-Science Dichotomy." *American Journal of Medicine* 82 (1): 107–11.

———. 1997. "From Biomedical to Biopsychosocial." *Psychotherapy and Psychosomatics* 66: 57–62.

Fries, James F. 1995. *Arthritis: A Take Care of Yourself Health Guide for Understanding Your Arthritis*, 4th ed. Reading, MA: Addison-Wesley.

Gawain, Shakti. 1995. *Creative Visualization: Use the Power of Your Imagination to Create What You Want in Life*, rev. ed. San Rafael, CA: New World Library.

Goldberg, R. T., W. N. Pachas, and D. Keith. 1999. "Relationship Between Traumatic Events in Childhood and Chronic Pain." *Disability and Rehabilitation* 21 (1): 23–30.

Grady, Denise. 1997. "Doctors Urged to Admit Mistakes." *New York Times,* 9 December.

Hadler, Nortin M. 1997. "Fibromyalgia: La Maladie est Morte. Vive le Malade!" *Journal of Rheumatology* 24 (7): 1250-51.

Hassan, W. 1996. "Methotrexate and Liver Toxicity: Role of Surveillance Liver Biopsy." *Annals of the Rheumatic Diseases* 55 (5): 273-75.

Henricksson, C. M. 1994. "Longterm Effects of Fibromyalgia on Everyday Life." *Scandinavian Journal of Rheumatology* 23: 36-41.

Hilfiker, David. 1984. "Facing Our Mistakes." *New England Journal of Medicine* 310 (2): 118-22.

Hoffman, Catherine, Dorothy Rice, and Hai-Yen Sung. 1996. "Persons with Chronic Conditions: Their Prevalence and Costs." *Journal of the American Medical Association* 276 (18): 1473-79.

Hudson, James I., and Harrison G. Pope, Jr. 1995. "Does Childhood Sexual Abuse Cause Fibromyalgia?" *Arthritis and Rheumatism* 38 (2): 161-63.

Joynt, Robert J., ed. 1980. *The Challenge of the Biopsychosocial Model.* Supplement to *Psychosomatic Medicine* 42 (1: II).

Kabat-Zinn, Jon. 1990. *Full Catastrophe Living: Using the Wisdom of Your Body and Mind to Face Stress, Pain, and Illness.* New York: Delta.

Kavanaugh, Arthur F. 1996. "Fibromyalgia or Multi-Organ Dysesthesia?" Letter to the editor, *Arthritis and Rheumatism* 39 (1): 180-81.

Kennedy, Maura, and David T. Felson. 1996. "A Prospective Long-term Study of Fibromyalgia Syndrome." *Arthritis and Rheumatism* 39 (4): 682-85.

Kidd, Bruce L. 1996. "Methotrexate and Liver Toxicity: Role of Surveillance Liver Biopsy, Conflict Between Guidelines for Rheumatologists and Dermatologists." *Annals of the Rheumatic Diseases* 55 (5): 273-75.

Kilborn, Peter T. 1999. "Ambitious Effort to Cut Mistakes in U.S. Hospitals." *New York Times,* December 26.

Kohn, Linda T., Janet M. Corrigan, and Mocla S. Donaldson, eds. 1999. *To Err Is Human: Building a Safer Health System.* Advance copy. Committee on Quality of Health Care in America, Institute of Medicine, National Academy of Sciences. Washington, DC: National Academy Press.

Kübler-Ross, Elisabeth. 1969. *On Death and Dying.* New York: Collier Books, Macmillan.

Lazarou, Jason L., Bruce H. Pomeranz, and Paul N. Corey. 1998. "Incidence of Adverse Drug Reactions in Hospitalized Patients: A Meta-Analysis of Prospective Studies." *Journal of the American Medical Association* 279 (15): 1200-1205.

Leal-Cerro, A., J. Povedano, R. Astorga, M. Gonzalez, H. Silva, F. Garcia-Pesquera, F. F. Casanueva, and C. Dieguez. 1999. "The Growth Hormone (GH)-Releasing Hormone-GH-Insulin-like Growth Factor-1 Axis in Patients with Fibromyalgia Syndrome." *Journal of Clinical Endocrinology and Metabolism* 84 (9): 3378-81.

Ledingham, J., S. Doherty, and M. Doherty. 1993. "Primary Fibromyalgia Syndrome—An Outcome Study." *British Journal of Rheumatology* 32: 139-42.

Levanthal, Lawrence J. 1999. "Management of Fibromyalgia." *Annals of Internal Medicine* 131 (11): 850-58.

Lovallo, William R. 1997. *Stress and Health: Biological and Psychological Interactions*. Thousand Oaks, CA: Sage.

Mannerkopi, K., T. Kroksmark, and C. Ekdahl. 1999. "How Patients with Fibromyalgia Experience Their Symptoms in Everyday Life." *Physiotherapy Research International* 4 (2): 110–22.

Martin, Paul. 1997. *The Sickening Mind: Brain, Behaviour, Immunity and Disease*. London: HarperCollins.

Mazzuca, Steven A., Rudy Yung, Kenneth D. Brandt, Robert D. Yee, and Barry P. Katz. 1994. "Current Practices for Monitoring Ocular Toxicity Related to Hydroxychloroquine (Plaquenil) Therapy." *Journal of Rheumatology* 21 (1): 59–63.

Medi-Span, Inc. 1995. Patient medication information sheets.

Melzack, Ronald, and Patrick D. Wall. 1965. "Pain Mechanisms: A New Theory." *Science* 150 (3699): 971–79.

Neeck, Gunther, and Walter Riedel. 1999. "Hormonal Perturbations in Fibromyalgia Syndrome." *Annals of the New York Academy of Sciences* 876: 325–38.

Pear, Robert. 1999. "A Clinton Order Seeks to Reduce Medical Errors." *New York Times*, 7 December.

Pecukonis, Edward V. 1996. "Childhood Sex Abuse in Women with Chronic Intractable Back Pain." *Social Work in Health Care* 23 (3): 1–16.

Potter, Brian. 1993 "Hydroxychloroquine." *Cutis* 52 (4): 229–31.

Quinter, John L., and Milton L. Cohen. 1999. "Fibromyalgia Falls Foul of a Fallacy." *Lancet* 353 (9158): 1092–94.

Radomsky, Nellie A. 1995. *Lost Voices: Women, Chronic Pain, and Abuse*. New York: Harrington Park, Haworth.

Redleaf, Angelica, with Susan A. Baird. 1998. *Behind Closed Doors: Gender, Sexuality, and Touch in the Doctor/Patient Relationship*. Westport, CT: Auburn House.

Roenigk, Henry H., Jr., Robert Auerbach, Howard I. Maibach, and Gerald D. Weinstein. 1988. "Methotrexate in Psoriasis: Revised Guidelines." *Journal of the American Academy of Dermatology* 19, pt. 1: 145–56.

Rossy, Lynn A., Nancy Dorr, Kristofer J. Hagglund, Julian F. Thayer, Matthew J. McIntosh, John E. Hewett, and Jane C. Johnson. 1999. "A Meta-Analysis of Fibromyalgia Treatment Interventions." *Annals of Behavioral Medicine* 21 (2): 180–91.

Russell, Anthony S. 1995. "Fibromyalgia: A Historical Perspective." *Journal of Musculoskeletal Pain* 3 (2): 43–48.

Schaefer, Karen Moore. 1995. "Struggling to Maintain Balance: A Study of Women Living with Fibromyalgia." *Journal of Advanced Nursing* 21 (1): 95–102.

———. 1997. "Health Patterns of Women with Fibromyalgia." *Journal of Advanced Nursing* 26 (3): 565–71.

Schwarz, Marcus J., Michael Spath, Hanns Muller-Bardorff, Dieter E. Pongratz, Brigitta Bondy, and Manfred Ackenheil. 1999. "Relationship of Substance P, 5-hydroxyindole Acetic Acid and Tryptophan in Serum of Fibromyalgia Patients." *Neuroscience Letters* 259 (3): 196–98.

Shorter, Edward. 1994. *From the Mind Into the Body: The Cultural Origins of Psychosomatic Symptoms*. New York: Free Press.

———. 1995. "The Borderland Between Neurology and History: Conversion Reactions." *Neurologic Clinics* 13 (2): 229–39.

Smythe, Hugh A., and H. Modolfsky. 1977. "Two Contributions to Understanding of the 'Fibrositis' Syndrome." *Bulletin of Rheumatic Diseases* 28: 928–31.

Soderberg, S., B. Lundman, and A. Norberg. 1999. "Struggling for Dignity: The Meaning of Women's Experiences of Living with Fibromyalgia." *Qualitative Health Research* 9 (5): 575–87.

Starlanyl, Devin, and Mary Ellen Copeland. 1996. *Fibromyalgia Syndrome and Chronic Myofascial Pain Syndrome: A Survival Manual*. Oakland, CA: New Harbinger.

Stoeckle, John D., and Andrew Billings. 1987. "A History of History-taking: The Medical Interview." *Journal of General Internal Medicine* 2 (2): 119–27.

Taylor, Mary Lou, Dana R. Trotter, and M. E. Csuka. 1995. "The Prevalence of Sexual Abuse in Women with Fibromyalgia." *Arthritis and Rheumatism* 38 (2): 229–34.

Taylor, Robert B., ed. 1998. *Family Medicine: Principles and Practice*. 5th ed. New York: Springer-Verlag.

Tierney, Lawrence M., Stephen J. McPhee, and Maxine A. Papadakis, eds. 1996. *Current Medical Diagnosis and Treatment 1997*. Stamford, CT: Appleton and Lange.

Tobkes, A. I., and H. J. Nord. 1995. "Liver Biopsy: Review of Methodology and Complications." *Digestive Diseases* 13 (5): 267–74.

United States Department of Commerce. 1998. *Statistical Abstract of the United States, 1998*. 118th ed. Washington DC: DOC.

United States Pharmacopeial Convention, Inc. 1996. Patient medication information sheets.

Walker, Edward A., et al. 1995. "Psychiatric Diagnoses and Sexual Victimization in Women with Chronic Pelvic Pain." *Psychosomatics* 36 (6): 531–40.

Walker, Edward A., David Keegan, Gregory Gardner, Mark Sullivan, David Bernstein, and Wayne J. Katon. 1997. "Psychosocial Factors in Fibromyalgia Compared with Rheumatoid Arthritis: II. Sexual, Physical, and Emotional Abuse and Neglect." *Psychosomatic Medicine* 59 (6): 572–77.

Walling, Mary K., et al. 1994. "Abuse History and Chronic Pain in Women: I. Prevalences of Sexual Abuse and Physical Abuse." *Obstetrics and Gynecology* 84 (2): 193–99.

Weil, Andrew. 1995. *Spontaneous Healing: How to Discover and Enhance Your Body's Natural Ability to Maintain and Heal Itself*. New York: Knopf.

Weintraub, Michael I. 1995. "Chronic Pain in Litigation: What Is the Relationship?" *Neurologic Clinics* 13 (2): 341–49.

Wilson, Jean D., Eugene Braunwald, Kurt J. Isselbacher, Robert G. Petersdorf, Joseph B. Martin, Anthony S. Fauci, and Richard K. Root, eds. 1991. *Harrison's Principles of Internal Medicine*. 12th ed. Vol. 2. New York: McGraw-Hill.

Winfield, J. B. 1999. "Pain in Fibromyalgia." *Rheumatic Diseases Clinics of North America* 25 (1): 55–79.

Wolfe, Frederick. 1994. "When to Diagnose Fibromyalgia." *Rheumatic Diseases Clinics of North America* 20 (2): 485–501.

———. 1997a. "The Relation Between Tender Points and Fibromyalgia Symptom Variables: Evidence That Fibromyalgia is not a Discrete Disorder in the Clinic," *Annals of the Rheumatic Diseases* 56 (4): 268–71.

———. 1997b. "The Fibromyalgia Problem." *Journal of Rheumatology* (24) 7: 1247–49.

Wolfe, Frederick, et al. 1990. "The American College of Rheumatology 1990 Criteria for the Classification of Fibromyalgia." *Arthritis and Rheumatism* 33 (2): 160–72.

Wolfe, Frederick, Kathryn Ross, Janice Anderson, I. Jon Russell, and Liesi Hebert. 1995. "The Prevalence and Characteristics of Fibromyalgia in the General Population." *Arthritis and Rheumatism* 38 (1): 19–28.

Wu, Albert W., Thomas A. Cavanaugh, Stephen J. McPhee, Bernard Lo, and Guy P. Micco. 1997. "To Tell the Truth: Ethical and Practical Issues in Disclosing Medical Mistakes to Patients." *Journal of General Internal Medicine* 12 (12): 770–75.

Index

This index includes primarily items from the general discussions of medicine, gender, and illness cultures in the problematique and conclusion. From the ethnographic chapters, it includes only personal names and concepts and special terms not introduced elsewhere. It covers only general discussions of these terms, not how they play out in the medical narrative.

abuse, emotional and verbal: definition, 299; in doctor-patient relationship, 38, 299–301, 320, 333n64; gendered aspects of, 300, 320; medical effects of, 300–301; as source of chronic pain, 300. *See also* biomedical rhetorics, dangers of

abuse, physical and sexual: chronic pain syndromes, connection to, 321, 343n59; fibromyalgia, connection to, 187–88, 321, 343n59

abuse, self-, 203–4

acute illness, 20, 34, 294, 296, 298

adolescent development, girls', 42, 44–45

agency, women's. *See* women's agency, theory of

amelioration, discourse of, 28–29. *See also* discourses of medicine

American College of Rheumatology (ACR), criteria for classification of fibromyalgia, 276–77

anger: mind rehearsal of, 47, 339n2 (Ch. 5); muting of, 44–46, 308; politics of, 46–47, 335n90. *See also* femininity; feminism

arthritis: age and gender differences in, 317–18, 343n50; prevalence of, 325n2

auto-ethnography: and autobiography, difference from, 51; as cultural and political critique, 51–55; definition, 5, 51, 337n114; insights of, 312–13; intellectual and political significance of, 53–55, 312–13; limitations of, 54–55; in medical anthropology, 337n121; and solipsism, avoidance of, 52–53. *See also* emotion; ethnography; situated (positioned) truths; "vulnerable writing"

Balshem, Martha, 309–10

Baszanger, Isabelle, 25, 326n3, 333n68, 334n74, 337–38n1

Behar, Ruth, 55, 337n125

"benevolent paternalism," 332n54

biomedical model, 27, 297–98; dangers of, 30, 36, 294, 298–99. *See also* discourses of medicine; self, patient

biomedical rhetorics, dangers of: for patient, 34, 299–301; for physician, 34

biomedicine. *See* medicine, scientific

biopsychosocial model, 301–2, 341n6 (Conclusion)

blame, self-: escape routes from, 51; trap of, 50, 253. *See also* illness cultures; medicine, alternative

blame-the-victim models of illness, 50–51. *See also* chronic illness; illness cultures; medicine, alternative

bodily identity. *See* identity, bodily

"body-cure," 294. *See also* medicine, scientific

Breines, Wini, 339n6 (Ch. 4)

Brison, Susan, 332n56

Brown, Lyn Mikel, 41, 42, 44, 308, 334–35n77, 335nn83, 85, 90

Cassell, Eric J., 31, 35, 299, 305

Christie, Agatha, 313

chronic back pain: physical and sexual abuse, connection to, 321

chronic conditions, general: age distribution of, 325n1; definition, 325n1; prevalence in U.S. of, 3, 325n1; U.S. health care resources devoted to, 341n10. *See also* chronic illness

chronic disease. *See* chronic illness

chronic fatigue syndrome, 9, 49, 317

chronic headache conditions: gender distribution of, 317; physical and sexual abuse, connection to, 321

chronic illness: causes in lifeworld of, 298; dangers of biomedicine for, 20, 30, 33–34, 294, 296–301; definition and sources of, 325n1; and dependence on doctor, 17; emotional oscillations and vulnerability in, 33–34; fluctuation and vagueness in symptoms of, 30; fragile sense of self in, 35; gender

chronic illness *(continued)*
differences in, 317; healing of through whole-person change, 298; medical stories of, 30; pervasiveness of, 20; probability of poor diagnosis, prognosis, and treatment of, 30–31, 330n37; psychosocial stress and, 30–31, 321; social isolation and, 17, 34; struggles with mind-body issues in, 50. *See also* biomedical rhetorics, dangers of; "longing for organicity"; suffering
chronic pain. *See* pain, chronic
chronic pelvic pain: physical and sexual abuse, connection to, 321
class: medical authority and, 309–11
"clinical expertise," 328n17
clinical manufacture of illness, 24–25, 36; fibromyalgia as example of, 296–98. *See also* constructionist perspectives on medicine
clinical medicine: "dense pragmatic perspective" on, 25; four phases of, 26–27; as kind of laboratory science, 25, 304–5, 328n12. *See also* patient construction; persuasion; storytelling; treatment (phases of clinical medicine)
"clinical science," 328n17
"clinical tales," 23. *See also* storytelling
Cohen, Milton L., 313–16
compliance, patient, 39–46; as factor in women's oppression, 44; rhetorical production of, 113–14; roots of in gender identity, 46–47. *See also* doctor-patient relationship, gender dynamics of
constructionist perspectives on medicine, 23–25, 303–5. *See also* clinical manufacture of illness; facts, medical
Cornwall, Patricia, 6
crime fiction. *See* mystery stories
crime metaphors, uses of, 314–15. *See also* metaphor, medical
Cross, Amanda, 6

depression: biomedical practice as cause of, 176–77; ethic of care, connection to, 45
diagnostic-treatment grid, 88
diary, medical, 12
difference: inner, 40, 309, 335n85; social, 39, 309, 335nn83, 90
DiGiacomo, Susan M., 53, 337n121
discourses of medicine, 20, 27–29, 298–99, 307. *See also* drug discourse
diseasing of social life, 3
doctor-patient relationship, gender dynamics of, 6, 37–48, 308–9, 318–320, 327n3, 331n46, 333nn63, 64, 68,

334n69. *See also* compliance, patient; resistance, patient; women's agency, theory of
"doing gender," 43, 46, 335n86. *See also* identity, gender
drug discourse, 90–93

Ehrenreich, Barbara, 318
emotion: dichotomy with reason, artificiality of, 55; "outlaw," 56; of patient, 334n76; role of in knowledge creation, 55, 312; socially constructed character of, 55; as source of critical theory, 55–56; writing about, 55–56
Engel, Beverly, 299
Engel, George L., 301–2, 341n6 (Conclusion). *See also* biopsychosocial model
English, Deirdre, 318
epidemic of chronic pain, 3, 49, 325n1
epistemic invalidation, 94–95, 300, 338n1 (Ch. 2). *See also* biomedical rhetorics, dangers of
epistemology of care, 87, 93–95
"ethic of care," 44–45, 142, 334–35n77. *See also* adolescent development, girls'; femininity; psychomedical perspective; relationship-first approach
ethnograhic materials, 11–13
ethnography, 5, 39: classic, narrative devices in, 313; definition, 51; medical, in anthropology and sociology, 337n113
"experience-near" accounts, 53, 312. *See also* auto-ethnography

Fam, Adel G., 281
facts, medical: human construction of, 23, 303–5. *See also* constructionist perspectives on medicine
femininity: dominant scripts on, 42–43; 1950s codes of, 141–42; and the pleasant self, 42, 44–46, 249–50; psychodynamics of in biomedical encounter, 44–46, 308; psychological costs of, 45; and the relational self, 42, 44, 334–35n77; socialization into, 339n6 (Ch. 4). *See also* depression; gender training; identity, gender
feminism: backlash against, 320, as producer of resistant self, 43; scripts on, 43, 46–47, 142, 309; as source of empowerment and political action, 43–44, 46, 309; success of in challenging power, 309. *See also* identity, gender; resistance, general; resistance, patient

Fenstermaker, Sarah, 43
fibromyalgia: age distribution of, 9; bio-medicine of, 8–11, 276–80, 315–16; causes of, organic, 9, 315, 326n8; causes of, psychosocial, 9, 320–22, 326n8; chronicity of, 9, 187–88; clinical manufacture of, 296–98; as construct, 315; dangers to society of inappropriate diagnosis of, 271–72; definition, 10; depression in, 188; diagnosis of, 276–80, 315–16; gender distribution of, 9; gender theory of, 249–50; history of, 9–10; iatrogenic production of, 280, 296–98; nonprogressive nature of, 9, 338n3 (Ch. 3); and pain, subjective experience of, 10–11; pain modulators in, 278; physical and sexual abuse, connection to, 321; popular interest in, 10, 315; prevalence of, 9; and "psychiatric disorder," 188; psychosocial roots of, 249–50; secondary form of, 281; skepticism about, 10, 315–16, 342nn35, 38; social construction of, 24; specialists in, 10, 315–16; symptoms of, 8–9, 278; syndrome nature of, 316; treatment of, 9; and women, historical and social implications for, 51, 315–22. See also "fibromyalgic," as subject position; gender theory of chronic pain; tender points
fibromyalgia syndrome (FMS). See fibromyalgia
"fibromyalgic," as subject position, 306–7
fibrositis, 10
fictions, medical, 23
"fight like a girl," 174
Fisher, Sue, 38, 333n68
Foucault, Michel, 4, 19, 25, 43, 329n25; limitations of approach to medicine, 329n25
fragmentation, of patient, 35, 298–99
Frank, Arthur W., 323

"gate control theory of pain," 337–38n1, 338n3 (Ch. 3)
Gawain, Shakti, 217–22, 224
gender, of physician, 327n3; and physician's values, 320
gender identity. See identity, gender
gender theory of chronic pain, 245–46, 249–50, 293, 295
gender training, 115, 142. See also femininity
genre. See autho-ethnography; ethnography; writing
Gilligan, Carol, 41, 42, 43, 44, 47, 308, 334–35n77, 335nn83, 84, 85

Gilligan model of feminine identity, 42–43; critique of, 42, 334–35n77
Gilman, Charlotte Perkins, 316–17
"girl games," 175
Goffman, Erving, 35, 305
"good patient," 113, 338n1 (Ch. 3); construction of, 114
Gorovitz, Samuel, 330n41
Grafton, Sue, 6
Gulf War syndrome, 3, 49

Hadler, Nortin M., 342n38
Haraway, Donna J., 54, 293
Harding, Sandra, 54, 293, 327–28n12
Hekman, Susan J., 42, 43, 335nn79, 80
Hilfiker, David, 331n45, 332n55
Hippocratic oath, 4, 26, 34. See also myths of medicine
hysteria, 318
"hysterical epidemics," 49. See also "women's disease"

iatrogenic illness, 30, 320, 327n8. See also medical mistakes
identity, bodily, 35–36; medicalization of, 305–7, 316–22, 323–24; "normal," 35, 306; shame about, 35, 294; "spoiled," 35, 305–7; "stigmatized," 35
identity, gender, 21; Brown, Gilligan, and Jack on, 41–46; contradictory character of, 43, 308, 335n85; and "discursive" self, 41–42, 308; and feminine self, 21, 42; and feminist self, 21; multiple nature of, 43, 308; processual nature of, 43, 308; role of in emotion, relationships, and politics, 41, 47, 308; as "situated accomplishment," 43; theories of, 41–44, 307–9, 335n80. See also "doing gender"; femininity; feminism; Gilligan model of feminine identity
Illich, Ivan, 330n41
illness communities, 324
illness cultures, 21, 48–51, 294–95. See also medicine, alternative
illness memoirs. See storytelling: by the ill
inner disruptions, patient experience of, 19, 34–37, 298–301. See also self: colonization of
inner world, of patient, 40–41
interpellation, 332n58
"intimate adversaries," 39
irritable bowel syndrome: gender distribution of, 317; physical and sexual abuse, connection to, 321

Jack, Dana, 41, 42, 45, 308, 339n2
(Ch. 5)
Jaggar, Alison M., 55–56

Kabat-Zinn, Jon, 215–17, 221
Keller, Evelyn Fox, 32
Kevorkian, Jack, 319
Kleinman, Arthur, 20, 30, 36, 53, 294,
299, 327n9, 330n37, 331n43, 338n3
Kleinman, Joan, 53
Knorr-Cetina, Karin D., 25
Kubler-Ross, Elizabeth, 234

Latour, Bruno, 25
Layne, Linda L., 337n121
"life as a work of art," 217–18
"lifeworld" of patient, 30
Light, Donald, Jr., 331n42
literary selves, split: analytic advantages
of, 52–53; S./I distinction, 16, 52
Locke, David, 22, 23, 25, 32, 304, 327–
28n12
"longing for organicity," 50, 336n108
Lupton, Deborah, 334n76

MacIntyre, Alasdair, 330n41
Mahoney, Maureen A., 47
managed care: dangers to patient of, 37,
319; and entrepreneurial physicians,
338n2 (Ch. 3)
Martin, Emily, 39
mechanistic model. See metaphors,
medical
medical biography, 115
medical chart, functions of, 12–13
medical gaze: definition, 4, 326–27n2;
history of, 19; shifts in, 325–26n3
medical mistakes: in chronic illness,
30; and clinician, interests and values
of, 30–31, 331n43; difficulties admitting, 331n45; disappearance from
view of, 23; disclosure of, 4; and
"error-ridden" character of medicine,
31, 34; patient contribution to, 16;
physician "management" of, 330–
31n42; prevalence of, 30, 330n41,
330–31n42; responsibility for, 36–
37, 272–73; sources of, 29–31, 292,
330n40. See also clinical manufacture
of illness; iatrogenic illness; National
Academy of Sciences report on medical
mistakes
medical reform, 16, 301–3, 324; barriers
to, 272–73; role of storytelling in,
323–24
medical whodunit, 5–6
medicalization: alternative to, 323–24;

dangers of, 315–22, 323; and desire
for diagnosis, 316, 342n39; of identity,
305–7, 316–22, 323–24; by ill persons,
334n71; loss of cultural riches due to,
323; of pain, 315–22; of psychosocial
problems, 20. See also identity, bodily;
self, patient
medicine, alternative: core ideas in, 212–
13; cultural blame associated with,
49–50, 294; limitations of, 49–50,
213, 224, 294–95; mind-body relationship in, 48–49, 294; "mind-cure"
in, 294; popular culture of, 6, 21, 48–
51; seductions of, 49, 294; similarities
to scientific medicine of, 49; strengths
of, 212–14, 294; support given biomedicine by, 294–95; therapies of,
341n3 (Conclusion). See also blame-
the-victim models of illness; psychological theories of illness
medicine, Ayurvedic, 29, 48, 294
medicine, Chinese, 29, 48
medicine, holistic. See medicine,
alternative
medicine, scientific, 6, 14–15, 18–20,
292; as apparatus of social control, 20,
27; as contaminated by social and cultural forces, 20–21; darker side of, 7;
discursive practices in, 27–29, 31–34,
305–7; and disruption of patient's
mind and emotions, 19, 23–24, 305–7;
masculinist nature of, 320, 327n3;
material practices in, 27; mind-body
duality in, 49; mystique and myths of,
4, 19, 20, 26, 292–96; neglect of disease causation and structural sources
of pain by, 49, 320–22; overstatement
of individual control by, 49; partnership relations in, 4, 21, 266; performative nature of, 305; physician empathy
in, 21, 331n46; productivity of, 18;
power of over patient's sense of self,
52, 305–7, 313, 318; radical material-
ism in, 29, 36; reductionistic nature
of, 49, 327n9; reform of, 301–3; similarities to alternative medicine of,
49; strengths of, 29, 36, 307, 318–
19; tools of, 18; worldview of, 297–
98. See also biomedical rhetorics,
dangers of; clinical medicine; constructionist perspectives on medicine; discourses of medicine; inner disruptions,
patient experience of; "medicine-as-
art"; "medicine-as-science"; metaphors, medical; rhetorics, of medicine;
"scienceness" of medicine
"medicine-as-art," 328n17

"medicine-as-science," 328n17
metaphors, medical: body as machine, 18–19, 297–98; clinical work as laboratory science, 25, 304–5; crime-related, 314–15; cultural tendency to create, 48; illness as moral flaw, 48; medicine as repair, 18; physician as mechanic, 18; role in medicine of, 19
"mind-cure," 294. See also medicine, alternative
"mindfulness meditation," 215–17
Mishler, Elliott G., 327n7
Mitchell, S. Weir, 316, 317, 320, 342n42
Mizrahi, Terry, 331n42
moralization of illness. See psychological theories of illness
Morris, David B., 323
Munt, Sally R., 313
mystery stories: facts and fictions in, 313; feminist, 313–15; medical, 5–6; uses in anthropology of, 314–15
mystique of medicine, 4, 26, 292. See also myths of medicine
myths of medicine, 19, 26, 292; dangers of belief in, 292–96; how kept mythic, 20

narrative. See stories; storytelling
National Academy of Sciences report on medical mistakes, 30, 302; limitations of scope, 302
neurasthenia, 316, 318, 320
Nichter, Mark, 334n71

objectification, discourse of, 28–29. See also discourses of medicine
ontological invalidation, 94–95, 300, 338n1 (Ch. 2). See also biomedical rhetorics, dangers of
ontology of care, 87, 93–95
Oudshoorn, Nelly, 25

Paget, Marianne A., 31
pain, acute. See acute illness
pain, chronic: cultural meanings of, 323; as cultural problem, 322; and desire for diagnosis by sufferers of, 50, 316; epidemic spread of, 3, 49, 325n11; as feminist issue, 317–18; gender differences in, 317–18; political protest against medicalization of, 324; socio-political roots of, 316–22; structural sources of, 316–22. See also arthritis; chronic fatigue syndrome; chronic illness; fibromyalgia
pain, medicalization of. See medicalization
pain, productivity of, 55, 323–24

pathologization, discourse of, 28–29. See also discourses of medicine
patient construction (phase of clinical medicine), 27, 28–29, 35. See also clinical medicine
performance of scienticity, 305. See also rhetorics of medicine
personhood. See self
persuasion (phase of clinical medicine), 27, 32–34. See also clinical medicine; rhetorics, of medicine
pharmacological philosophy, 87–95
Pipher, Mary, 335n90
pleasantness: costs of, 45; physical symptoms and, 249–50; as product of chronic illness, 17; as product of gender socialization, 17, 249–50. See also depression; gender theory of chronic pain
"postbiomedical" discourses, 6–7
"postfeminist" era, 320
post-traumatic stress disorder, 24
power, in medical encounter. See doctor-patient relationship, gender dynamics of
practice approaches to science, 23–25
problem with no name, 322
psychological theories of illness: blame the victim, tendency to 48, 49–50; health crusading, ties to, 48
psychological therapies: for chronic pain, 250, 295. See also gender theory of chronic pain
psychomedical perspective, 45–46
psychoneuroimmunology, 286, 336n103

quantification, discourse of, 28–29. See also discourses of medicine
Quintner, John L., 315–16

Radomsky, Nellie A., 321
Rapp, Rayna, 39
rebellion, against biomedical power, 15–16, 169, 174–75, 309
relational self. See "ethic of care"; femininity
relationship-first approach, 45–46. See also "ethic of care"; femininity
resistance, general: discursive forms of, 43; ethnic and class differences in, 335n90; feminist discourse as source of, 43; openly political forms of, 43
resistance, patient, 39–40, 46–47, 163, 309–11, 333–34n68; friendships as vehicle for, 163; limits on by feminine self, 308; re-narrativization of the self as form of, 313; roots of in identity,

resistance, patient *(continued)*
47, 308–9; silent forms of, 47, 163;
as source of political action, 44; storytelling as mode of, 323–24; tactics of,
47; variation of by inner difference of
multiple selves, 40, 308–9; variation
of by social difference of race and class,
39; writing as form of, 163. *See also*
doctor-patient relationship, gender
dynamics of; feminism; silence; voice
rest cure, 342n42. *See also* Mitchell,
S. Weir
rhetorical tactics, 113–14
rhetorics, of medicine, 20, 31–34, 304,
328n16; conversational analysis approach to, 328n16; dangers for chronic
patient of, 33–34; emotionally coercive
character of, 292; error-camouflaging
effects of, 25, 31–32; Foucauldian approach to, 328n16; "official," 32;
performative aspect of, 305; "personal,"
32. *See also* abuse, emotional and verbal; biomedical rhetorics, dangers of
rhetorics, of science: in rhetoric of medicine, 32–33, 304; and "truth," 22

Sacks, Oliver, 23
science, making of: human error in, 22,
304; inexact methods in, 22, 304;
interests of scientist in, 22, 305; technical error in, 22; values of scientist in,
22, 305. *See also* practice approaches
to science; truths, scientific
science-as-practice, 25, 328n12. *See also*
clinical medicine
"scienceness" of medicine, 19, 23–25,
303–5
self: colonization of, 313; cultural
sources of, 53; "discursive" character
of, 41–42; disruption of sense of, 35–
36, 305–7; essential nature, critique of,
42; re-narrativization of, 313; renewal
of, 286; trauma to, 332n56. *See also*
identity, gender; self, patient; suffering
self, patient: biomedical diminishment
of, 52, 298–99, 305–7; death of, 306;
medicalized nature of, 305–7; reconstruction of, 15–16, 286. *See also*
medicine, scientific; self
self-narrativization. *See* auto-ethnography
self-reflexivity. *See* auto-ethnography
sexual politics, 38–40, 320
Shorter, Edward, 336n108
Showalter, Elaine, 49–50, 315, 325n1
sign, of illness: contrasted with symptom,
330n35

silence, 47, 320, 321, 323–24; ethnic differences in, 335n83; political and psychological advantages of, 47; powerlessness and pathology, distinguished
from, 47; storytelling as antidote to,
323–24. *See also* doctor-patient relationship, gender dynamics of; resistance, patient; voice
situated (positioned) truths, 312–13
Smythe, Hugh, 282–83
social construction of illness. *See* constructionist perspectives on medicine
somatization, of psychosocial stress, 250,
253. *See also* gender theory of chronic
pain
Sontag, Susan, 48–49, 336n100;
limitations of *Illness as Metaphor*,
336n100
"spoiled" identity. *See* identity, bodily
"spontaneous healing," 214–15
Stein, Howard F., 338n1 (Ch. 3)
Stevens, Patricia E., 333n64
stories: alternative, 293; compelling nature of, 23; good and bad, 29; social
structural (gender theory of chronic
pain), 293. *See also* storytelling
storytelling: by the ill, 323–24, 336–
37n112; medical, 19, 23, 29–31, 292,
293–96; scientific, 21–23, 293; as
source of better medical practice,
323–24
storytelling (phase of clinical medicine),
27, 28–29, 36. *See also* clinical
medicine
Strauss, Anselm L., 327n11
stress: and symptoms, 321; among
women, increase in, 321
subjectivity. *See* self; identity, gender
suffering: dehumanization by medical
and social sciences of, 53, 338n3; due
to medical intervention in the self, 35
symptom, of illness: contrasted with sign,
330n35
symptomization, of psychosocial stress,
250, 253
syndrome, characteristics of, 3

tender points: in diagnosis of fibromyalgia, 277–79, 315–16; problems in
interpretation of, 278, 315–16; problems in measurement of, 277–79. *See
also* fibromyalgia
Todd, Alexandra Dundas, 38, 39
"tolerization," of patient to drug, 87,
90–91, 85–99
Traweek, Sharon, 25

treatment (phase of clinical medicine), 27. *See also* clinical medicine
truths: anthropological, 54; medical, 4, 292–93; scientific, 21–22. *See also* auto-ethnology; rhetorics, of medicine; science, making of

voice: ethnic differences in, 335n83; expression of through bodily symptoms, 321; in medical encounter, 12, 21, 37–39, 308–9, 320; and power, 12, 320; recovery of ill persons', 323–24
"voice of medicine," 327n7
"voice of the lifeworld," 327n7
"vulnerable writing," 55, 312, 337n125. *See also* auto-ethnography; emotion

Weil, Andrew, 214–15, 224
Wendell, Susan, 338n1 (Ch. 2)
West, Candace, 43
Witkin, Georgia, 321
Wolfe, Frederick, 281, 342n36
women's agency, theory of, 41–48,

307–9. *See also* doctor-patient relationship, gender dynamics of
"women's disease," 315–22
women's health movement: critique of physician abuse and medical paternalism, 37–38, 300, 307; history of, 37, 333n62
women's movement: and political action, 324; role of Charlotte Perkins Gilman in, 316–17; and scripts of femininity, resistance to 43; and scripts of feminism, identification with, 43. *See also* identity and power
women's psychology, 41–46
writing: anthropological, 51–55, 311–15; feminist, 51–55, 313–15. *See also* auto-ethnography; ethnography; mystery stories
Wu, Albert W., 332n55

Young, Allan, 24

Zimmerman, Don H., 43

Designer: Nola Burger
Compositor: Integrated Composition Systems
Text: 10/13 Sabon
Display: Franklin Gothic
Printer and Binder: Sheridan Books, Inc.